For Love and Money
Care Provision in the United States

Nancy Folbre, editor

Russell Sage Foundation ◆ New York

The Russell Sage Foundation

The Russell Sage Foundation, one of the oldest of America's general purpose foundations, was established in 1907 by Mrs. Margaret Olivia Sage for "the improvement of social and living conditions in the United States." The Foundation seeks to fulfill this mandate by fostering the development and dissemination of knowledge about the country's political, social, and economic problems. While the Foundation endeavors to assure the accuracy and objectivity of each book it publishes, the conclusions and interpretations in Russell Sage Foundation publications are those of the authors and not of the Foundation, its Trustees, or its staff. Publication by Russell Sage, therefore, does not imply Foundation endorsement.

Library of Congress Cataloging-in-Publication
For love and money : care provision in the United States / Nancy Folbre, editor.
   p. cm.
 Includes bibliographical references and index.
 ISBN 978-0-87154-353-0 (pbk. : alk. paper) 1. Caregivers—United States. 2. Social service—United States. 3. Home care services. 4. Caregivers—United States. I. Folbre, Nancy.
 HV40.8.U6F67 2012
 362'.0425—dc23

                    2012014044

Text design by Suzanne Nichols.

RUSSELL SAGE FOUNDATION
112 East 64th Street, New York, New York 10065
10 9 8 7 6 5 4 3 2 1

Contents

About the Authors

NANCY FOLBRE is professor of economics at the University of Massachusetts Amherst.

SUZANNE BIANCHI is Distinguished Professor of Sociology at the University of California, Los Angeles and Dorothy Meier Chair in Social Equities.

LAURA BRASLOW is Ph.D. candidate in sociology at the Graduate Center of the City University of New York.

PAULA ENGLAND is professor of sociology at New York University.

JANET GORNICK is professor of political science and sociology at the Graduate Center of the City University of New York and director of the Luxembourg Income Study.

CANDACE HOWES is Barbara Hogate Ferrin '43 Professor of Economics at Connecticut College.

CARRIE LEANA is George H. Love Professor of Organizations and Management and director of the Center for Health and Care Work at the University of Pittsburgh.

KRISTIN SMITH is family demographer at the Carsey Institute and research assistant professor of sociology at the University of New Hampshire.

DOUGLAS WOLF is professor of public administration and Gerald B. Cramer Professor of Aging Studies at Syracuse University.

ERIK OLIN WRIGHT is professor of sociology, Vilas Distinguished Professor, and director of the Havens Center for the Study of Social Structure and Social Change at the University of Wisconsin–Madison.

Authorship and Acknowledgments

We have assigned primary authorship of the chapters in this book on the basis of major contributions, seniority, and alphabetical order. However, the collaborative inputs into each chapter far exceeded those typical of edited volumes, and in a very real sense this book was coauthored by all the contributors. We are all members of the Working Group on Care Work sponsored by the Russell Sage Foundation, and we have benefited from regular group meetings and the wise guidance of an excellent program officer, Aixa Cintrón-Vélez.

We gratefully acknowledge the helpful suggestions from two early reviewers of our manuscript, Ruth Milkman of the Graduate Center of the City University of New York and Judith Seltzer of the Department of Sociology at the University of California, Los Angeles.

Members of the Advisory Committee on the Future of Work at the Russell Sage Foundation also provided valuable feedback. Two anonymous reviewers helped us improve the final version.

Several graduate students provided excellent research assistance, including Jooyeoun Suh and Anastasia Wilson of the University of Massachusetts Amherst and Rob Callaghan and Dave Monaghan of the City University of New York Graduate Center. Elise Nahknikian provided indispensable editorial assistance. Thanks to all.

Introduction

Nancy Folbre

Care represents a distinctive form of work with important implications for living standards, economic opportunities, and quality of life. Primary responsibility for the care of children, the frail elderly, and people experiencing sickness or disability has traditionally been assigned to women, reinforcing the economic significance of gender (Blau, Brinton, and Grusky 2006). As market provision of care services has increased in the United States in recent years, women have continued to play a predominant role. Low-income African American and immigrant women are heavily overrepresented in the most poorly paid care jobs, and they face particularly serious problems balancing the demands of paid employment and family care.

But everyone is affected by the organization of care work. All of us begin life as helpless infants, and most of us require assistance during periods of sickness and infirmity before we die. People who take responsibility for the unpaid care of family members and friends often reduce their participation in paid employment and experience pay penalties, incurring substantial lifetime earnings losses (Waldfogel 1997; Budig and England 2001), and workers who enter care occupations typically pay a penalty in reduced earnings (England, Budig, and Folbre 2002).

Whether paid or unpaid, care work is often shaped by moral obligations, social norms, and personal preferences that greatly complicate its remuneration. Families, communities, and government policies all provide forms of implicit or explicit insurance for care over the life cycle. The distribution of these costs remains complex, contested, and often unclear. Family care work often creates benefits for society as a whole that are not captured by family members. For instance, when parents successfully rear children, employers and taxpayers are able to claim a share of the future returns on the human capital created (Folbre 2008a). When adult children are able and willing to care for elderly parents, costs to public health insurance systems for nursing home expenses are reduced (Wolf 1999). Yet our economic accounting systems do not measure, much less credit, unpaid family care.

As family stability has declined and paid employment among women has increased, both public and market provision of care services has expanded, creating new economic anxieties and raising pointed questions: Why do women continue to do most care work, both unpaid and paid? Who provides care for our most vulnerable dependents, and at what cost? How do paid care workers—especially those employed in low-wage jobs caring for children, the frail elderly, and people with disabilities—fare compared to other workers? How do unpaid and paid care combine to shape the process of economic development and the distribution of well-being? How effective and equitable are public policies toward care of children, people with disabilities, and the frail elderly in the United States?

This book, the joint effort of interdisciplinary researchers, addresses these questions from a vantage point of particular concern for low-income families and low-wage workers. We provide an overview of care provision in the United States, with a special focus on the problems emerging in the interactive care of children, the frail elderly, and people with disabilities outside of the more studied arenas of health care and education. We break with the traditional intellectual division of labor by examining both unpaid and paid care within a unified framework and emphasizing their joint contribution to economic well-being. This unified framework holds important implications for social theory and public policy.

CARE POLICY DILEMMAS

Some of the most vital social policy debates of the last twenty years reflect underlying ambivalence regarding both the definition of care work and appropriate rewards for performing it. Consider the following three care policy dilemmas that span the fields of child care and adult care.

1. *Our current cash and tax assistance programs for low-income parents consider care work to be "work" only when it is conducted for pay.* Temporary Assistance to Needy Families (TANF) imposes strict paid work requirements and time limits on people (primarily single mothers) receiving assistance, whether or not recipients have access to subsidized child care to facilitate their employment. Receiving a wage for caring for someone else's children is considered work, but caring for one's own children is not. The Earned Income Tax Credit (EITC), essentially a work- and income-tested family allowance, provided a subsidy of as much as $5,028 to a single mother of two earning between about $12,000 and $15,000 in 2009.[1] No earnings, no subsidy. Note that if two single mothers, each with two children under the age of five, exchanged babysitting services, swapping children for eight hours a day, five days a week, and paying one another the federal minimum wage of $7.25 an hour, they could both take full advantage of this credit, receiving a total of more than $10,000 for providing essentially the same services they would provide their own children. In other words, caring for a nonkin child for pay counts as work, but caring for your own does not.

2. *Adoption of policies to reallocate federal and state spending from nursing homes to home- and community-based care has been slowed in many states by fears that this move will increase the demand for services and that family members and friends currently providing unpaid care will "come out of the woodwork" and request remuneration.* Numerous studies show that both the frail elderly and people suffering from disabilities prefer consumer-directed home- and community-based services to institutionalization (Congressional Budget Office 2004; Howes 2010). Such programs offer some cost-saving potential.[2] But nursing home care is financially

attractive to budget-strapped states, not only because it offers some economies of scale for the care of individuals with particularly intense needs, but also because the generally low quality of Medicaid-funded nursing homes (exacerbated by the high percentage of residents with dementia) discourages many eligible recipients from taking advantage of the care to which they are entitled. Furthermore, subsidies for home- and community-based services sometimes enable people to hire family members who need market income and might not otherwise be able to provide care services (Howes 2004, 2005). Many policymakers are uncomfortable with the thought of paying for services that they think should be provided free of charge—even when many families cannot actually afford to provide them (Simon-Rusinowitz et al. 2005).

3. *Despite widespread agreement that foster care is preferable to institutionalization for many children and adults whose families cannot adequately care for them, public subsidies for foster care remain low, especially when provided by kin. Cultural norms dictating that family care should always be motivated by love, not money, contribute to the fear of attracting foster families "for the wrong reasons."* The supply of foster care for children who have been removed from their homes as a result of abuse or neglect is inadequate (Doyle and Peters 2007). Low levels of public support for foster care help explain the shortfall. The monthly subsidies provided to foster parents have primarily been determined by considering the cost of food, clothing, and shelter for children, ignoring the cost of care time (Folbre 2008a). Foster children placed with relatives often receive less government help than those placed with nonkin, even though they tend to be more economically disadvantaged (Geen 2003). Oregon pioneered the development of foster care for adults, but even that state sets reimbursement rates lower for kin than for nonkin (Mollica et al. 2009, 23). Many families that would like to provide foster care for a friend or family member cannot afford to do so.

"Crowding Out"Versus Penalizing Care

These three care policy dilemmas illustrate the tensions that have intensified as public subsidies for care provision have increased. Public subsidies provide a necessary safety net and contribute to the development of human capabilities. On the one hand, they provoke fears of weakening family obligation in ways that discourage or "crowd out" private effort. On the other hand, public subsidies for care provision reduce the economic costs of family care and can increase its efficacy as well as its supply.

The concern that payment for services once provided in the home might corrupt or displace intrinsic motivation is not entirely misplaced. However, we should also be concerned about the possibility that increase in the cost of fulfilling family obligations will discourage family and community commitments. Traditional restrictions on women's participation in paid employment once guaranteed a large supply of labor for family care. Women have typically been assigned greater social responsibility for family members than men, even at the cost of developing their own capabilities. Both economic development and collective mobilization have loosened those restrictions, reducing gender inequality. But these historical shifts have also increased the cost and stress of family care.

Fear of "crowding out" affects women more directly than men. Most single parents are women who face economic difficulties because the father of their children is not significantly contributing to family support. Most of the indigent elderly in need of care are women because women typically live longer, are more likely to survive their spouse, and have lower savings and pension benefits than men. Furthermore, the main providers of foster care—including kin foster care—are women.

Low-income families are particularly vulnerable. They often have a higher ratio of dependents to wage-earners than middle- and high-income families, leaving their wage-earners with greater caregiving responsibilities as well as a greater need for market income. With low wages and little savings, these families often find it difficult to meet the needs of sick or elderly family members. Single mothers with little education often work at jobs with nonstandard hours, making it difficult for them to find adequate child care. When a child or other family member needs urgent care, these mothers are forced to leave their jobs, contributing to a pattern of unstable employment that lowers their earnings. A recent study shows that low-wage white women experience a greater percentage lifetime reduction in earnings as a result of motherhood than high-wage white women (Budig and Hodges 2010).

The transition to an increasingly market-based economy highlights a growing disjuncture between the private costs and public benefits of care provision that bears particularly heavily on women. The gender division of labor in care proves difficult to renegotiate, weakening marriage-based or long-term commitments. This coordination problem may help explain why the "gender revolution" has slowed, perhaps even stalled (Gerson 2010; England 2010; Esping-Anderson 2009b). It also helps explain the need to rethink public policies toward care provision.

OVERVIEW OF THE BOOK

This book explores the theoretical dilemmas of care provision and provides an empirical overview of both unpaid and paid care of children and adults needing personal assistance (primarily people with disabilities and the frail elderly) in the United States. We offer estimates of the value of unpaid care time that help place unpaid and paid care in a common context. This provides a basis for an analysis of care policy and consideration of two pressing policy problems: the lack of adequate support for family care and the uneven quality of both jobs and services in the paid care sector.

Scholars disagree on the very definitions of "care" and "care work." Chapter 1, "Defining Care," addresses these conceptual issues head on. It reviews the extensive literature on unpaid and paid care work and establishes the definitions of care work that we apply in the remainder of the book. It outlines measures of the need for care, making a case for joint consideration of the current and projected needs of children, people with disabilities, and the frail elderly. It explains how institutional diversity and motivational complexity contribute to serious problems with both the level and the quality of care provision.

Measurement problems arise at the outset of this discussion. Unpaid or informal care is typically assessed by survey questions that ask respondents to report either episodes of caregiving or the amount of time they devote to specific types of care. Paid care workers are typically designated by occupational and industrial classifications that have evolved in often overlapping and arbitrary ways. Differences in definition, time period, and survey design often lead to inconsistent estimates. Discussion of these more technical issues is provided in the appendix ("Measuring Care Work").

Chapter 2, "Motivating Care," explores the "for love and money" theme in more detail, focusing on the importance of intrinsic prosocial motivation and emphasizing the cultural construction of values, norms, and preferences. In general, normative change in recent years has been associated with greater emphasis on extrinsic rewards—the money nexus. Considerable evidence suggests that intrinsic rewards based on prosocial motivations such as altruism continue to play a crucial role. Indeed, in many ways the relationship between unpaid and paid care provision echoes cultural tensions between moral responsibility and pecuniary reward. We also look at how women's traditional specialization in care provision has been reinforced by external constraints, including cultural norms.

Chapter 3, "Unpaid Care Work," makes the best possible use of existing data to construct an empirical picture of unpaid care provision in the United States. A review of research based on many different sources of data describes the demographic context of care for children and adults needing personal assistance. An analysis of pooled data from the American Time Use Survey (ATUS) from 2003 to 2008 reveals the average temporal burden of unpaid work that takes the form of direct interactive care of others or indirect support for such care. It then focuses more narrowly on interactive care for children and adults, examining important gender- and age-based differences and comparing time devoted to children with time devoted to caring for or helping adults. The final section of this chapter examines the economic and emotional burdens of care, asking how they are distributed by gender, race, and class.

Chapter 4, "Paid Care Work," begins with an overview of industries and occupations in which care services are provided, then narrows to a consideration of two specific occupational clusters engaged in child care and adult care. Both quantitative and qualitative analyses show that wages and working conditions in these occupations are problematic, often making it difficult for workers to strengthen or maintain their intrinsic motivation and leading to high turnover rates that reduce continuity and quality of care (IOM 2008; Helburn 1995). Furthermore, low-quality jobs make it difficult for those who engage in them to sustain healthy family and community development.

Chapter 5, "Valuing Care," explores differences between the cost of care and its larger value to society. The cost of unpaid care often remains invisible. When families pay someone to provide care for a dependent family member, they report expenditures (and workers report wages), unless the transaction takes place under the table. But when families provide care themselves, the costs of their own time and work effort go uncounted. The resulting inconsistencies distort comparisons of living standards within households, across households, and among countries. The value of unpaid care can be estimated by asking what it would cost to purchase care of comparable quality. However, both unpaid and paid care contribute to the development of human capabilities and health, yielding benefits to society as a whole that are not captured by market prices. Many estimates of the public benefits of care services substantially exceed estimates of their costs, demonstrating the important role that government can play in providing greater support for care work.

While some scholars and advocates have analyzed the impact of public policies on parts of the care landscape, ranging from unpaid care of children to paid care of adults, relatively little attention has been devoted to public policies affecting care provision as a whole. Chapter 6 provides a systematic inventory of such policies in the United States, followed in chapter 7 by a critique of their inadequate and uneven impact. Disparities based on class, race-ethnicity, and geography remain glaring, with unfortunate consequences for our neediest and most dependent citizens. Many middle-class families, lacking access to child care and early childhood education subsidies and required to spend down their assets in order to gain eligibility for Medicaid-funded nursing home assistance, also remain vulnerable. High-income families are in a better position to balance work-family needs, but they too experience unnecessary risk and stress.

Our policy assessment provides a bridge to one of our most important conclusions: public policies should provide increased support for both unpaid and paid care work, helping individuals gain the flexibility they need to balance family responsibility with paid employment. In the child care arena, we need to make it easier for families to take leaves or reduce their hours of paid employment, but we also need to improve the quality and accessibility of child care and early education. In the adult care arena, we need to make it easier for people with disabilities and the frail elderly to obtain adequate care within their own homes and communities, but we also need to improve the quality of institutional care.

Chapter 8 summarizes our research and policy recommendations. Our picture of the care sector as a whole explains why improved care provision is a necessary—though not sufficient—condition for gender equality. It also strengthens the case for increased public investment in care provision. We urge other scholars to join us in developing a more detailed agenda for policy-relevant research on care for the most vulnerable members of our society.

NOTES

1. See Center on Budget and Policy Priorities, "Policy Basics: The Earned Income Tax Credit," http://www.cbpp.org/cms/?fa=view&id=2505 (accessed June 2, 2010).

2. Research suggests that long-term care in the community is less expensive than nursing home care; see, for instance, Summer (2005). However, comparisons may not be entirely accurate because (1) states build overly restrictive cost controls into home care programs; (2) nursing home residents may have more intense care needs; and (3) the value of informal care provided in the home and community should be factored in (see discussion in chapter 5). For more discussion of these issues, see PHI (2003).

Chapter 1

Defining Care

Nancy Folbre and Erik Olin Wright

While scholarship on care work has burgeoned in recent years, most researchers tend to specialize in analysis of either unpaid care provided within families or paid care provided through wage employment, overlooking similarities and synergies between the two. Quantitative studies often lump care work in with other low-wage jobs, understating the significant impact of intrinsic motivation and the importance of personal attachment. Qualitative studies, on the other hand, seldom explain the links between the distinctive nature of care and measurable outcomes such as pay, working conditions, and care outcomes. Research on care also tends to accumulate in silos determined by different constituencies (children, people with disabilities, or the elderly) or by different sites of care provision (households, public institutions, or for-profit firms).

In this chapter, we lay the theoretical foundations for a more unified approach to care policy. First, we explain what we mean by care work and discuss its distinctive features. Building on previous research, we define "interactive care" as work in which concern for the well-being of the care recipient is likely to affect the quality of the services provided. We define "support care" as work that enables interactive care, and "supervisory care" as on-call availability to provide interactive care when needed. Although emotional attachment does not enter our definition of care work, we argue that it often plays a crucial role in the development of concern for the well-being of care recipients.

Second, we argue for a unified focus on the provision of care for children, individuals with disabilities, and the frail elderly. Most empirical assessments of adult need for nonmedical care are based on the difficulty that individuals have performing various actions defined as "activities of daily living." We argue that assessments of care needs should be extended and improved to encompass care for children as well as adults. We also summarize some important reasons why the need for care is likely to increase in coming years.

Third, we emphasize the institutional diversity and motivational complexity of care work. Most people who receive care rely on both unpaid and paid caregivers, funded in a number of different ways and provided in a number of settings, ranging from care recipients' own homes to public institutions to for-profit businesses. Institutional diversity is accompanied by motivational complexity. As Viviana Zelizer (2005) observes, we have a tendency to assume that care is motivated either by love or by money and that these two different motivations represent "hostile worlds." That is, paying money for care undermines love, so care provided for love should not be paid; similarly, care provided for money does not and should not entail love. Like Zelizer, we challenge this view, emphasizing the ways in which love and money often combine and intersect, sometimes (though not always) in complementary ways. This perspective leads us to reject a common usage of the term "commodification" as a pejorative term applied to any service provided for money, implying that such service is stripped of emotion or concern for others. Instead, we emphasize the ways in which a mismatch between the needs of care recipients and care providers can emerge in either unpaid or paid care.

The growth of public policies designed to provide social safety nets has sometimes been described as a process of "defamilialization" (Esping-Anderson 1999). But in many ways public care policies involve "refamilialization"—providing more support for the care of children, individuals with disabilities, and the frail elderly within the home and community. As Gøsta Esping-Anderson (2009b, 104) now emphasizes, "There is a widespread belief that externalizing family responsibilities will jeopardize the quality of family life and undermine familial solidarities. All available evidence points towards the exact opposite conclusion."

The rubric of "refamilialization" also encompasses a number of other care policies: efforts to improve the quality of paid care services so that they come closer to meeting the idealized standards of family care; efforts to improve conditions of wage employment to ensure that all workers have sufficient money and time to devote to their family, friends, and community; and efforts to revise concepts of family obligation to move toward greater gender equality.

THE DISTINCTIVE FEATURES OF CARE

Interactive care—whether paid or unpaid—represents a distinctive form of work. Unlike the idealized consumers portrayed in standard economics textbooks, care recipients often lack the competence, information, or time required to make good choices. Unlike standard products, care services are heterogeneous, emotionally intense, and often person-specific. "Outputs" are often coproduced by paid employees, family members, and care recipients themselves: teachers collaborate with parents and children to improve child outcomes, and home care providers collaborate with medical experts, family members, and the individuals they assist.

Motivations for care provision reach far beyond the extrinsic rewards traditionally emphasized by economists (wages, benefits) or sociologists (social approval) to include prosocial motivations that offer intrinsic rewards, such as the gratification of helping others or a genuine desire to make the care recipient better off. Care preferences are shaped by the organization of care work itself. Prolonged personal interaction with those who need care often leads to emotional attachment to them. Care preferences are also shaped by cultural traditions and institutional structures (Bowles 1998). Moral obligation seems stronger—and exchange motivation weaker—than for other kinds of work. Both worker motivation and the structure of interactions between care providers and recipients influence service quality. This complex personal and institutional environment mediates all efforts to improve the productivity of care work, including application of new information technologies.

Care services share another common characteristic: they are often person-specific, customized services whose quality is difficult to measure and monitor (Folbre 2008b). Traditional assumptions of consumer sovereignty do not hold, in part because the recipients are often either very young or have reduced cognitive abilities as a result of sickness or old age. When care consumers lack the information or power to choose among competing providers (as is often the case when people enter a nursing home), quality of care can deteriorate to dangerously low levels (Eika 2009).

Family members are not always altruistic. They sometimes default on their obligations, raising the problem of family failure. Many single mothers receive little assistance from the fathers of their children. Husbands and wives negotiating commitments to children and siblings negotiating commitments to their parents often confront strategic dilemmas that can lead to inefficient outcomes (Lundberg and Pollak 2003). For instance, spouses may be reluctant to make a decision that lowers their future earnings because they cannot be sure that the other spouse will fully compensate them or insure them against increased economic vulnerability. Adult children may be reluctant to take an elderly parent into their home because they fear that siblings may default on their responsibilities and free-ride on their efforts. In today's complex and often blended families, which may include stepchildren and informal cohabitation, family obligations are often poorly defined.

Willingness to provide mutual aid in meeting care responsibilities represents an important social asset. Too often, however, this willingness is treated as a natural and inexhaustible resource. Mutual aid is susceptible to burnout and withdrawal. Community groups can help coordinate individual actions by specifying rules for cooperation and imposing sanctions on free-riders (Ostrom 1990). In the absence of such rules and sanctions, voluntary commitments can impose high costs that undermine altruistic norms and preferences (Bowles 1998). Offering explicit, per-unit payment can also undermine such norms and preferences. However, basic reciprocity and reward have a positive effect on cooperation (Frey 1998).

Both the willingness and ability of family members depend in part on the resources at their command and vary substantially by race, ethnicity, and class, as well as by gender (Gerstel and Sarkisian 2008). As the next chapter emphasizes, cultural norms based on gender have a powerful effect (England 2005). Biological predispositions may also differ: women's tendency to "tend and befriend" may increase their social resilience, but make them economically vulnerable (Taylor 2002). The gender pay gap is explained in part by women's continuing responsibilities for family care as well as their disproportionate concentration in paid care occupations (England, Budig, and Folbre 2002). African American and immigrant women are overrepresented in many low-paid care occupations (Duffy 2005; Howes 2002).

Family living standards are affected by both purchased and family-provided care. Conventional measures of poverty and inequality focus on market income alone, providing an incomplete picture of resources such as time available to care for children and other family members (Folbre 2008a, 2008c). Families maintained by women alone face particularly serious problems meeting their care needs. Inequality in access to care services can have even more profound consequences than inequality in market income. Children who lack the sustained attention of concerned parents, teachers, and health care providers often fail to thrive. Sick and elderly individuals who feel neglected often become depressed and demoralized in ways that worsen their health. Care shapes the development of human capabilities and the quality of life from birth to death.

Emerging problems in care provision are linked to other social trends, such as changes in household structure and community ties (McLanahan 2004; Putnam 2000). Increasing wage inequalities, persistent unemployment, and racial-ethnic differences complicate the care landscape. Globalization, deunionization, immigration, and job restructuring have created new problems for the low-wage workforce (Appelbaum, Bernhardt, and Murnane 2003). A focus on care work provides both a new lens for examining these trends and a potentially unifying framework for building political coalitions to address them.

Our approach to care work emphasizes complex institutional and organizational interactions that cannot be explained simply as the result of individual choices. We believe that individuals try to make the best of what they can get. However, we put less emphasis on individual choice than on coordination problems. We emphasize the impact of social norms, group identity, strategic dilemmas, and collective action, placing these in the context of an analysis of the care sector of the economy as a whole.

DEFINING CARE WORK

In this book, we distinguish three types of care work: interactive care activities, support care activities, and supervisory care or "on-call" responsibilities. The first two categories encompass activities that are typically assessed by time use surveys or occupational designations. The third category, supervisory care, represents a responsibility that often constrains work activities—being available or "on call" to interrupt other activities and provide interactive care—but is not itself an activity. A good example of this category is the need for a caregiver to be close by when a young infant or an individual with profound disabilities is sleeping. Our definitions apply to both unpaid and paid care work, departing from the usage typical of many time use studies that equate care with unpaid work in the home (Razavi 2007; Budlender 2008).

We define *interactive care* as activities in which concern for the well-being of the care recipient is likely to affect the quality of the services performed in interaction with that person.[1] Face-to-face, hands-on care, where care providers and recipients know one another by name, often falls into this category. We use the term *support care* to describe services undertaken to enable interactive care. Time devoted to housework, meal preparation, and administration or management of care provides the infrastructure necessary for more personal interaction. These tasks, which Mignon Duffy (2011, 19) terms "nonnurturant care," can be performed in an impersonal way. Yet they often influence the quality of interactive care.

The distinctions among these three types of care activities reflect our desire to highlight work with a relational and emotional component but also to recognize the significance of related activities of support and supervision. From a broad perspective, virtually all activities can be said to affect care provision.[2] Similarly, one could argue that virtually all activities, including care, are inputs into agriculture or manufacturing. Our categorization, however, calls attention to both the labor process and the direct beneficiary of services provided. Our distinction between interactive and support care resembles that made in conventional labor force statistics between occupation (defined in terms of what people do, such as management or clerical work) and industry (defined in terms of the end-product of work, such as manufacturing or health services).

This categorization provides the framework for later empirical discussion. In chapter 3, we tally the unpaid time devoted to interactive and support care and time devoted to supervisory care of children. (Few data are available on supervisory care of adults.) In chapter 4, we tally the number of individuals employed in interactive care occupations and in support care industries. Together, these chapters provide a quantitative assessment of both unpaid and paid care activities, drawing a picture of care provision as a "sector" of the economy that spans both the family and the market. Chapter 5 compares the relative magnitudes of unpaid and paid care work in terms of labor hours and market prices and also explains why their social value is likely to exceed their market value.

Harry Braverman (1975) used the term "labor process" to call attention to struggles between employers and workers over the exercise of skill and autonomy in paid employment. The labor process has often been defined in terms that seem more applicable to the production of goods than of services, with little attention to gender differences. But the term calls attention to the lived experience of work and highlights the qualitative features of interactions among care managers, care providers, and care recipients. Interactive, support, and supervisory care are often blended in care work and sometimes even combined in the same job.

The labor process of care is often characterized by intrinsic motivation (van Staveren 2001; Jochimsen 2003). Both Kari Waerness (1987) and Arnaug Leira (1994) emphasize the extent to which care departs from traditional definitions of work as an activity performed only for pay. This, in itself, is not distinctive. Many other types of work provide intrinsic satisfaction, or what economists term "compensating differentials." What is distinctive is the prosocial form that intrinsic motivation often takes in care work—concern for the well-being of those who are the primary beneficiaries.

Some care theorists suggest that family care is so intensely personal and emotional that it should not be termed "work" (Jochimsen 2003; Himmelweit 1999).

Even paid care often retains its personal quality, resisting "complete commodification" (Gardiner 1997). However, we emphasize, like Emily Abel and Margaret Nelson (1990, 4), that work can encompass both affective relations and instrumental tasks. Other scholars support this view. Indeed, Madonna Harrington Meyer, Pam Herd, and Sonya Michel (2000, 2) emphasize that it is important to recognize care as a form of work, lest it be construed merely as a voluntary gift.

Francesca Cancian and Stacey Oliker (2000, 2) define caring as a combination of feelings and actions that "provide responsively for an individual's personal needs or well-being, in a face-to-face relationship." Similarly, Mignon Duffy (2011) describes "nurturant care" as an activity that demands more than mere performance of emotional labor. Airline stewardesses are trained to make passengers feel welcome, reassured, safe, and willing to follow orders in the event of an emergency (Hochschild 1983). Likewise, sales personnel are instructed to behave in ways that will create some emotional resonance with customers, such as using first names. However, genuine care work often entails genuine emotional engagement rather than mere surface acting.

Emotional engagement is difficult to observe, much less measure, and differences among workers—and even among different episodes of care provided by the same worker—are likely. Concern for the well-being of a care recipient may not be ubiquitous or even completely necessary. Concern alone does not guarantee the delivery of high-quality services—skill also matters. In fact, concern can be taken too far, becoming intrusive when it disrespects the emotional autonomy of a care recipient. Nonetheless, concern for the well-being of a care recipient is *likely* to affect the quality of the services performed.

Few care transactions resemble the stylized exchanges that take place in ideal markets, in which consumers know what they want and can exercise considerable choice. Many care recipients—especially children and the mentally infirm—lack the autonomy required to hire, fire, or even evaluate their caregivers. They rely on a third party, whether a family member or an employer, to perform those tasks on their behalf. But third parties cannot easily monitor the quality of the care provided. Therefore, they prefer to hire a caregiver who does not need to be closely watched. A caregiver's intrinsic concern for the care recipient's well-being provides some quality assurance. Especially for individuals who lack autonomy, the ideal caregiver is one for whom the needs of the care recipient are "transparent" and take precedence over other demands (Kittay 1999).

Our definition of care emphasizes the nexus between work motivation and outcomes rather than the characteristics of the people receiving care. Therefore, we disagree with those who exclude activities that involve "meeting a need that those in need could not possibly meet themselves" (Bubeck 1995, 183). Even the most autonomous among us experience periods of dependency when we rely on the kindness of others. Most of us are interdependent, providing and receiving care from friends and family. The exchange of care services among adults shapes both daily routines and quality of life.[3]

But while we begin with a broad definition of care, we agree with other scholars on the importance of "dependency" work (Kittay 1999). Children, individuals with disabilities, and the frail elderly are often unable to meet all of their needs on their own. Care work often goes beyond fulfillment of basic needs to develop the capabilities of its recipients—their health, their mental abilities, or skills that will be useful to themselves and others. The work of nurturing children at home or teaching them in school develops their productive capabilities. We do not commonly conceive of caring for adults as a similar form of investment, but in fact such care also maintains existing human capital as well as slowing its inevitable (at least with current medical technology) depreciation. Care work also fosters human relationships that encourage trust and reciprocity.

Our definition of interactive care emphasizes concern for a care recipient's well-being, not their happiness. A teacher's job is to educate students, not necessarily to make them smile. Doctors and nurses aim to improve health in the long run, not just comfort in the short run. Therapists try to help people learn to cope with their problems, not always to cheer them up. Even competent adult consumers may not be the best judges of quality when purchasing services designed to increase their capabilities rather than meet their immediate needs.

Our definition of interactive care work based on the likely implications of concern for care recipients does not paint a bright line between what is interactive care work and what is not (as later chapters will show). But it does provide a reasonable criterion for arraying different kinds of jobs along a continuum, ranging from those in which genuine concern is likely to be consequential to those in which it is probably irrelevant. Care of young children, individuals with profound disabilities, and the frail elderly lies at the most consequential end of the spectrum. At the other end are paid jobs that involve little human interaction or concern for others in order to be effectively performed. In between lie a range of services—both paid and unpaid—in which concern for the well-being of others may sometimes play an important role.

EMOTIONAL ATTACHMENT
AND PERSON-SPECIFIC SKILLS

Concern for the well-being of others, which economists tend to describe as "altruistic preferences," can take a rather general form based on abstract moral principles. However, in practice, altruistic preferences are often person-specific, formed through a process of emotional attachment. Furthermore, many of the skills required to improve the well-being of others are person-specific. As a result, long-term relationships often improve care outcomes. Emotional connection itself—the feeling of being "cared for"—provides direct benefits to many care recipients.

While we do not include emotional attachment and person-specific skills as part of our *definition* of interactive care work, we emphasize that they are likely to play an important role in the development of effective concern for care recipients. This is rather obvious in the case of family care. Young monkeys raised with ample food but no physical affection fare worse than those raised with insufficient food but ample nurturance. Infants who lack a stable relationship with a committed caregiver often fail to thrive. Studies of the determinants of human happiness reveal that relationships with family and friends exert a greater positive impact than pecuniary factors such as wealth and income (Layard 2005).

Evidence of the negative effects of disruptive or abusive family environments, the incidence of domestic violence, and high rates of family dissolution on children's development show that we cannot take the quantity or quality of family care for granted. We should not treat families as though they are homogenous units, or assume that they are sites of perfect altruism. Good family care is not always forthcoming, and individuals often break their promises. If we view family commitments as implicit contracts, we can describe many cases in which individuals literally default on their contractual obligations, like individuals who fail to repay a loan.

Conventional economic models of home production assume easy substitutability between money and time (Gronau 1977). In the real world, money and time are not always substitutes. Wealthy parents can hire a nanny to take on some care responsibilities. But if they delegate too much to a nanny, they may fail to develop meaningful or reciprocal relationships with their children. A husband who works overtime at the office can send his wife flowers and buy her jewelry to make up for the fact that he is never home for dinner. Such trade-offs often fail to satisfy. Legal restrictions on slavery, prostitution, and organ sales suggest that there are some things money should not buy, even if it can (Radin 1996).

Money cannot buy love, and love often requires face time, physical contact, interaction, engagement, and visible commitment. Love offers intrinsic rewards, but also limits choices. Emotional attachment has a downside—it can increase vulnerability and limit substitutability among care providers. Even if parents are abusive, social workers may be hesitant to remove a child from the home for fear that separation will be even more harmful. A woman who is the victim of spousal abuse may be reluctant to press charges because she prefers abuse to indifference.

Emotional attachment and person-specific skills are relevant to the world of paid as well as unpaid care. As Deborah Stone (2000a, 99) puts it, "At some point almost all caregivers use the word 'love' to describe their feelings toward some or all of their clients." Most individuals interviewing a direct care provider for a job tending children, individuals with disabilities, or frail elders will choose someone who they believe has some affinity, even affection, for the person to be cared for. They also hope to find someone who will develop a reliable, mutually satisfying long-term relationship with that person. Consumers (or clients, or patients, or students) seeking direct care often hope for some degree of emotional engagement—at least enough to guarantee respect, affection, and concern: "It may not matter who . . . picks up your rubbish bag in the street but it does matter who wipes your bum . . . and that ought to be the same person day in and day out because it's a very personal service and you have to trust that person" (Wistow et al. 1996, 29).

Personal networks can provide information that improves the quality of all transactions in which the quality of services is difficult to ascertain (Granovetter 2005; Dimaggio and Louch 1998). Personal relationships are particularly important in care work because positive emotional engagement strengthens altruistic preferences and often encourages people to help one another (Batson 1990). Reported satisfaction with medical care is strongly related to the emotional content of interaction, which may actually improve health outcomes. Indeed, the positive effects of believing that one is being cared for may help explain so-called placebo effects in which patients report benefits from sugar pills or surgery that has not actually taken place (Thompson 2005). Individuals with disabilities and frail elders often experience a high risk of social exclusion, and the relationships they develop with caregivers can help them stay connected.

Both parents and students often try to win the affection of teachers, recognizing that this may affect the level of effort that is forthcoming. Students benefit from developing their emotional intelligence—the ability to sense when they need help and to obtain such help by collaborating with others (Goleman 1995). Teachers try to develop these skills in their students, as well as those more easily measured on standardized exams. The quality of an output such as health or skill often depends more on the relationship between care provider and recipient than on the individual characteristics of either. Child care providers must cajole and convince children to cooperate. Teachers must motivate students to do their homework. Doctors and nurses, as well as elder care workers, must persuade patients to change their eating or exercise habits or to take medication.

Peer effects also come into play. The number of other children and the type of behavior they engage in affects the quality of child care at least as much as the credentials of the provider. A mentally healthy elderly person in a nursing home where a high percentage of residents suffer from dementia is likely to be adversely affected. Individuals with disabilities can feel stigmatized when they are segregated from others. Students learn from others students; selective schools and colleges can charge higher tuition than institutions with identical teaching staff in part because parents recognize the value of such peer effects (Winston 1999).

The outputs of care work are often multidimensional. One aspect of teacher performance can be measured by changes in students' scores on standardized exams. But such measures do not capture the extent to which a teacher succeeds in instilling motivation or independent problem-solving skills. Likewise, hospital performance cannot be accurately measured by the speed with which patients exit the hospital, because the care process matters (Shih and Schoenbaum 2007). Effects on long-run physical and mental health, though difficult to isolate, can countervail short-run cost savings.

The central role of emotional attachment and person-specific skills means that disruptions of care relationships can have adverse consequences. Most studies of paid child care and elder care call attention to the negative effects of high turnover rates among staff (see the discussion in chapter 4). Similarly, changing schools frequently can lower young children's chances of academic success, and transitions between hospitals, nursing home facilities, and home often pose difficulties for those receiving medical care. Expanded scope for consumer choice offers important benefits but can also undermine continuity of care. "Consistent assignment" of caregivers offers tangible benefits.[4]

The complex subjective and emotional content of paid care work helps explain why it is often helpful to give paid care workers a strong voice in the organization of their work and to encourage "job crafting" that facilitates effective collaboration (Leana, Appelbaum, and Shevchuk 2009). In addition to helping improve the efficacy of care provision, worker participation can help protect workers from endemic occupational hazards such as emotional burnout and compassion fatigue.

CARE NEEDS

The individuals who need care most are those unable to care for themselves. Infants and young children clearly fit this category, with age a fairly good predictor of their capabilities for self-care. Not all elderly people need care from others, but they tend to become somewhat dependent as they reach advanced age. Non-elderly individuals with disabilities also represent a large percentage of those in need of assistance. Fertility decline in the United States has helped free up time for mothers to participate more extensively in paid employment. However, it has also reduced the number of adult children—as well as the number of siblings—available to help aging family members.

Projecting Needs

Measures of dependency are often simply based on a standard numerical definition—the ratio of the population under the age of fifteen and over the age of sixty-five to that in the so-called working ages between sixteen and sixty-four. Worldwide, this ratio was about 0.6 in 2002. That is, for every working-age person there was about six-tenths of one person in an age group likely to be characterized by dependency.

The dependency ratio calls attention to the similar claims that the young and old make on the working-age generation, with important implications for change over time. As average fertility declines and life expectancy increases, the average age of the population tends to increase. Fewer children require care, but more adults at the opposite end of the life cycle may become needy, making the initial "demographic dividend" yielded by fertility decline a demographic liability as the ratio of elderly to the working-age population increases.

However, the simple dependency ratio does not provide an accurate measure of care needs, for two reasons. First, care needs differ substantially across age groups. One useful refinement of this ratio weights the number of individuals under age seven and those over age seventy-five twice as heavily as other children and elderly, because these individuals are likely to impose a greater temporal burden (Razavi 2007). But more research is needed to more precisely determine the relationship between age and expected care needs. The incidence of disability is not always age-related and sometimes reflects the uneven impact of medical technology (such as improved treatment of battlefield wounds or advances in neonatal care), which reduces mortality but increases morbidity.

As life expectancy increases, the probability of suffering a chronic health problem such as congestive heart failure, dementia, or Alzheimer's disease goes up. Increased obesity in the United States is associated with a number of chronic health problems in old age, including diabetes. Improvements in medical technology have made it more likely that premature babies will survive, but increased survival rates have, sadly, also brought increases in the likelihood of disability at birth. Many other disabilities afflict individuals in the working-age population. Notable among these are the disabilities resulting from HIV infection, a chronic disease that has become more widespread over the past thirty years. Even more recently, war-related traumas (both physical and psychological) have also increased care needs for working-age adults in the United States.

Needs Assessment

Most efforts to determine the type and quantity of care to which individuals other than children are entitled through a publicly funded service program set criteria based on some minimum level of problems with self-care. A common standard for public assistance to people with disabilities or those who are elderly is based on need for assistance with activities of daily living (ADLs), such as eating or toileting, and instrumental activities of daily living (IADLs), such as shopping or paying bills (for further discussion, see the appendix).

Estimates of the size of the population needing long-term care are often based on assessments of ADLs. Eligibility for many federal and state programs, especially those entailing institutional services, is based on the need for help with multiple ADLs. The definition of "long-term" in the phrase "long-term care" often goes unspecified. Individuals who are recuperating from a temporary injury or illness are clearly not included. But definitions are based on the potential need for long-term care rather than actual utilization of it—that is, someone can receive "long-term care" for a very short period of time. In fact, long-term care may often be provided for fewer years than the putatively "short-term" care provided to children. Standard definitions of long-term care exclude healthy children, even though children under the age of five clearly need assistance with many ADLs, and those under the age of eighteen typically need assistance with IADLs.

Need-based measures are only approximate. They are not always defined in comparable ways and are likely to be subject to some reporting bias (see the more detailed discussion in the appendix). The level of need for help with ADLs may vary. One person may need only to have his food cut up for him; another may need to be spoon-fed. Also, the level, type, or frequency of care that we "demand" from ourselves when we have the capacity to meet those demands may be more or less than the amount that society judges us to "need" if we are unable to provide for our own needs. Someone able to bathe herself is free to go for days without bathing, for instance, yet if she loses that capacity she may be supplied with a helper who will provide a daily bath. Similarly, someone may "supply" care in response to a caregiver's perceptions of the care recipient's needs rather than the care recipient's own "demands." It seems quite likely that, in many cases, the care recipient's views and the care provider's views about the nature and quantity of care that is needed are quite different.

If the services we are examining were provided only in a market, we might describe this as a potential mismatch between the supply and demand. However, concepts of supply and demand apply only in a limited way here. Many of those with the greatest need for care, such as young children and adults with severe cognitive impairments, have limited ability to express a demand for it. Their needs are met through a combination of social obligation and altruistic commitment—if they are met at all. For these reasons, we generally speak of care needs rather than demands, and of care provision rather than supply.

Children's Care Needs

In 2010 the majority of mothers who had children under age five living with them worked for pay (see the more detailed discussion in chapter 3). Among those who were employed, about 33 percent of their children were in organized care (day care centers, nursery or preschools, federal Head Start programs, and kindergarten–grade schools), 30 percent were cared for by a grandparent, and about 29 percent received care from another parent.[5] About 19 percent were cared for by a non-relative, either in their own home, in another person's home, or in family day care. Grade schoolers age five to fifteen who lived with an employed mother were cared for in a similarly complex array of settings. In 2010 about 6.4 percent were in organized care, 17 percent were cared for by a grandparent, and 25 percent received care from another parent. The father's participation was typically greatest when mothers were employed on a non-daytime shift.

Many children of non-employed mothers—about 12 percent—also spend time in organized care, although most do not have a regular care arrangement other than parental care: 15 percent were cared for by grandparents, 3 percent by another parent, and 3 percent in more informal care settings. We use the term "early childhood education and care"—shortened to ECEC—to encompass two types of organized care: "child care" programs, which are primarily intended to provide substitutes for parental care, and "early education" programs, such as Head Start and pre-kindergarten programs, which have an explicit educational purpose (see the more detailed discussion in chapters 6 and 7).

As of September 2008, about one-half of one percent of all children under age eighteen nationwide were part of the foster care system (for more details, see chapter 6). Most of these children were placed with foster families, and about one-quarter with relatives other than parents or guardians. About four times as many children live in informal care arrangements with kin other than their parents, without formal assistance from the foster care system.

Between 13 and 18 percent of all children have one or more special health care needs.[6] Prevalence is consistent across income levels, but varies by race-ethnicity—from a high of 18 percent among mixed-race children to 15.5 and 15.0 percent among non-Hispanic whites and blacks, respectively, to 8.3 percent among Hispanic children and 6.3 percent among Asian children (U.S. Department of Health and Human Services/HRSA 2007; Rosenbaum 2008).

Adult Care Needs

In 2007 approximately 13.7 million adults required assistance with either ADLs or IADLs (see the more detailed discussion in chapter 3). Of these, 6.6 million needed enough assistance to qualify for publicly funded long-term services and supports, if they met the income and asset qualifications. Only 1.8 million of those actually lived in nursing facilities; another 1.6 million persons received paid care in home- and community-based settings. But most care—84 percent of all 21.5 billion hours of non-institutional personal assistance—was provided in the home by unpaid family and friend caregivers (LaPlante, Harrington, and Kang 2002). Despite their documented need, only 33 percent of older adults, 18 percent of adults with disabilities between the ages of eighteen and sixty-four, and 68 percent of adults with intellectual and developmental disabilities (ID/DD) received paid help in any venue.

People with disabilities represent a significant share of the total population in need of care. About half the individuals needing assistance who live in communities (rather than institutions) are non-elderly (including children with developmental or physical disabilities) (Kaye, Harrington, and LaPlante 2010). Even among those who meet the narrow definition of needing help with two or more ADLs, more than 45 percent are non-elderly. In an analysis of the 1994 Disability Supplement to the National Health Interview Survey (NHIS), Lois Verbrugge and Li-Shou Yang (2002) found that 7 to 9 percent of adults had a disability that began before age twenty and another 20 to 30 percent experienced the onset of their disability before the age of forty-four. These younger adults have care needs that are both similar to and very distinct from those of older adults who have not spent the majority of their life living with a disability. For example, the former are far more likely to live independently and to rely on caregivers who come to their homes to bathe, dress, and help them go to work.

Among the older population, the prevalence of disability declined during the 1980s and 1990s, and there is some evidence that this trend continued into the early 2000s (Manton, Gu, and Lamb 2006). The less severe form of disability codified as being unable to perform IADLs showed consistent declines during the 1990s. The more severe form of disability associated with inability to perform ADLs showed declines during the mid and late 1990s, both in the prevalence of reported difficulty with these tasks and in the use of help from others (Freedman et al. 2004).

However, the growing prevalence of obesity and diabetes at younger ages may have alarming implications for the older population of the future (Institute of Medicine 2007). Recent research suggests that we may already have experienced a reversal, since 2000, in the trend toward lower prevalence of disability at older ages (Fuller-Thomson et al. 2009; Seeman, Merkin, and Karlamangla 2010). In any case,

FIGURE 1.1   /   Institutions Providing Care

Households/Families

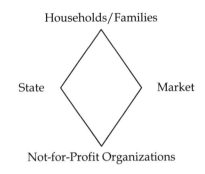

State

Market

Not-for-Profit Organizations

Source: Authors' figure based on Razavi (2007).

rapid growth in the share of the population over age seventy-five could easily offset gains from declining rates of disability and associated care needs.

INSTITUTIONAL DIVERSITY AND MOTIVATIONAL COMPLEXITY

Care services can be provided by many different kinds of institutions, including families, neighborhoods, the state, the market, and nonprofit organizations. These are sometimes pictured in terms of a care "diamond," as in figure 1.1. In theory, the diamond could be divided up into component parts representing the relative importance of these types of institutions in care provision. However, the state plays a central role not just as a provider of care but also as arbiter, enforcer, and regulator of many care responsibilities (Razavi 2007). For instance, family law defines obligations to care for kin, and labor law and work-family reconciliation policies regulate market providers.

Unpaid and paid care intersect with different institutional forms, as indicated in table 1.1. We denote care as "unpaid" when it is not paid on a per-unit basis, but it may be implicitly paid in the sense that it is rewarded by personal reciprocity or by public support in the form of direct subsidies or tax benefits. Indeed, the boundary between unpaid and paid caregivers is sometimes permeable, since income-sharing within families often represents a form of remuneration for services provided. Individuals can care for themselves directly or through purchase of services. Family and friends can provide unpaid or paid services or both. Nonprofit organizations can mobilize volunteers to provide unpaid care or raise money to pay caregivers. Insurance firms provide support for some types of care provision through, for instance, long-term care insurance.

Community provision of care—whether in the form of assistance from friends and neighbors or from nonprofit charitable organizations—often supplements

TABLE 1.1 / Paid and Unpaid Care by Sources of Support

	Unpaid Care	Paid Care
Individual	Self-care	Privately hired care workers
Family or friends	Volunteers	Informally reciprocated or formally paid care workers
Nonprofit organizations	Volunteers	Direct funding of paid care workers
Insurance firms	—	Direct funding of paid care workers
State or public sector	Tax deductions and credits for dependent care	Direct or indirect funding of paid care workers

Source: Authors' summary.

family care. However, its availability and reliability are sometimes tenuous. Some communities are able to mobilize more resources for care than others. Unfortunately, those most in need of mutual aid may live among those least able to provide it. As Stacey Oliker (2000, 182) puts it, poverty may "undermine the material and moral capacities of networks of exchange."

The state or public sector provides support for both unpaid and paid care. This can take several different forms: support for family caregivers in the form of tax deductions or tax credits; direct services provided by government employees, as in public kindergartens and schools; subsidies for market-based services, as in child care subsidies; and Medicare and Medicaid payments to hospitals and private nursing homes. Public provision of care services is often framed as a social safety net for those unable to meet their needs in any other fashion. But coverage is often inadequate and uneven, with large variations across states (see the discussion in chapter 7).

Both unpaid and paid care provision can be provided in different sites, as indicated in table 1.2. Unpaid care is not restricted to the home but is often delivered by friends and family members in hospitals, nursing homes, or schools in the form of volunteer activities. Likewise, paid care is not restricted to institutions but can take place in individual households. Wage-earners are the direct providers of paid care, but they work in environments largely shaped by owners and managers.

Each of these institutional sites of care is characterized by distinctive strengths and weaknesses and influenced by the sources of support described in table 1.1. Unpaid care in one's own home or the home of a family member or friend is often considered the "gold standard." Surveys of nursing home workers regarding institutional quality sometimes include a question such as, "If your mother needed care, would you recommend this nursing home to her?"[7] On the other hand, families sometimes fail to provide adequate care for dependents, and the burdens of family care can be very unevenly distributed. A substantial percentage of parents in the United States raise children with no assistance from another coresident biological

TABLE 1.2   /   Sites of Paid and Unpaid Care Provision

Households	Institutions
Care recipient's own home	State-run facilities
Home of a family member or friend	Nonprofit facilities
Home of a foster care provider	For-profit facilities

Source: Authors' summary.

parent. Family members are not always equally willing to care for a child or adult with a disability, and daughters often feel more responsibility than sons for care of frail elderly parents. Both the level and quality of care that individuals receive in their home depend on a combination of factors: personal resources, intrafamily negotiation, and the level of public support.

Institutions directly financed and run by the state, such as public schools, are often quite variable in quality, as are institutions that enjoy indirect subsidies from the state, like child care agencies. For-profit provision of care services can create temptations to cut costs in ways that lower quality, especially in care services for vulnerable populations (Cancian 2000). Low levels of public subsidy for services provided for profit appear to compound quality problems, as indicated by a large literature pointing to deplorable conditions in Medicaid-financed nursing homes (Eika 2009; U.S. General Accountability Office 2003; Diamond 1992). Federal and state regulations also exert a powerful effect. One comparative study of the quality of child care centers, for instance, found that differences in state regulatory regimes had larger effects on measurable quality than differences between for-profit and nonprofit firms (Helburn 1995).

Institutional diversity offers advantages, creating a portfolio of alternatives that provide an effective safety net. Modes of care provision are typically mixed: most families combine their own child care with care and education provided in the public sector or purchased in the market; many nursing homes in the United States are for-profit institutions that rely heavily on reimbursements from the federal government through Medicaid. However, serious problems with care provision often emerge from the interface between different modes of provision. Families may lack the flexibility they need to adjust the demands of paid employment to provide family care, and they may not receive adequate public support for the care they do provide. Public support may crowd out private support, and vice versa. Family caregivers and paid caregivers may not get the support and training they need in order to communicate and work together effectively.

As British researcher Clare Ungerson (1997, 377) puts it, "The social, political, and economic contexts in which payments for care operate and the way in which payments for care are themselves organized are just as likely to transform relationships as the existence of payments themselves." Considering the characteristics of care work raises questions of institutional design that are more complex than the answers to binary questions such as "paid or unpaid"?

MATCHING NEEDS AND MOTIVATIONS

A first step in challenging the conventional polarity between love and money lies in describing combinations of intrinsic and extrinsic motivation. A standard economics textbook assumption is that providers supply paid labor only in return for income. Reliance on extrinsic motivation also describes individuals who supply unpaid labor because they will be sanctioned if they do or only out of some exchange motivation—such as anticipated future payback. But intrinsic motivations can modify or soften the impact of extrinsic motivations, as with many types of service work that are characterized by an important role for trust, identity, and emotion (Levy and Murnane 2004). In care work, strong intrinsic motivations may even override or dominate extrinsic rewards. We unpack the concepts of extrinsic and intrinsic motivation in more detail in the following chapter.

A second step is to examine the needs of care recipients. Standard economics textbooks assume that they know what they need and how to get it ("consumer sovereignty"). We consider two other alternatives: consumers may lack the information necessary to accurately determine their own needs, or they may benefit from a sense that a provider is motivated by genuine concern for their well-being.

The matrix in figure 1.2 illustrates several possible combinations of worker motivations and consumer needs based on the intersections of these categories. Cell 1 represents the intersection of textbook assumptions for both workers and consumers. Exchanges of this type conform to the stylized impersonal exchange of worker and consumer, as if "the buyer and the seller were in plastic bags" (Hyde 1983, 10). At the opposite end of the diagonal, cell 9 represents the combination of factors particularly relevant to high-quality interactive care. Care recipients need assurance that the provider cares about their personal well-being, and care workers are strongly motivated to provide care on this basis. This intersection can occur in both unpaid and paid care, though we might expect it to be especially common in unpaid care provided within the family and the community.

Many variations lie between these two extremes. Cells on the diagonal of the figure reflect some complementarity between the needs of consumers and the motivations of workers. For instance, in cell 5 consumers lack perfect information, but workers with at least some intrinsic motivation (such as norms of professional responsibility) are likely to provide it whether they are paid to do so or not. Cells off the diagonal represent a potential mismatch between consumers and workers. For instance, in cell 7 consumers may be unable to clearly ascertain or express their needs, and workers motivated only by extrinsic rewards may not be willing to help them. A child may dislike going to kindergarten because the teacher does not create a welcoming environment. A frail elderly person may resent the hurried manner of a home health care worker and retaliate by refusing to cooperate in taking medicine. A patient in a clinic may be on the verge of

FIGURE 1.2 / The Complex Range of Consumer Needs and Provider Motivations

Needs of Consumers	Motivations of Providers		
	Extrinsic motives only	Strong extrinsic motives and weak intrinsic motives	Weak extrinsic motives and strong intrinsic motives
Certain of own impersonal needs	1. Transactions in idealized competitive market	2. Some transactions in markets; some transactions in the family and the community	3. Some transactions in markets; many transactions in the family and the community
Uncertain of own needs as a result of information problems	4. Some transactions in markets	5. Some transactions in markets; some transactions in the family and the community	6. Some transactions in markets; many transactions in the family and the community
Benefiting from sense that provider is motivated by genuine concern for consumer's personal well-being	7. Some transactions in markets	8. Some transactions in markets; many transactions in the family and the community	9. Some transactions in markets; many transactions in the family and the community

Source: Authors' summary.

revealing a health problem but lack the confidence to confide in an unsympathetic nurse.

This approach to possible mismatches between the needs of care providers and care recipients differs from the traditional Marxian critique of commodification because it implies that mismatches can occur in both paid and unpaid care. Paid care is not necessarily characterized by the absence of intrinsic motivation, and unpaid care is not necessarily characterized by its strong presence. Intrinsic motivation probably plays an important role in many jobs, but is especially important in high-quality care provision.

SUMMARY

We believe that the development of a more unified approach to care provision can aid in the design of public policies. In particular, we argue that the conventional "love versus money" frame offers a simplistic picture of the interaction among different institutional forms of care, overlooking important similarities and complementarities between unpaid and paid care work. We need to challenge the view that public care provision necessarily contributes to "defamilialization" and show how it can contribute to "refamilialization." We need to recognize the problems that can arise in all forms of care work, along with the need to coordinate them in a more effective way.

Both women and men tend to choose care occupations in part because they consider them socially worthwhile (Stone 2000a; Satterly 2004, 37). They respond to and help develop norms of appropriate behavior. They hope to gain the respect and appreciation of both their employers and those they care for in return for their hard work. They often bond emotionally with those they care for, becoming even more altruistic over time. However, these sources of intrinsic prosocial motivation can be undermined by economic stress, poor working conditions, or an inability to deliver effective care due to inadequate training or institutional roadblocks. A closer look at motivations for care helps explain the importance of both reforming public policies and expanding care research.

NOTES

1. We considered using the terms "direct care" instead of "interactive care" and "indirect care" instead of "support care." But this nomenclature would be confusing because the term "direct care" is frequently used in policy discussions today to refer to the care of people who are elderly or disabled, excluding the care of children. Further, the adjective "interactive" conveys our emphasis on the personal and often emotional character of certain care activities.

2. For instance, Maren Jochimsen (2003, 11) defines care as activities aimed at "the long-term maintenance, sustenance, and repair of these physical and social relationships which are indispensable for continuing human existence in a social context."

3. The process of finding life partners and developing stable and satisfying relationships with them requires considerable effort, for instance, and many market services, ranging from speed-dating to couples therapy, aim to help meet such needs. Problems of "self-care" deserve consideration, especially in a world in which an increasing proportion of adults live alone. Activities such as eating, drinking, bathing, and grooming are socially necessary. People who cannot feed themselves or engage in other activities of daily living are considered disabled and require the assistance of other person. Grooming and manicuring services are often purchased in the market, suggesting that we should consider them productive activities when performed at home. Obesity, lack of exercise, and other health problems indicate that people do not always care for themselves as well as they should.

4. See, for instance, the Nursing Home Quality Campaign, "Fast Facts: Consistent Assignment," http://www.nhqualitycampaign.org/files/factsheets/Consumer%20Fact%20Sheet%20-%20Consistent%20Assignment.pdf.

5. U.S. Census Bureau, "Table 1a: Childcare Arrangements of Preschoolers Living with Mother, by Employment Status of Mother and Selected Characteristics: Spring 2010." Available at: "Child Care: Who's Minding the Kids? Child Care Arrangements 2010," http://www.census.gov/hhes/childcare/data/sipp/2010/tables.html (accessed December 21, 2011).

6. The 2005–2006 survey of the federal Health Resources and Services Administration (HRSA) puts the estimate at 13.9 percent, or 10.2 million children under the age of eighteen with special health care needs (U.S. Department of Health and Human

Services/HRSA 2007). The National Survey of Children with Special Health Care Needs, using a broader definition, finds that 19 percent of children—14.1 million—in 2007 who were less than eighteen years of age had special health care needs. The broad definition of children with special health care needs (CSHCN) is "children who have or are at increased risk for a chronic physical, developmental, emotional or behavioral condition and who also require health and related services of a type or amount beyond that required by children generally," as specified in Title V Maternal and Child Health Program (Johnson 2010).

7. Personal communication, Marta Szebehely, Department of Social Work, Stockholm University, June 2009.

Chapter 2

Motivating Care

Paula England, Nancy Folbre, and Carrie Leana

T he simple contrast between doing something for love and doing something for money conceals enormous variation in the forms that intrinsic
and extrinsic motivation can take, as well as the ways in which these forms
can be combined. "Love" can represent many different types of motivations: a
sense of moral obligation, a social norm of responsibility, a general concern for
other people, or a very specific concern for the well-being of a specific person.
"Money" can also represent many possibilities: a weekly paycheck, a share of
someone's income, an expected bequest, or future payback for an informal service rendered. What are the implications of these distinct motivations for care
provision? Where do they come from? Why do they seem to differ between men
and women? How do these distinct motivations interact, and how might they
be affected by the organization of care work itself?

In this chapter, we review and synthesize the interdisciplinary research that
addresses these theoretical questions. Although we review the relevant empirical
evidence, much of the literature on these topics is speculative, allowing us only to
offer hypotheses needing further research. First, we build on the discussion in the
previous chapter to offer a more detailed taxonomy of motivation, making analytical distinctions between extrinsic and intrinsic motivations for giving care and
emphasizing the importance of intrinsic motivations that are "prosocial" or based
on concern for others. Second, we discuss possible biological and social sources of
prosocial motivation. Third, we summarize a number of reasons why women tend
to specialize in care provision, ranging from extrinsic factors such as discrimination and social pressure to intrinsic factors such as internalized preferences for care
resulting from biology, early socialization, or regular participation in care work.
Fourth, we explore an apparent trade-off between love and money—reasons why
prosocial motivations to provide care may carry an economic penalty. Finally, we
explore the labor process of care, emphasizing that the organizational structure

and design of care work may affect extrinsic and intrinsic rewards and the quality of the services provided.

A TYPOLOGY OF EXTRINSIC AND INTRINSIC MOTIVATIONS

Several subcategories of extrinsic and intrinsic motivation are relevant to the supply of unpaid and paid care services and the quality of the care provided. When work is extrinsically motivated, it is performed because of a desire to gain external rewards or to avoid punishments. Such rewards can take many forms, ranging from pay and benefits to the approval of others. As we describe in more detail later in the chapter, extrinsic motivation can also result from restrictions on alternatives to doing care work. Intrinsic motivation derives from the workers' own preferences and priorities. It may be based on the pleasure or sense of accomplishment a worker gets by doing the work itself. Alternatively, intrinsic motivation may grow out of prosocial concerns for the welfare of others. Such prosocial concerns can be conceptualized as both a trait (a person's general disposition to help others) and a state (temporarily induced by a particular situation or context, such as being made aware of others' suffering).[1]

These types of motivation are conceptually distinct but often work in concert, as when a care worker takes a job for pay (extrinsic motivation) but also out of a desire to help other people (intrinsic prosocial motivation). However, we believe that prosocial motivations are most relevant to explaining why people engage in care work and describing how well they perform in care jobs. Research has shown that there is little about the actual *doing* of care work that is in itself inherently interesting or pleasurable, independent of the prosocial aspects of the work such as helping others. Indeed, care work is hard work, involving large measures of both physical and emotional labor, and although the caregiver may derive pleasure from the outcome of her efforts (for example, a patient regaining health), the process of doing the work is more often described as difficult, frustrating, and even dirty.[2] As we discuss in later chapters, however, intrinsic motivation in care work could be improved through strategic redesign of care jobs. Table 2.1 summarizes our typology of motivations.

Common treatments of extrinsic motivation center on traditional incentives like pay and benefits. Extrinsic motivation can also arise from restrictions on other activities.[3] For example, the worst-paying care jobs attract some workers who take them simply because they cannot get a better-paying or more appealing job, owing to low skill levels or discrimination based on sex, race, national origin, or citizenship status. Sex discrimination in labor markets has increased the supply of women to both paid and unpaid care work by restricting access to other jobs, paying women less than men for equal work in male-dominated jobs (Reskin and Roos 1990; Bergmann 1986). If women cannot get predominantly male jobs, more of them will end up in female-typed paid care work. When sex discrimination lowers women's wages, couples are more apt to assign women primary responsibility for family care.

TABLE 2.1 / Motivations for Provision of Care Services

Extrinsic Motives

Response to physical coercion or restriction of other alternatives

Expectation of direct payment or other rewards (or avoidance of penalties)

Expectation or hope of social approval or indirect or postponed rewards such as reciprocity

Intrinsic Motives

Enjoyment of the activity or labor process itself

Prosocial Intrinsic Motives

Conformity to caring norms because they are taken for granted or part of one's identity

Values that involve a moral obligation or duty or that flow from a sense of calling or love for others in the abstract

A desire to contribute to the happiness or well-being of a specific person

Source: Authors' summary.

Women who enter a male-dominated, noncare profession—like men who enter a female-dominated care profession—may be perceived as a less attractive dating or marriage partner as a result.[4] Some empirical research based on surveys of college students based on personal ads supports this hypothesis (Badgett and Folbre 2003). Taking a higher-paying job may actually put a woman at an economic disadvantage if it reduces her chances of finding a husband. High-earning men in the United States today are likely to marry potentially high-earning wives (Sweeney and Cancian 2004). But this correlation may arise simply because neighborhoods and schools are increasingly segregated by class (England 2004).

Another type of extrinsic motivation for family care work is the expectation of, or hope for, reciprocity, especially from one's children. Economists tend to describe such expectations in instrumental terms, as anticipated rewards. Sociologists are more likely to interpret them as effects of social norms. The urge to provide family care may derive from taken-for-granted expectations or from a conscious attempt to gain the approval or avoid the disapproval of family and peers. For example, if women are expected to provide much of the child and elder care in families, they may face serious disapproval for delegating it to others, while men may face disapproval for eschewing employment in favor of full-time unpaid care. Men aspiring to work in paid care jobs, such as kindergarten teacher or nurse, may be mocked as effeminate when they announce their intentions.

Prosocial motivations for care include norms that have been internalized as tacit assumptions or as personal preferences. Sometimes norms are sufficiently taken-for-granted that they are not articulated. For example, most of us do not stop to think about whether it is appropriate for a parent to send a child out to work for pay at age ten; if asked, we would probably say that doing so would be harmful, but mostly we do not give it any thought. Sometimes particular norms (articulated or tacit) support important parts of our identities and are fiercely defended if challenged. Conformity to norms of masculinity, for instance, may help explain why men tend to eschew care work, whether paid or unpaid.

Another type of prosocial motivation is embodied in moral values that specify giving care as an obligation or duty. For example, parents may believe that they have a moral duty to care for their children, and adult children may believe that they have a moral duty to repay that care when their parents need assistance in old age (Ibarra 2010, 130). Earlier, we discussed caring out of the expectation of reciprocity as an example of extrinsic motivation. Here, we point to the possibility that internalized values may motivate care even when there is no expectation of future reward.

Some care work—both paid and unpaid—is seen by those who do it as a calling that represents a source of deep personal meaning (Bellah et al. 1985; Hall and Chandler 2005). Certified nursing assistants often describe their line of work in these terms (Mittal, Rosen, and Leana 2009). The pleasure of altruism is sometimes described as a "warm glow" derived from the process of giving itself (Andreoni 1990). Prosocial motivation to care may take a general or abstract form as a desire to help the needy. Alternatively, it may be rooted in concern for the well-being or happiness of a specific person—the form of altruism most commonly identified as love.[5] Most of us love our spouses, partners, children, and/or parents, as well as feeling some obligation to care for them. Paid care workers often develop affection for the particular people they care for as well.

Acknowledging the importance of prosocial motivation does not imply that the ideal care worker is selfless, or that extrinsic rewards such as pay and benefits matter less to them than to other workers. A romantic view of the altruistic care worker can deflect attention from the demoralizing effects of low extrinsic rewards and even serve to justify low wages (Folbre and Nelson 2006). Similarly, efforts to enhance intrinsic motivation through better work design can help reduce high turnover problems among nursing home aides, but it is not an adequate solution (Bishop et al. 2008). Most care workers need decent pay and working conditions to adequately care for themselves and their own family members, and as we discuss in later chapters, extrinsic and intrinsic rewards can complement each other.

In real-world situations, a mix of motivational forms is often at play. For example, maternal care of children may be motivated by a blend of genuine care for the children's well-being and happiness, taken-for-granted norms about the roles of women and men in the family, and a desire for approval. People may go into teaching, elder care, child care, medicine, or the clergy because they place an abstract value on helping others that they experience as a calling, and they may go on to really care about the happiness and well-being of specific charges once in the job. These prosocial motives will be combined with concerns about extrinsic factors such as compensation: some of the people who initially choose a care occupation also expect to be paid well and may choose between care jobs on the basis of pay or even leave the care work profession if the pay is too low.

The assistance that adult children often provide to their elderly parents also may combine prosocial and extrinsic motivations. This assistance may be motivated by both altruistic concern for the parent's well-being and a strongly held, internalized sense of reciprocal obligation. Alternatively, such assistance may result from extrinsic motivations, such as direct expectations of payback, including a possible gift or bequest from the parents (Bianchi et al. 2008). These motivations may combine in a variety of ways. For instance, a demonstration effect may come into play in which second-generation adults help their parents both because they love them and because they want to demonstrate good behavior to their own offspring, who may be more likely to help them at some point in the future as a result (Cox and Stark 2005).

Individuals who place great importance on helping others may be more likely to enter caring occupations, although little research has focused explicitly on this issue. Paid care workers often tend to position themselves as advocates for their clients, patients, or students. For instance, teachers often resist high-stakes testing because of fears that it could undermine broader educational goals, not merely because it pits them against one another in assessments of relative performance (Amrein and Berliner 2002). Similarly, the Nursing Code of Ethics stipulates that "the nurse promotes, advocates for, and strives to protect the health, safety, and rights of the patient."[6] Some major nursing unions consider mandatory staffing ratios in hospitals their highest priority because they believe such ratios help protect the quality of care (Lowes 2010). In sum, prosocial motivations shape collective identity and action as well as individual choices.

SOURCES OF INTRINSIC MOTIVATION

Attention to the overlaps and interactions among different types of motivation raises important questions about how motivations are formed and how they change over time. Answers to these questions appear to be converging toward an interdisciplinary synthesis. Traditional economic models typically take preferences as a given, focusing instead on how people respond to differences in income and prices (Becker and Stigler 1977). Although these models do not assume that individuals have identical preferences, they typically devote far more attention to group differences in skill to explain different outcomes.[7] In contrast, approaches based on experimental, behavioral, and institutional economics often call attention to differences in preferences, including altruism. Similarly, sociologists generally emphasize the social construction of norms and values, examining the ways they may be shaped by institutional arrangements. Evolutionary biology suggests that natural selection exerts a powerful influence on individual predispositions to provide care, and a growing number of behavioral economists, sociologists, and psychologists are exploring this possibility.

Biology and Care Preferences

Evolutionary biology emphasizes natural selection. While perfect selfishness may promote individual survival, evolution favors reproductive success or fitness. Genes are passed on by individuals who reproduce offspring, who in turn survive long enough to reproduce. Natural selection clearly encourages altruism toward close kin who share genes, but what about altruism toward others?[8] Some contemporary evolutionary biologists argue that selection takes place on the group as well as on the individual level (Sober and Wilson 1998). Groups that successfully promote in-group altruism and solidarity—treating all members of the group as though they were kin—may be more likely to survive environmental stress or military attack than other groups. This possibility has important implications for motivations for care. Psychologist Shelley Taylor (2002, 217) argues that adult caregiving and responses to strangers rely on attachment bonds similar to those felt between parent and child. The hormone oxytocin, present in both men and women but especially in lactating women, helps elicit the disposition to care not just for one's own child but also for strangers, with a positive impact on trust (Kosfield et al. 2005).

Evolutionary arguments about gender differences in dispositions hinge on differences in the factors determining men's and women's reproductive success. Sperm are more plentiful and less biologically costly to produce than eggs. Women lose their reproductive capacity at an earlier age than men. Mothers, but not fathers, must gestate for nine months and often breast-feed to successfully reproduce. Since fathers invest less in individual offspring than mothers, they have less to lose from abandoning or neglecting a child (Trivers 1972). Evolutionary theorists assert that these asymmetries help explain why, in many species, females bond more quickly with offspring and devote more energy and resources to the next generation than males do (Hrdy 1999; Trivers 1972; Daly and Wilson 1983). Biologists also study how differences in ecological niches may promote or discourage paternal care and resource sharing and how female parenting effort may take the form of bargaining with males for increased support of offspring—bargaining that may prove costly in terms of their own economic welfare (Low 2000).[9]

These evolutionary pressures may also have implications for the broader development of male and female preferences. Male reproductive fitness is affected by the number of females impregnated, and physical strength becomes an advantage for males competing with one another in winner-take-all games that reward risk-taking behavior. If they fail to mate, no amount of willingness to help nurture offspring will help pass on their genes. Selection for parental effort places females in strategic environments more likely to reward cooperation. With no shortage of potential mates, they face substantial long-term risks of being unable to raise highly dependent offspring to maturity (Buss 1996).

Evolutionary theory provides an explanation for conflict, as well as complementarity, between men and women. All organisms face a trade-off between resources they can devote to their own well-being and those they devote to reproduction—a trade-off especially relevant to our species, since we have developed means of separating sex from reproduction. Parents sometimes devote fewer resources to their offspring than those offspring desire, and sibling rivalry can be intense. A parent who shifts the costs of successfully raising offspring toward another parent can generate a higher number of offspring, increasing his or her own reproductive fitness.

Evolutionary views about biological sources of gender differences in preferences related to care excite intense controversy among feminist theorists, particularly when they are deployed in support of arguments that movements toward gender equality are impossible or harmful (Browne 1999). Biological predispositions toward the development of certain preferences may indeed reduce malleability, lending support to the claim that preferences can be taken as a given. However, predispositions to develop certain preferences do not preclude malleability.

Sex differences among humans are not extreme. The distribution of men's and women's characteristics overlaps substantially (Hyde and Linn 2006). Historical changes in women's roles have been dramatic, suggesting that social and economic forces exert a significant impact. Finally, and most importantly, inherited predispositions do not provide a rationale for limiting women's options or absolving men from responsibility to provide care. But one need not believe (and we do not) that preferences are unchangeable in order to use insights from evolutionary theory or to fruitfully explore the effects of sex-specific hormones on behavior.

Social Formation of Intrinsic Motives

Social scientists offer an array of models of how norms, values, and preferences are developed, with implications for how gender differences arise. Some psychologists focus on children mimicking adults or on adult reinforcement of children's behavior. Some aspects of temperament are inherited, and some temporally stable traits become fixed at an early age (Pinker 2008). On the other hand, some psychologists emphasize substantial plasticity into adulthood (Dweck 2008).

Sociologists often trace norms and values to structural or institutional roots. For example, Melvin Kohn shows how one's occupation affects various value orientations, including whether one emphasizes autonomy or obedience in socializing one's children (Kohn 1989; Kohn and Schooler 1983). Similarly, providing unpaid or paid care for others may create or strengthen empathy. Workers may "acquire sentiment" for their clients, their fellow workers, or even their employers (Akerlof 1982). Such sentiments seem especially strong among those who provide direct care. As one grandmother who became involved in caring for her grandson put it: "I didn't expect this and I didn't want it, but my heart's involved now."[10] Paid caregivers often describe a similar process: "I love them. That's all, you can't help it" (Stone 2000a, 99).

Do people who perform caring jobs develop more caring preferences? The answer to this question has important implications for our understanding of gender differences. If prosocial motivation is enhanced by doing care work, then any forces other than preferences that propel women into care work will reinforce the gender division of labor. For example, if mothers care for their children because they earn lower wages than fathers, or if women enter caring occupations because their access to other jobs is restricted, both women's and men's preferences are shifted in a direction that reproduces these choices even if relative wages shift or barriers to job choice are removed. Biological differences between men and women complicate this dynamic but do not eliminate it. If preferences for care are even partially a result of doing care work (rather than simply what brings people into such work), then assigning men greater responsibility for care would be likely to increase their preferences for care to some extent.

Culturewide beliefs about men's and women's abilities sometimes influence gender differences in preferences. For instance, social psychologist Shelley Correll (2004) randomly assigned students to two groups, telling one group that both sexes had been shown to be equally good at a test and the other group that men were better at it. This false information affected individual students' belief in their own abilities. Students who believed that they were worse at math expressed less preference to take the math courses needed to pursue a career in engineering or other technical fields. The results imply that stereotypic beliefs—as well as challenges to them—can influence preferences.

The stereotypic belief that women are better at care work probably encourages women to choose care-oriented careers and discourages men from doing so. Despite a long-term shift toward support for equal opportunity for women, beliefs in "gender essentialism"—the idea that women and men naturally have different skills and interests—have persisted (Charles and Bradley 2009; Charles and Grusky 2004). These beliefs influence the fields of study and jobs that individuals find meaningful, reinforcing gender differences.

Since the 1980s, sociological models of culture have focused less on values and preferences and more on tacitly assumed ways of doing things, or "toolkits" (Swidler 1986). These are not explicitly and passionately held values about what is right and wrong, or consciously held preferences, but assumptions that are often taken for granted. People may act in conformity with expectations simply to make sense to other people, "doing gender" even in the absence of sanctions for failure to do so (West and Zimmerman 1987).

Although economists have traditionally expressed little interest in the formation of norms and preferences, a growing literature based on institutional, behavioral, and experimental approaches has brought them to center stage. Both norms and preferences can sometimes be interpreted as functional solutions to market failure or contracting problems. For example, as mentioned earlier, parents may not be able to contract with children to provide support for them in old age. Children, obviously, cannot contract with their parents to raise them with care. Private insurance arrangements designed to provide protection against ill health or disability may not be efficient because the least vulnerable individuals can opt out.[11]

In the face of such contracting problems, groups may intentionally or unintentionally instill altruistic preferences in their members. As already discussed, altruism can strengthen solidarity, a particular advantage in the face of intergroup conflict (Choi and Bowles 2007). Since altruism can be costly for individuals, groups that develop ways of persuading—or pressuring—people to sacrifice can offer collective benefits. Social coercion may solve the free-rider problem, inducing people to sacrifice individually for the group.[12] A certain amount of docility may facilitate contributions to public goods—as when soldiers follow orders to participate in battle (Simon 1990, 1992).

These economic models posit a strong role for group selection in cultural evolution (Sober and Wilson 1998). Groups that successfully inculcate the caring preferences or enforce the caring norms may "outcompete" others. Unlike older functionalist theories in sociology, this group selection approach does not assume that everyone benefits equally. Indeed, within-group inequalities may determine who is taught to be docile and caring and who is not. Both individuals and groups may act in conscious or unconscious ways to develop or defend normative rules that serve their interests (Knight 1992). The powerful may seek to inculcate altruistic norms and preferences in those less powerful.

An extension of this model suggests that patriarchal institutions have forced women to overspecialize in care provision (Folbre 2006a; Folbre and Braunstein 2001). Much of the current feminist literature on care emphasizes the ways in which inflexible and inertial institutional arrangements extend well beyond external constraints to internalized values. Diemut Bubeck (1995, 181) describes an "interlocking set of constraints and practices that channels women into doing the bulk of care that needs to be done in any society." Scott Coltrane and Justin Galt (2000, 36) argue that the belief that women are the obvious choice for parental care work "masks relations of power and inequality." Hilary Land and Hilary Rose (1985) have developed the concept of "compulsory altruism."[13] Beneath the colorful language lies the analytic proposition that social arrangements create or reinforce caring preferences that are costly to individuals but beneficial to society as a whole.

Changing Gender Norms

Women still do the majority of paid and unpaid care work, as the next two chapters will document. Yet the gender segregation of work has changed substantially, as have norms about gender, although it is hard to determine the causal linkages. Interestingly, the pace of change in both is uneven. For instance, women's employment increased dramatically in the United States between 1960 and 1995. At that point, however, the percentage of women working for pay leveled off, then dipped slightly in the early years of this century, prompting some observers to exaggeratedly proclaim that an "opt-out revolution" was under way (England 2010). A similar pattern can be observed in occupational sex segregation, which declined rapidly between 1970 and 1990, then slowed. Most of the change has come from women entering traditionally male jobs rather than men entering traditionally female jobs (England and Li 2006; England 2010).

Many studies of gender attitudes show that men are typically seen as more competent (both generally and in male-typical pursuits, though not in female-typical pursuits), while women are seen as nicer and warmer, what psychologists often call "communal" (Fiske et al. 2002; Spence and Buckner 2000; Conway, Pizzamiglio, and Mount 1996). Until the mid-1970s, psychologists routinely treated masculinity and femininity as two opposite poles: one could be more masculine only by being less feminine (Beere 1990). This approach was largely displaced by Sandra Bem's (1974) conceptualization, in which people could rank high on masculine traits, high on feminine traits, androgynous (high on both), or low on both. She championed a conceptualization of gender in which masculine and feminine preferences were no longer seen as oppositional. But even the less gender-restrictive Bem Sex Role Inventory, which bases what is called "feminine" or "masculine" on what student respondents say is expected of men and women in our society, sees care as feminine and competition as masculine. Characteristics seen as feminine include "affectionate," "sensitive to the needs of others," and "eager to soothe hurt feelings." Those seen as masculine include "ambitious," "competitive," and "individualistic."[14]

Sociologists use attitudinal surveys to assess change over time. The General Social Survey (GSS), administered on a regular basis in the United States since 1972, asks many questions designed to trace changes in norms regarding women's behavior but pays relatively little attention to men's behavior. The wording of these questions, as well as the responses to them, link femininity with care and reflect the assumption that care represents a moral obligation but not an achievement. For instance, the GSS asks, "Do you strongly agree, agree, disagree, or strongly disagree with the following: It is much better for everyone if the man is the achiever and the woman takes care of the home and family." The implicit assumption in this question—that taking care of home and family, however well done, is not an achievement—is seldom acknowledged.

Attitudes most resistant to change concern the movement of women out of their traditional child care provider roles. Consider four questions that represent an indicator of egalitarian gender attitudes: whether working mothers can have as warm and secure a relationship with their children as non-employed mothers, whether women should take care of the home, whether preschoolers suffer if their mothers are employed, and whether men are better politicians than women. Both men and women tend to express much stronger concerns about women reducing their commitments to children (the first three questions above) than about women competing successfully with men (the last question).[15] In other words, there is more agreement that bad things happen if women become less caring toward dependents than about gender equality in the non-household realm. Unfortunately, women's commitments to dependents often prevent them from becoming politicians, participating in voluntary organizations (Herd and Harrington Meyer 2002), or competing successfully with men in other arenas.[16]

A large sociological literature documents significant shifts in both men's and women's attitudes in a more egalitarian direction since the 1960s (Mason, Czajka, and Arber 1976; Mason and Lu 1988; Thornton and Freedman 1979; Thornton, Alwin, and Camburn 1983; Twenge 1997). The egalitarian trend, however, reversed during the 1990s as attitudes became more traditional; they moved back in the egalitarian direction after 2000. Current attitudes are no more egalitarian than they were in the mid-1990s (Cotter, Hermsen, and Vanneman 2011). Concerns about the well-being of dependents could help explain this slowdown.

Some economists study people's preferences by inferring them from their behavior under controlled conditions, rather than inferring preferences based on what people say they want. Experimental studies that offer highly stylized, controlled choices suggest that women on average are more generous and trusting than men, particularly in interactions with other women (Eckel 1998; Eckel and Grossman 2001). This may help explain why a higher proportion of women enter care work, though the experiments do not directly examine this hypothesis. Men appear to be slightly more prone to opportunistic or greedy behavior, arguably making the average man less suitable for care work than the average woman (Simpson 2003). Experimental work by psychologists offers a related finding—that men are more likely to ask for or demand higher wages or rewards, and therefore more likely to receive them, suggesting a greater sense of entitlement than women have (Babcock and Laschever 2003). However, it is important to remember that differences in average behavior should not be generalized to apply to all men and women (Hyde and Linn 2006).

How much of the disproportionate representation of women in unpaid and paid care work is explained by gender differences in internalized norms, values, or preferences?[17] The evidence suggests that such gender differences have a small but significant effect. Although most economists ignore preferences as explanations, economist Randall Filer (1983) shows that preferences measured with psychological items, some of which he labels "tastes" and some of which he calls "affective human capital," explain some gender differences in occupation and wages. Women's greater interest in working with and helping people explains a modest amount of the gender gap in pay, probably operating through their choice of occupations (Fortin 2008). Studies using longitudinal survey data show that youth who preferred a more female-typed occupation at age fourteen to twenty-one were more likely to work in one over ten years later, net of other factors; however, gender differences in these initial occupational aspirations explain only a small fraction of the gender difference in later occupational placement and pay (Okamoto and England 1999; Marini and Fan 1997).

In sum, research suggests that women tend to express more altruistic and caring preferences than men, but that these differences do not fully explain existing levels of occupational segregation. Social norms have shifted, with far more Americans supporting paid employment and equal opportunities for women today than in the 1960s. Yet recent stalling of the "gender revolution" makes clear that there is nothing inexorable or automatic about egalitarian change (England 2010).

THE COSTS OF CARING

"I need no shackles to remind me, I'm just a prisoner of love."[18] As these lyrics and those of many other songs attest, love is often experienced as an exquisite but painful form of bondage. The sensation of being constrained by one's affections is often a more general one, applying to the ties that bind us to family, to friends, and more generally to our fellow creatures. However poetic their effects, these constraints also have economic relevance. Women's specialization in family care channels their efforts into a product that cannot easily be bought, sold, traded, or bargained over. While it may (or may not) increase their personal satisfaction, it clearly increases their economic vulnerability. Specialization in paid care work often carries an economic penalty (England et al. 2002).

Just how expensive are values and preferences that emphasize care for others? Although we can't answer this question decisively here, we believe it is important to pose it. Some gender differences in behavior do not have significant direct economic consequences—such as differences in hairstyle or wardrobe. But specialization in care is quite costly, for a number of reasons. The time that women spend out of the labor force caring for family members substantially lowers their lifetime earnings and reduces their economic security, especially if they divorce (Bergmann 1981; Duncan and Hoffman 1988; Rose and Hartmann 2004). It may also lower their bargaining power within marriage (Lundberg and Pollak 1993). As Eva Kittay (1999, 49) puts it, "By virtue of caring for someone who is dependent, the dependency worker herself becomes vulnerable." Paid care work is also costly. Empirical research that examines the impact of entering caring occupations, while controlling for other factors, including personal characteristics, finds a pay penalty (England et al. 2002; Budig and Misra 2009). Care jobs pay less than others requiring equivalent amounts of skill or education. They even pay less than other professions that employ a similar preponderance of women (see later discussion in chapter 4).

Individual dispositions or personality characteristics can affect wages by leading people into or away from certain types of occupations. Workers earn less in jobs where they identify with their employer's mission (François 2000, 2003), which is likely to be the case in jobs that involve caring for others. People who say that they have a desire to work with and help people have lower earnings (Fortin 2008). "Masculinity," defined by interest in typically masculine activities, inhibition of tender emotional expressiveness, and lack of fearfulness, has a positive effect on earnings (Filer 1981). "Machiavellianism," or a willingness to engage in behaviors that involve manipulating others in one's own interest—a personality characteristic that is seemingly the opposite of caring—has a positive effect on earnings for people in high-ranking occupations (Bowles, Gintis, and Osborne 2001; Osborne 2000). The effects of such socioemotional personality traits on earnings are large, comparable to the effects of education and experience.

A preference for caring developed as a result of caring activities, which might be called endogenous altruism, can also be costly. An emotional attachment to their students, patients, or charges may discourage workers from demanding higher wages or changes in working conditions that would benefit them but that might adversely affect care recipients. By contrast, owners, employers, and managers in care industries are less likely than care workers to come into direct contact with care recipients and may be more likely to engage in cost-cutting strategies without experiencing negative emotional consequences themselves. Owners and managers often seem to depend on their workers' willingness to sacrifice for their clients—expecting workers to respond to cutbacks in staffing levels, for instance, by intensifying their efforts or agreeing to work overtime. These aspects of prosocial motivation may be good for care recipients, at least in the short run, but they penalize workers who develop caring preferences.

THE LABOR PROCESS OF CARE

With the historical rise of wage labor and women's employment, more care work has moved from the family to the market. The implications of this transition for the quality of care services received by children, disabled adults, and elders depend on how care work is organized—particularly on how this organization affects motivations to provide care (Folbre and Weisskopf 1998; Folbre and Nelson 2002).

The Central Importance of Motivation

Organizations that attract workers with a public service motivation or a calling often enjoy improved performance (François 2000, 2003). This is hardly surprising, since intrinsic motivation should improve performance in any job by ensuring that workers perform even when they are not being monitored. Indeed, prosocial motivation affects many of the noncognitive traits that economists now term "soft skills," such as ability to cooperate with others. This probably explains why employers often rank attitude as more important than specific skills or academic background (Duncan and Dunifon 1998; Bowles, Gintis, and Osborne 2001). When workers are motivated to care, they provide higher-quality services and are more satisfied with their jobs (Uttal and Tuominen 1999; MacDonald 1996). Prosocial motivation may be particularly important to quality performance in care work, which often involves task ambiguity and multitasking, factors that make close monitoring of workers difficult (Holmstrom and Milgrom 1991; Kreps 1997).

The difficulty of measuring output in care services makes it difficult for employers to implement performance-based rewards that incentivize quality care. When performance in some tasks is more easily measured than others, performance-based rewards focus on these tasks, inducing employees to reallocate effort away from less easily measured parts of the job (Holmstrom and Milgrom 1994). Over time this may cause workers to focus less on unrewarded but potentially important tasks. For example, the higher valuation of research over teaching in many universities, which stems in part from the relative ease of measuring publication, has shifted pecuniary incentives away from teaching, discouraging the devotion of time and effort to that activity.

Workers are most likely to develop genuine altruism for specific care recipients when turnover is low enough, staffing levels high enough, and assignments stable enough to allow them to interact repeatedly with the same clients on the job. Consistent interaction often leads to emotional attachment, which in turn is likely to increase the quality of care. Repeated interaction among individuals encourages empathy, which, in turn, improves the likelihood of cooperation (Dovidio, Allen, and Schroeder 1990).

The effect of pay on intrinsic motivation remains an important topic of debate. Some economists argue that low pay in care jobs helps screen out workers who care only about money (Heyes 2005). Others argue that it does not necessarily have that effect (Folbre and Nelson 2006; Taylor 2007). Early laboratory experiments on intrinsic and extrinsic motivation showed that applying extrinsic rewards (pay) to inherently interesting tasks decreased intrinsic motivation (Deci 1971). Other studies found that offering payment for volunteer activities can have a demotivating effect. If the offer of pay is withdrawn, subjects become less willing to do the activity without pay than they had been before pay was offered (Frey 1998; Kohn 1990).

However, such results do not support a simplistic crowding-out interpretation, for two reasons. First, the well-known psychological phenomenon of "loss aversion" may explain why motivation is reduced after pay is given and then withdrawn (Fehr and Falk 2002, 715).[19] Second, crossing the highly charged symbolic divide between things that are done entirely for free and those done for money has been shown to have different implications than simply increasing the monetary reward. Indeed, evidence suggests that, once payment has been introduced, higher payment is associated with greater effort (Gneezy and Rustichini 2000).

The effect of payment on motivation depends partly on how workers interpret the form of the payment. Extrinsic rewards that are seen as punitive or controlling tend to reduce intrinsic motivation for a task, while those that are seen as acknowledging tend to increase it. Controlling rewards are coupled with close supervision or other processes that raise questions about the subjects' abilities and threaten their self-esteem, while acknowledging rewards send the message that the subject is trusted, respected, and appreciated (Deci and Ryan 1985, 2000; Frey and Jegen 2001). Thus, if rewards are seen as acknowledging, they may "crowd in" rather than "crowd out" intrinsic and prosocial motivation. This is consistent with one interpretation of George Akerlof's (1982) gift exchange model—that some employers pay above market wage to take advantage of workers' belief that they should reciprocate a generous employer. Although none of the experiments cited here have focused on care work, their implication seems to be that increasing the extrinsic motivation for care work by raising pay would strengthen prosocial motivation as well, as long as the rewards were seen by the workers as acknowledging their contribution.

The Organization of Paid Care Work

Concern for the well-being of care recipients is a central aspect of employment in paid care and has significant implications for care quality. One study of nursing assistants in nursing homes found five related reasons why employees stay in these jobs: (1) being called to service; (2) religious or spiritual motivation; (3) patient advocacy; (4) personal relationships with patients and their families; and (5) escape from difficult home lives (Mittal, Rosen, and Leana 2009). Those who had done the job longest reported that they derived emotional satisfaction and personal strength from providing care to others. When that care was directed toward patients with whom they had formed strong emotional bonds, their motivation to remain was even stronger. Many also found meaning in the intimate nature of the work, which they described as being essential to quality care. They described themselves as caring deeply for their patients and acting as informal, sometimes invisible advocates for them in an otherwise impersonal system. Such expressed motivations underscore the shared priorities of the givers and receivers of paid care.

Despite extensive regulation of health and safety issues in many direct care occupations, the ability of management to script and monitor care work is limited by the need for worker improvisation and autonomy. The quality of care provided to recipients by care workers may be directly related to the extent to which care workers are allowed to be flexible on the job and to call upon their own judgment and creativity to respond to the changing and often unpredictable needs of care recipients. Low-wage care jobs tend to be procedurally regimented, with rules regarding everything from personal hygiene (such as frequency of hand washing) to procedures for providing the most intimate aspects of care. Yet care workers must often exercise discretion in carrying out their day-to-day work, particularly in regard to quality-of-life issues such as care recipients' dignity, privacy, and autonomy. Every day, care workers make small and large decisions regarding their personal interactions with the individuals they care for, including how to protect their dignity when assisting them in bathing and toileting. Such challenges loom especially large in nursing homes, where the majority of residents' interpersonal interactions take place with paid care workers rather than family or friends (Burgio et al. 1990; Burgio and Bourgeois 1992).

Work discretion is the freedom that individuals have to implement essential tasks. It is the cornerstone of intrinsic work motivation and an area where management practice can make a big difference in terms of workers' motivation to provide high-quality care. When employees feel a sense of personal control, they are motivated to perform their jobs well—perhaps even exceptionally well—because doing so creates a sense of personal mastery and satisfaction. Discretion has long been recognized as a primary source of intrinsic work motivation, particularly in highly demanding jobs. It has also been shown to enhance workers' feelings of agency, fostering greater innovation and extra-role behavior at work (Karasak 1979; Hackman and Oldham 1980; Spreitzer and Sonenshein 2003). Discretion can have cognitive as well as motivational effects, allowing more effective on-the-job learning. Evidence suggests that workers can develop tacit knowledge that allows them to make better day-to-day decisions and enact more efficient work processes (Leana and Florkowski 1992; Wagner et al. 1997).

Care work often entails collaboration with others—both with care recipients, who must often be motivated to cooperate, and with fellow workers. Teachers, nurses, child care workers, and adult care workers (except those working in the care recipient's home) typically work in conjunction with peers and with other individuals with highly variable skill sets. Research on work organization points to the need to balance the cognitive gains that collaboration brings against the potential for diffusion of responsibility. The classic literature on teamwork points to the advantages of collaboration when "two heads are better than one," but at the same time warns of costly process losses because of coordination problems (Thompson 2003).

Work relationships based on trust and a shared sense of purpose can enhance organizational performance because individuals are more willing to subordinate immediate individual goals to collective purposes (Leana and van Buren 1999). Teamwork and cross-functional learning can pay off in improved service quality (Hodson 2008; Adler, Kwon, and Heckshur 2008). Individuals can learn better work practices through informal observation and by seeking the advice of their peers—training mechanisms that are often far more effective than formal programs or individual trial-and-error learning. Collaboration with others at work can also provide important social support, which may decrease feelings of "iso-strain"—the isolation and strain often reported by care workers and common in jobs with high demands, low control, and little interaction with peers (Karasak and Theorell 1990). Thus, the effects of work organization and management practice that simultaneously encourage worker autonomy and collaboration can provide important benefits.

SUMMARY

Many different types of research suggest that intrinsic motivation plays a vital role in care work and that prosocial motivation is uniquely central to the provision of high-quality care. At the same time, norms and preferences supporting altruism and care are highly gendered, encouraging women to take on care responsibilities. The process of doing care work reinforces these preferences. Discrimination and social expectations also channel women into care work. Because unpaid care tends to reduce time and effort devoted to paid work, and because jobs involving care often pay badly, norms and preferences for care are costly. In the language of collective action, men can "free-ride" on women's caring preferences and thus have some incentive to reinforce them.

We do not know to what extent differences between women and men are shaped by biological versus social factors. However, we do know that social factors play an important role and that the gender division of labor has proved historically malleable. Social forces that reinforce gendered norms of care or inculcate caring preferences more strongly in women than in men perpetuate gender inequality. Both individual and cultural renegotiation of gender asymmetries in norms and preferences of care is now under way. It seems likely that women will continue to challenge the notion that they should take greater responsibility than men for the care and support of dependents.

The notion that care work should be provided for love rather than money has often served to legitimate gender inequality. What we know about motivation to provide care does not support a simplistic model in which money crowds out pro-social motivation; nor does it suggest that care provided out of love is always superior to care provided at least in part for pay. Rather, it demonstrates the importance of the institutional and personal contexts in which care is provided. The central policy problem is how to combine love *and* money in equitable and efficient ways. Before addressing this problem, we turn to a detailed empirical examination of both unpaid and paid care work and a critical inventory of existing care policies.

NOTES

1. Some psychologists, including Adam Grant (2008), treat prosocial motivation as distinct from intrinsic motivation. Our decision to treat it as a subset of intrinsic motivation reflects our effort to develop an interdisciplinary approach, as well as a sense that this nomenclatural distinction does not have substantive implications for our discussion here.
2. See Mittal, Rosen, and Leana (2009) for a description.
3. Even more extreme examples of extrinsic motives for care come from the historical record. For example, slave women had to care for the slave owner's children and other family members on penalty of physical beatings or death. In some societies, legal restrictions on women's employment force women to specialize in unpaid care work for their families. Husbands' historical legal right to beat their wives probably kept some women in the service of their families. Sexual services have sometimes been coerced on pain of physical punishment. In contemporary affluent societies, however, simple employment discrimination represents a much more common barrier. The cumulative effect of past and present discrimination based on sex and race helps explain why women of color and immigrants are disproportionately represented in low-wage paid care work (Glenn 2010).
4. For more on rewards to following gender norms in marriage markets, see Mason and Lu (1988), Goldscheider and Waite (1991), Fisman et al. (2006), and Badgett and Folbre (2003).
5. Feminist theorist Seyla Benhabib (1987) provides a thoughtful discussion of the distinction between holding a generalized value about obligation to a nonspecified other and caring about specific others.
6. See "Code of Ethics for Nurses," http://nursingworld.org/MainMenuCategories/EthicsStandards/CodeofEthicsforNurses (accessed January 5, 2011).
7. Gary Becker's *Accounting for Tastes* (1996) could be considered an important exception. Becker explains that preferences for "specific commodities" can change in response to an individual's experiences and social environment. But Becker theorizes an extended utility function that specifies how past experiences determine the amount of utility an

individual obtains from specific commodities. He treats these extended preferences as exogenously given and unchanging.

8. The evolutionary logic behind care of adults with permanent serious disabilities or the elderly has not been well explored, perhaps because such behavior is less common in species other than our own. It is difficult to see why such behavior would be genetically selected for, since resources devoted to the care of those who can no longer reproduce do not contribute to reproductive success. However, the ability to make and enforce binding contracts could provide a link. Parental ability to invest in children may be enhanced by their ability to contract for reciprocal care in old age. Public provision of social insurance can also have this effect, lowering the lifetime costs and risks of making commitments to children.

9. Differences in economic organization provide a clear analogue. Thus, we might expect to see considerable variation across different societies at different points of time in the extent to which fathers contribute to the cost of raising children.

10. Associated Press, "Feds Study Grandparents as Caregivers," *New York Times*, June 4, 2002.

11. In more technical terms, "adverse selection" comes into play.

12. Rational choice theorists differ in whether they see group enforcement processes as changing preferences or merely inducing compliance with norms because they change incentives. However, in order for the group to successfully solve the first-order free-rider problem, its members must solve the second-order problem of what motivates group members to use resources to create the incentives for others to obey. This suggests to us that intrinsic motivation is necessary to the process.

13. The concept of "compulsory altruism" could also be interpreted as a form of "internalized oppression." Note that libertarians sometimes use the term to decry the requirement that citizens pay taxes for welfare or requirements of national service, as in the discussion of Ayn Rand in Howard Gold, "Atlas's Achilles Heel: Commentary: Revisiting the Ideas of Ayn Rand," MarketWatch/*Wall Street Journal*, June 12, 2010, http://www.marketwatch.com/story/revisiting-the-ideas-of-ayn-rand-2010-06-12 (accessed January 7, 2011).

14. Sandra Bem and her students listed two hundred personality traits that were masculine or feminine, but neutral in social desirability. They listed another two hundred traits considered either socially desirable or socially undesirable. Students rated each trait (x) by answering the following question: "In American society, how desirable is it for a man (or woman) to be x." The twenty most "feminine" traits, the twenty most "masculine" traits, the ten most neutral (for gender) undesirable traits, and the ten most neutral desirable traits make up the Bem Sex Role Inventory.

The complete list of masculine traits is: acts as leader, self-reliant, aggressive, self-sufficient, ambitious, strong personality, analytical, willing to take a stand, assertive, willing to take risks, athletic, competitive, defends own beliefs, dominant, forceful, has leadership abilities, independent, individualistic, and makes decisions easily. The complete list of feminine traits is: affectionate, loves children, cheerful, loyal, childlike, sensitive to needs of others, compassionate, shy, does not use harsh language, soft-spoken, eager to soothe hurt feelings, sympathetic, tender, flatterable, understanding, gentle, and warm.

15. See the End of the Gender Revolution? website, http://www.bsos.umd.edu/socy/vanneman/endofgr/default.html (accessed January 20, 2011).

16. Pamela Herd and Madonna Harrington Meyer (2002) also argue, however, that "civic engagement" should be reconceptualized to include unpaid family care.

17. This question is related to—but not exactly the same as—the question of how much women's specialization in care work originates on the supply side of labor markets, because supply-side explanations may focus on either skills (human capital) or preferences. Economists generally hypothesize that gender differences in wages and occupations result from differences in human capital rather than preferences. Gary Becker (1993), for instance, argues that very small biological differences between men and women, such as women's superior ability to care for very small infants, lead to a process of cumulative specialization that widens gender differences in productivity in the home. These differences lead, in turn, to gender differences in productivity in the labor market as women gain less experience and thus less human capital. Because women supply less labor to the market, they earn lower wages, which in turn reinforces their specialization in family care. Furthermore, when they combine family and market work, the effort they devote to family care may lower their energy for and commitment to market work. Solomon Polachek (1981) argues that women, anticipating these arrangements, choose occupations with little penalty for time out of employment for child care. Paula England (1982) shows, however, that the occupations in which women are concentrated do not have a lower penalty for time out of employment. This suggests a role for discrimination, but could also be consistent with differences in men's and women's preferences.

18. "Prisoner of Love," music by Russ Columbo and Clarence Gaskill, with lyrics by Leo Robin, was published in 1931 and made famous by Perry Como; it was also recorded by the Art Tatum–Lionel Hampton–Buddy Rich trio in 1955 and by the Ink Spots and Ray Price. Other songs with the same name have been written and performed by David Bowie and also by the rock group Spear of Destiny.

19. The term "loss aversion" refers to the phenomenon in which individuals appear to react more strongly to a loss than to an equivalent gain. That is, the pain they feel at losing $1,000 is greater than the pleasure they gain from winning $1,000, even when the loss or gain is over the same range.

Chapter 3

Unpaid Care Work

Suzanne Bianchi, Nancy Folbre, and Douglas Wolf

C are for family members is a central feature of the human life cycle. Most of us are tenderly cared for as children and hope to be tenderly cared for in old age. In between, most of us provide some care for family members and friends. Current descriptions of unpaid care work tend to focus on one particular demographic group. In this chapter, we examine unpaid care for children, both healthy and with disabilities, and for adults who need personal assistance (because of age-related or other disabilities), emphasizing the features common to both. We discuss both the economic and health correlates of providing care to others.

We focus on three questions. First, how is the social context that surrounds the provision of unpaid care changing? We provide an overview of the historical and demographic factors that affect the supply of unpaid care work from family members, paying particular attention to changes in women's paid work and changes in the gender division of labor in the home, family structure, and changes in the composition of the population requiring care. Second, how much unpaid care is provided in the United States? We provide an empirical overview of unpaid care provision in the United States, reviewing survey measures from previous studies of the number of hours of care that children and adults receive and the number of hours of care that adults provide. We use the American Time Use Survey (ATUS) to derive new estimates of the total amount of unpaid care provided. Third, what are the challenges that families face in providing adequate care for members, and how do these vary by gender, class, and race-ethnicity? Some households have the time or money to attend to family care needs, but the families that need care most are often the least able to provide it.

THE DEMOGRAPHIC CONTEXT

Changes in the structure of employment, family composition, age, and health of the U.S. population have affected both the supply of and demand for care over the past fifty years. Three trends are particularly noteworthy:

- Women's participation in paid employment has grown substantially, reducing the number of hours available to women—who have traditionally been the primary caregivers—to provide unpaid care to family members. This has led to an increase in expectations that men should collaborate in the care of both children and the elderly.
- Today's much higher rates of family disruption may have weakened norms of obligation and feelings of emotional attachment.
- The combination of fertility decline, the aging of the population, and health trends suggests that the need for unpaid care of adults will increase relative to unpaid care of children. This has implications for both the timing of unpaid care over the life cycle and the relative caregiving roles of women and men.

Women's Employment

The increase in women's labor force participation over the last half of the twentieth century has had a significant impact on provision of unpaid family care (Casper and Bianchi 2002). Mothers and daughters are still on the front lines of care-giving to children and older parents, but the time they allocate to paid and unpaid pursuits has shifted dramatically in recent decades. More children have employed mothers, and more adults engage in paid employment. Time constraints lead to a sometimes frenzied juggling of responsibilities.

The employment of mothers with children under age eighteen increased from 45 to 78 percent between 1965 and 2000, with the increase in full-year employment (fifty or more weeks) rising from 19 to 57 percent during the same period (Bianchi and Raley 2005, table 2.2). Mothers' employment rates leveled off in the late 1990s, causing some to argue that a slowdown or even retrenchment in the trend toward gender equality might be under way in the United States (Cotter, Hermsen, and Vanneman 2004; Sayer, Cohen, and Casper 2004), but the current widespread recession has ended the slight increase in "stay-at-home" mothers. The number of mothers who did not work outside the home declined from 5.6 million in 2006 to 5.3 million in 2008.[1]

Mothers return to work much sooner after the birth of a child today than in the past. Among all women having their first child in the early 1960s, only 10 percent were at work three months after the baby's birth. Subsequently, this percentage increased dramatically: it more than doubled between 1970 and 1990, followed by a smaller increase in the 1990s. By 2001–2002, this percentage had risen to 42 percent, and to 58 percent among women who had worked during their pregnancy. By one year after the birth, 64 percent of women were at work in 2001–2002, and 79 percent of those who had worked during their pregnancy were back at work (Johnson 2008).

Despite the increase in mothers' employment and earlier return to work after childbirth, many mothers still curtail employment to raise young children full-time, whereas fathers seldom do so. In 2007, 24 percent of couples with children under age fifteen had a mother who was out of the labor force for an entire year, presumably to care for children (Kreider and Elliott 2009). "Stay-at-home" fathers accounted for only 3 percent of families with children under age fifteen in 2007.

Married fathers have increased the amount of time they spend doing housework and child care (Bianchi, Robinson, and Milkie 2006). These fathers have been picking up some of the slack induced by the increasing paid work of married mothers. Yet fathers continue to be more likely than mothers to work long hours in paid employment, averaging forty-five hours per week in the labor market. Fathers' paid work hours (unlike those of mothers) are not responsive to the age of their children (Bianchi and Raley 2005). Fathers' long paid work hours are likely to be part of the reason why mothers in some families feel that they must curtail their hours of employment to focus on family caregiving.

About one-quarter of all households with children have only one parent present in the household. In 85 percent of these households, that single parent is the child's mother (Bianchi 2011). Single-parent households have fewer adults available to meet child care needs (Vickery 1977). Most single mothers do not have the option to drop out of the labor force or reduce their hours of employment in response to the needs of very young children unless they receive assistance from other family members, friends, or the government. The labor force participation rates of non-poor single mothers are much higher than those of married mothers, resembling those of men in the same age group. Since the welfare reforms of the mid-1990s, the United States has encouraged employment of poor single mothers rather than long-term reliance on welfare support. The labor force participation rates of poor single mothers receiving public assistance jumped from 30.5 percent to 45.8 percent between 1996 and 2001, before falling back somewhat to 39.3 percent by 2004 (Kim and Joo 2009).

Family Demographic Change

Family life has become more complex, less predictable, and less stable. Many fathers do not live with their biological children, and nonresident parents (usually fathers) typically devote little time to child care. As a result of the high rates of partnering and repartnering, the family system is more turbulent in the United States than elsewhere and women spend more time as lone mothers, rearing children without a father present, than their European counterparts (Cherlin 2009). Both nonmarriage and family disruption also complicate caregiving across generations, weakening both formal and informal ties of obligation.

Currently, about 40 percent of children in the United States are born outside of marriage (Hamilton, Martin, and Ventura 2009). Racial-ethnic differences are extremely large: about 28 percent of white children are born to unmarried parents, compared with 72 percent of African American children and 51 percent of Hispanic children (Hamilton, Martin, and Ventura 2009). Among mothers who were unmarried at the time of their child's birth, only 36 percent are living with the father when the child is five years old (17 percent have married and 19 percent live together) (Carlson and McLanahan 2010). Even among unmarried mothers who are cohabiting with the baby's father at the time of birth, only a little over half are still together by the time the child is five years old.

Divorce probabilities have not risen in thirty years, but remain high: only about half of married couples are still together at their twentieth anniversary (Goodwin, Mosher, and Chandra 2010). High rates of family dissolution mean that many children experience a series of stepparents as their parents divorce and repartner. Many of the children born to unmarried mothers will have weak ties to their fathers and paternal grandparents, a situation that is partially offset by stronger ties to maternal kin, particularly their maternal grandmothers (Nelson 2006; Bianchi 2006). Because divorce and unmarried childbearing tend to distance fathers and their children, the erosion of caring relationships between the generations can persist as children age into adulthood and older fathers become ill or frail (Cooney and Uhlenberg 1990). Later-life divorce appears to disrupt parent–adult child contact more often for older divorced fathers than for mothers (Shapiro 2003).

The rise in stepfamilies increases the number of individuals with family connections, but leaves the obligations associated with these connections poorly defined (Coleman and Ganong 2008; Cherlin 2009). Large racial and ethnic differences in family formation and dissolution suggest that care provision varies across groups, especially in reliance on extended family, "quasi-kin," and friends.

The growing share of elderly in the population is also altering the landscape of family caregiving. Declining disability prevalence at older ages may reduce the need for care from spouses and other family members. However, as discussed in chapter 1, a more realistic expectation is that the number of older people needing care will increase in coming years, with important implications for the timing and composition of unpaid family care. The renegotiation of traditional gender roles discussed in chapter 2, combined with a shift toward care of adults rather than children, may increase demands on men. In the United States, members of the baby boom generation, now reaching retirement age, have much smaller families than the ones they were born into: on average they have two children per family rather than their parents' three or four (Uhlenberg 2005). Smaller family sizes mean fewer siblings with whom to share responsibilities in dealing with family health care problems.

UNPAID CARE OF CHILDREN

Newborn babies and infants need constant care. As children progress to the toddler, schoolchild, and teenage stages, their care needs typically decrease as they acquire the physical capacity, skills, knowledge, and maturity to take care of themselves.

How Many Children Need Care?

There are around 75 million children under the age of eighteen in the United States, 50 million of whom are under the age of twelve.[2] A little over one-fifth of U.S. households include one or more children under age twelve. Currently, about 80 percent of U.S. women bear children, and the vast majority of adults provide at least some care for their own or their partner's children during the course of their lives. Further, a significant percentage of children age five and older—about 14 percent in 2004—suffer from some type of disability (Institute of Medicine 2007, 69). Although their needs vary considerably, most of these children require extra attention and effort. In 2009 about 1.7 percent of adults, or 3.9 million, reported that they had provided unpaid care to a child under the age of eighteen because of a medical, behavioral, or other condition or disability in the last twelve months (NAC/AARP 2009a, 12).

Children under age twelve spend an average of 120 hours a week, or 17 hours a day, in their own homes, according to the Child Development Supplement of the Panel Study of Income Dynamics (PSID).[3] Although paid caregivers may supervise children in their home and older children spend some hours in self-care, the majority of time that young children spend at home is time when an adult—usually a parent—is at home with them, or close by in case they need adult attention. While fathers have increased the amount of time they devote to children since the 1960s (from 2.5 hours per week in interactive child care in 1965 to 7.8 hours in 2008), mothers devote substantially more hours per week to interactive child care than fathers do: 10.2 hours in 1965, increasing to 13.9 hours in 2008 (Bianchi 2011, tables 1 and 2). The gender gap for total time spent with their children by married parents is narrower: 31 hours for fathers compared with 50 hours for mothers (Raley, Bianchi, and Wang, forthcoming).

Gender differences in single parenting contribute significantly to overall gender differences in time devoted to children. Although the number of coresident single fathers has increased since the 1970s, single mothers still account for the overwhelming majority (85 percent) of coresident single parents (Kreider and Elliott 2009).

Overall, about 32 percent of women's total adult years entail coresidence with biological children under age eighteen. (This calculation includes childless women, so the average is higher for women with children.) The comparable percentage for men is 20 percent. This is somewhat compensated by the fact that men often are the stepfathers or "social" fathers to other men's children when they remarry. On the other hand, men will spend 8 percent of their adult years living with stepchildren or other children compared with about 3 percent for women (King 1999). However, the quantity—and perhaps also the quality—of time spent parenting is lower for stepfathers than for biological coresident fathers (Hofferth et al. 2002).

Recent evidence suggests that children may be facing an increased risk of disability: activity limitations and associated risk conditions rose for children over the 1984 to 2004 time period (Institute of Medicine 2007). Care for disabled children is especially gendered. Disabled children are more likely than other children to live with single parents, especially mothers. Those who do not live with either biological parent are more likely to live in households headed by women (Cohen and Petrescu-Prahova 2006). Sadly, poor child health seems to increase the risk of divorce or separation for mothers, another factor contributing to greater maternal responsibility (Joesch and Smith 1997).

In addition to the many stepparents who care for children in blended families, many adults other than biological parents provide care. The percentage of children who live in their grandparents' home, while relatively small, has been rising over time (Casper and Bianchi 2002, figure 6.1). Estimates from the 2007 American Community Survey (ACS) suggest that about 6.2 million grandparents lived with grandchildren and that about 2.5 million were responsible for the care and support of those grandchildren (U.S. Census Bureau 2008a).

UNPAID CARE OF ADULTS WITH DISABILITIES AND THE FRAIL ELDERLY

A substantial amount of unpaid care is also provided to adults who need personal assistance as a result of disability or age. Data suggest that rates of disability are rising for non-elderly adults but declining for elderly adults (Institute of Medicine 2007). Close to 11 million adults who live in the community need long-term care, broadly defined as needing help with one or more activities of daily living (ADLs) or instrumental activities of daily living (IADLs). About 92 percent of these adults receive unpaid help (Kaye et al. 2010). Many of the approximately 1.8 million people in nursing homes also enjoy some assistance from family members, even though they are in the hands of paid caregivers. Disabled younger adults are often cared for by parents or siblings. For care recipients who are married, the informal caregiver is most often a spouse. For the unmarried elderly, many of whom are widows, adult children play an important role, with children who live near or with a parent tending to provide significantly more care than those who are geographically distant (Compton and Pollak 2009; McGarry 1998).

Care for adults with disabilities or chronic illness is often viewed as more onerous than care of children. The need for this type of care often represents an exogenous shock, one that is unexpected, difficult to anticipate, and perhaps related to sudden illness or recognition of a trajectory of increased dependency, such as when a spouse or parent is diagnosed with dementia or Alzheimer's disease. Research aimed at categorizing late-life patterns of functional change indicates that about 20 percent of the older population falls into a "persistently severe" disability category characteristic of dementia, while 15 to 19 percent experience "sudden" or "catastrophic" decline. Around 40 percent exhibit an intermediate pattern of persistent decline that plays out over a period of several months (Lunney et al. 2003; Gill et al. 2010). Caregivers typically find considerable satisfaction in helping others, but many also experience financial hardship and emotional stress (NAC/ AARP 2009b).

FIGURE 3.1 / Proportion of U.S. Adult Population Age Fifty and Over with a Parent or Spouse with Care Needs, by Gender and Age, 2002 to 2006

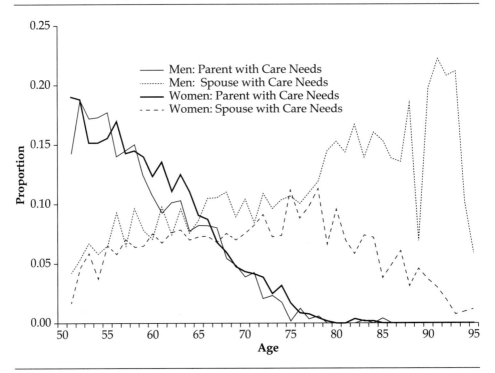

Source: Authors' calculations, based on pooled data from 2002, 2004, and 2006 waves of the Health and Retirement Survey (University of Michigan, various years, a). Respondents are coded as having a parent with care needs if they say that the parent (a) needs help with "basic personal needs like dressing, eating, or bathing," (b) cannot be left alone for one hour, or (c) according to a doctor has a "memory-related disease." Someone's spouse is coded as having care needs if either the spouse self-reports a "difficulty" with dressing, bathing, eating, and so on, or the spouse is in a nursing home.

Who Needs Care?

Adult need for care is influenced by disability, age, and the relationship between the caregiver and the care recipient. Although older adults are more likely than younger ones to require care, about one-half of those living in the community who need long-term care are non-elderly. The nursing home population, by contrast, is predominantly elderly (Kaye et al. 2010). Age is the most predictable determinant of the need for care, and it shapes demands on family members over their life cycle. Figure 3.1, based on data from the 2002 to 2006 Health and Retirement Study (HRS), shows patterns of care needs for adults from age fifty-one through age ninety-five. This figure shows both the proportion of men and women in each age group with at least one living parent needing care and the proportion with a spouse needing care.[4] An unknown percentage in each age group may have minor or adult children with special care needs, but that information is not included in the data. Between the ages of fifty and sixty-five, it is more common to have an older parent who needs help than to have a spouse who needs help. After age sixty-five, it becomes much less common to have parents in need of care simply because it becomes less common to have living parents.[5]

Somewhat surprisingly, older men are more likely than older women to have a spouse who needs care. Not many men survive into their nineties, but among those who do, 20 percent or more have a wife who needs help, while fewer than 5 percent of the women in this age group have a husband with care needs. These differences partly reflect the fact that men are less likely to become widowers than women are to become widows. Men in their nineties are therefore more likely to be married—and hence at risk of having a spouse who needs care—than women in their nineties. Moreover, the prevalence of disabling conditions is greater among women than among men. Overall, women's greater longevity puts them at greater risk of needing long-term care. One recent survey estimates that 62 percent of adults receiving unpaid care are women (NAC/AARP 2009a, 14).

Another useful measure estimates the number of potential caregivers available for each elderly person in need of care (Spillman and Pezzin 2000). Based on the 1994 National Long-Term Care Survey (NLTCS), 4.5 million of the 5.5 million chronically disabled elderly had a spouse or children, adding up to a total of 14.5 million potential spousal or child caregivers, or about 3.1 potential caregivers per potential care recipient. This ratio is likely to decrease in the coming decade, since the average number of adult children was at its peak when the 1994 NLTCS was collected.

Who Provides Unpaid Care and How Is It Shared?

Estimates of the number of informal caregivers vary widely. A 2009 survey conducted for the National Alliance for Caregiving (NAC) and the American Association of Retired Persons (AARP) reported that about 27 percent of all adults, or about 62 million people, had cared for an adult in the preceding twelve months (NAC/AARP 2009a).[6] However, the amount of time devoted to care varied substantially among caregivers and over time. Women provide the majority of care, however it is defined or measured (for further discussion, see the appendix). The survey found that 66 percent of caregivers were women (NAC/AARP 2009a, 14). Another study based on data from the 1999 NLTCS estimates that 71 percent of all "primary caregivers"—a category that includes in-laws, other relatives, friends, and neighbors—are female, including 59 percent of the caregivers who are spouses and 77 percent of those who are children of the care recipients (Wolff and Kasper 2006).

There are significant gender differences among siblings in the degree of involvement in providing care for a needy parent, and perceptions of inequity often become a source of distress (Ingersoll-Dayton et al. 2003). Married sons with no siblings are far more likely to provide parent care than those who have at least one sister (Wolf, Soldo, and Freedman 1996), and the monthly care provided by members of sibling groups with a parent needing care is reduced by about three hours per sister (Wolf, Freedman, and Soldo 1997). Recent research on sibling pairs confirms that availability of sisters reduces sons' contributions (Friedman and Seltzer 2010; Spitze and Trent 2006). Qualitative interviews suggest that some of the gender difference—though certainly not all—may be related to what brothers and sisters perceive as the correct approach to dealing with a parent's level of need. Brothers emphasize the importance of keeping parents self-sufficient, in part by waiting until a parent asks for help. Sisters emphasize the importance of anticipating need and addressing it in advance (Matthews 2002).

Elder care can involve a range of activities, including social calls and assistance with organizing, supervising, and financing paid care services. It also includes help with ADLs (which fits our definition of interactive care) and with IADLs such as housework, shopping, and money management (which fits our definition of support care). More than 54 percent of people age sixty-five and older living in the community with chronic disabilities receive help with IADLs only (Wolff and Kasper 2006). Similarly, a large majority of helpers assist only with IADLs (Wolf 2004).

However, many recipients receive help with both types of tasks, sometimes from different helpers. Adult children are more likely to help with ADLs, and spouses with IADLs (Wolf 2001). Most help with ADLs came from coresident rather than from non-coresident children; the opposite was true for at least some IADL tasks. For example, nonresident adult-child helpers provided more of the help with "getting around outside," travel beyond walking distance, and money management tasks. Evidence suggests that chronically ill midlife and older gay, lesbian, and bisexual adults rely heavily on friends as well as family for assistance (Muraco and Fredrikson-Goldsen 2011). On the other hand, some evidence suggests that the presence of HIV creates a "roadblock" to informal care provision, especially among less-educated African Americans (Moody et al. 2009).

How Much Care?

In view of the diverse needs to which caregivers respond and the wide range of tasks with which they provide assistance, it is not surprising that the time intensity of caregiving—measured in hours spent caring per period—is quite variable. One might expect that this variability would be amplified by the various approaches to counting caregivers (see the discussion in the appendix). Yet estimates of the average amount of time that caregivers devote to adults—between nineteen and twenty-four hours during a typical week—are remarkably consistent across a number of data sources, even when those data sources produce very different estimates of the *number* of caregivers.[7]

Average hours per week spent in caregiving is, however, a somewhat misleading and incomplete indicator, because the distribution of care hours is both highly variable and extremely skewed. The 2002 HRS data reveal that those caring for a spouse spent nearly 28 hours per week providing care, while those caring for parents or grandchildren averaged 10.4 and 9.1 hours per week, respectively. The NAC/AARP survey data show that 51 percent of caregivers reported spending eight or fewer hours a week on care activities; 22 percent spent nine through twenty hours, 13 percent spent twenty-one through forty hours, and 11 percent spent more than forty hours. This very unequal distribution of care work produces a high average value—nearly nineteen hours per week—although a majority of caregivers are providing eight hours or less a week.

Together, these findings suggest that a large number of informal caregivers spend modest amounts of time assisting spouses, parents, or other family members with fairly routine household or related tasks, while a smaller but very high-intensity group of caregivers spends large amounts of time providing assistance with these and other tasks, including hands-on personal care such as bathing, dressing, and feeding.

"Sandwich" Care

Relatively few individuals take on major responsibility for caring for parents while raising young children, but the combined effect of longer life expectancies and delayed childbearing is an increased likelihood that working-age adults will find themselves responsible for care of younger and older dependents at the same time (Pierret 2006; Spillman and Pezzin 2002). Depending on the definition of caregiving responsibilities, between 1 and 33 percent of women in their late forties and early fifties are providing care and support to children and parents simultaneously, with the best estimate that about 9 percent of women in this age group are "sandwiched" caregivers who are providing substantial amounts of care and support both to children and to parents.

Although sandwiched caregivers are a little less likely to be in the labor force than their peers who are not supporting two generations, labor force rates are high for both groups (72 percent versus 76 percent) (Pierret 2006). When they do care for both generations, employed sandwiched caregivers use many strategies to balance work and family demands (Neal and Hammer 2009). The most common strategy seems to be reducing the number of hours of work, which occurs almost twice as often for women as for men (31 percent of wives as compared to 17 percent of husbands). Nearly equal percentages of women and men refuse or limit travel (27 percent of wives and 23 percent of husbands), but women are much more likely to switch to a job that provides more flexibility or to decline or choose not to work toward a promotion. If someone is already caring for a child, the impact of also becoming a caregiver for an elderly person is unclear. But at least one recent study suggests that sandwiched caregivers report a lower quality of life than those with fewer care responsibilities (Rubin and White-Means 2009).

BOX 3.1 / Time Use Activities

We divide all reported activities into four major categories: paid work time, unpaid care time, self-maintenance, and leisure time. (Supervisory time is treated separately.)

- *Paid work* is time spent working for pay and traveling to and from paid work.
- *Unpaid care* is time devoted to activities such as child care, adult care, and the cleaning and maintenance of the home—activities that someone else could be paid to do on one's behalf—plus travel time associated with these activities. Volunteer work is also included in this category. Unpaid care can be divided into interactive or support care.
- *Self-maintenance* is time spent sleeping, bathing, tending to personal needs, and eating, plus the travel time associated with these activities.
- *Leisure* is time spent socializing, reading, watching TV, or engaging in sports or other recreation activities, plus the travel time associated with these activities.

ESTIMATES OF UNPAID CARE PROVIDED FOR CHILDREN AND ADULTS

An estimate of the average amount of time devoted to unpaid care for both children and adults can be generated by pooling data from recent American Time Use Surveys (ATUS) (see the appendix to this chapter). This type of estimate allows a "population" view of caregiving—including all adults who might have caregiving demands and combining time provided to the care of both children and adults. The ATUS asks respondents to report how many minutes of a selected day are spent directly on care activities as well as the amount of (sometimes overlapping) time that adults spend supervising children, during which they may be simultaneously involved in other activities.

Box 3.1 illustrates our broad conceptualization of time allocation. Time is divided into four broad categories: paid work, unpaid care activities, self-maintenance, and leisure or free time activities. Paid work includes not only hours of work but also time spent commuting. Self-maintenance is dominated by sleep but also includes personal care and eating. Leisure is a residual category that includes a diverse array of activities. The broad category of unpaid care includes interactive care of children and adults as well as what we term "support care" (see box 3.2). Interactive care activities include only those that require direct interaction with the recipient of care. Support care is one step removed, since it can be done without direct interaction with the care recipient and can benefit all household members, including oneself. Support care can take the form of housework or work in the community, such as volunteer efforts.

Supervisory care also plays an important role. Even though infants spend about half their time asleep, they wake up at unpredictable times demanding immediate

> BOX 3.2 / Unpaid Care Activities and Responsibilities
>
> *Interactive care* activities involve direct interaction with care recipients. They typically require personal contact and often require cooperation from the care recipient. Examples include feeding or dressing a child, reading aloud to or instructing a child, and feeding or bathing an adult with disabilities.
>
> *Support care* is care that supports interactive care but does not necessarily involve direct interaction with the care recipient. It may benefit other members of a household in addition to the care recipient. It includes two types of activities:
>
> 1. *Household support care* includes activities such as cooking, shopping, cleaning, and organizing the household.
>
> 2. *Social support care activities* are volunteer activities that provide assistance to others. Some probably include interactive care, but the data do not allow us to distinguish these.
>
> *Supervisory care* entails responsibilities for supervising or being available to someone who needs assistance, such as a small child who cannot be left alone or a sick person who may call out for help at unpredictable times.

attention, and young children cannot be left alone. The ATUS asks survey respondents to report the amount of time that a child under the age of thirteen was "in your care." We categorize the time reported in answer to this question as supervisory care, unless it coincides with interactive care (to avoid double counting).

Adults who are sick, disabled, or infirm also often need someone to remain nearby "on call" to help them take medication, be mobile, or obtain medical assistance. Needs for this supervisory care constrain the activities of unpaid caretakers, often making it necessary for them to purchase care services in order to engage in paid employment. Unfortunately for our purposes, the ATUS does not collect data on on-call care for adults.

Figure 3.2 pictures time use on an average day between 2003 and 2008, showing the total amount of time allocated by men and women to the four main categories of time use during a representative twenty-four-hour period. If we consider both paid work and unpaid care activities, men and women average about the same amount of time devoted to work—but men devote relatively more time to paid work, and women more time to unpaid care. More than 75 percent of both men and women perform at least some unpaid care (either support or interactive care) on an average day, with support care consuming considerably more time than interactive care.

Although both men and women provide more support care as they age—with people over sixty-five, many of whom are retirees, devoting the most time to it (see figure 3.3)—women consistently provide more than men. Time devoted to interactive care, however—a category that combines interactive care of children and interactive care of adults—varies less between men and women. Among those who devoted at least some time to an interactive care activity, men over age

FIGURE 3.2   /   Average Hours per Day, U.S. Adults Age Fifteen and Over, 2005 to 2008

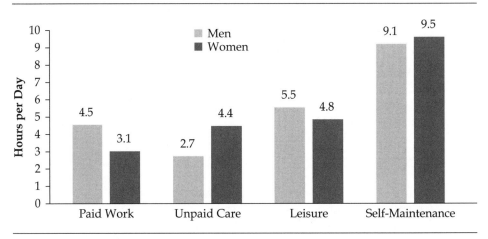

Source: Authors' calculations from the American Time Use Survey (U.S. Bureau of Labor Statistics, various years).
Note: Daily hours may not sum to twenty-four because of both rounding and omission of time use that remained unspecified.

FIGURE 3.3   /   Average Hours per Day Spent in Unpaid Care Activities by U.S. Adults Age Fifteen and Over, 2003 to 2008

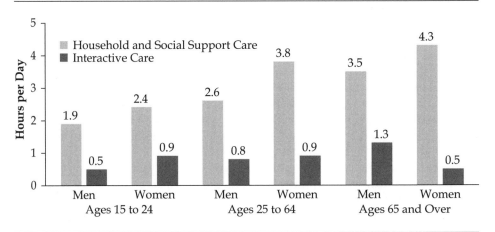

Source: Authors' calculations from the American Time Use Survey (U.S. Bureau of Labor Statistics, various years).
Note: Includes only respondents who devoted at least some time to unpaid care on the diary day.

TABLE 3.1 / Mean Daily Hours Devoted to Interactive Child Care and Adult Care, by Gender and Age of Unpaid Care Worker, 2003 to 2008

	Women		Men	
	Engaged in Activity on Diary Day	Mean Hours per Day Provided by Those Engaged in Activity	Engaged in Activity on Diary Day	Mean Hours per Day Provided by Those Engaged in Activity
Child care				
Age of care worker				
Fifteen to twenty-four	35.2%	1.9	18.8%	1.2
Twenty-five to sixty-four	48.7	2.4	33.6	1.8
Sixty-five and over	11.2	1.9	10.5	1.6
Adult care				
Age of care worker				
Fifteen to twenty-four	14.7	0.9	14.2	0.9
Twenty-five to sixty-four	14.3	1.2	12.7	1.3
Sixty-five and over	12.4	1.4	13.8	1.5

Source: Authors' calculations from the American Time Use Survey (U.S. Bureau of Labor Statistics, various years).

sixty-five devoted more time to interactive care than women in that age category. This is consistent with the findings from HRS data, reported in figure 3.1, that older married men provide more care for a spouse than older married women do.[8]

Disaggregating interactive care into two components—that provided for children and for adults—helps explain this pattern. Women under sixty-five are far more likely than men under sixty-five to engage in interactive care for children (see table 3.1), and the women who provide this type of care devote more time to it than the men who do the same. Among women age twenty-five to sixty-four, almost 50 percent devoted some time to interactive child care on the diary day, compared to little more than one-third of men, and the women who provided care spent 2.4 hours on it, compared to the men's 1.8.

Gender differences in interactive care for adults are strikingly small in every age category. The participation rate varies only from a low of 12.4 percent for women over sixty-five to a high of 14.7 percent for women age fifteen to twenty-four, with men of all age groups and women of other ages falling in between those two remarkably similar "extremes" (see table 3.1). The average amount of care provided ranged from 0.9 hours for both women and men in the youngest age group to 1.5 hours for men over sixty-five. This surprising finding may partially reflect the way in which adult care activities were defined by the American Time Use Survey (see further discussion later in the chapter).

TABLE 3.2 / Care for Household and Nonhousehold Children, by Gender and Age of Unpaid Care Worker, 2003 to 2008

	Household Child Care				Nonhousehold Child Care			
	Engaged in Activity on Diary Day		Mean Hours per Day Provided by Those Engaged in Activity		Engaged in Activity on Diary Day		Mean Hours per Day Provided by Those Engaged in Activity	
	Women	Men	Women	Men	Women	Men	Women	Men
Age of care worker								
Fifteen to twenty-four	68%	40%	2.4	0.8	46%	69%	0.4	0.6
Twenty-five to sixty-four	85	82	3.3	2.1	32	31	0.4	0.3
Sixty-five and over	16	20	0.4	0.3	90	93	1.4	1.3
Age of care worker								
Fifteen to twenty-four	32	24	0.2	0.2	73	80	0.7	0.8
Twenty-five to sixty-four	36	37	0.4	0.3	69	67	0.8	1.0
Sixty-five and over	27	39	0.5	0.7	76	65	0.8	0.8

Source: Authors' calculations from the American Time Use Survey (U.S. Bureau of Labor Statistics, various years).

Note: Includes only respondents who engaged in some child or adult care on the diary day.

Most people under age sixty-five who provide child care do so for a child living in their own household, but men age fifteen to twenty-four represent an important exception. Among those who provided child care on the diary day, 69 percent provided some care for a child not living in their household, perhaps because they were likely to be noncustodial fathers (see table 3.2). Of those sixty-five or over who provided child care—most of them for their grandchildren—90 percent or more were caring for a child who was part of another household. Even women in the prime child-rearing years who engaged in some child care were likely to spend some time caring for a non-household child—46 percent of women age fifteen to twenty-four and 32 percent of women age twenty-five to sixty-four (see table 3.2).

Those who provided care for an adult on the diary day were far more likely to care for an adult who was not living in their household than for one within it. This is true even for adults age sixty-five and older, suggesting that the elderly represent an important care resource for elderly relatives or friends who do not live in their own homes (see table 3.2). Among those over age sixty-five who provided

TABLE 3.3 / Daily Time Devoted to Specific Child Care Activities, by Gender and Age of Unpaid Care Worker, 2003 to 2008

	Physical	Developmental	Travel	Other
Engaged in specific activity, conditional on engaging in some child care activity				
Age fifteen to twenty-four				
Women	35%	20%	35%	10%
Men	16	19	58	8
Age twenty-five to sixty-four				
Women	33	25	28	13
Men	31	28	30	11
Age sixty-five and over				
Women	15	24	46	15
Men	6	19	63	12
Average minutes spent on specific activities by those engaging in some child care activity				
Age fifteen to twenty-four				
Women	44	31	23	16
Men	10	25	29	9
Age twenty-five to sixty-four				
Women	47	45	32	21
Men	25	39	24	17
Age sixty-five and over				
Women	17	38	29	27
Men	6	33	36	19

Source: Authors' calculations from the American Time Use Survey (U.S. Bureau of Labor Statistics, various years).

adult care on the diary day, 76 percent of women and 65 percent of men provided some care to an adult who was not a household member.

When adults engage in interactive child care, what exactly are they doing? Table 3.3 disaggregates child care activities into four categories: physical care (such as feeding or changing diapers), developmental care (such as reading aloud or actively playing with a child), travel with a child, and other activities. Specific interactive care activities vary by both age and gender. Women in both the youngest and oldest age groups who provided child care were more likely than men to provide physical care, while men were more likely to travel with children—probably ferrying them to activities. Women and men were about equally likely to engage in a developmental care activity. However, women devoted far more time, on average, to physical care, and considerably more time to developmental care. The older generation—both men and women, probably grandparents—were particularly likely to spend time traveling with children when they provided child care and devoted about as much time to this task as those in the prime parenting years.

The ATUS defines elder care differently from child care: it includes a category for "helping" that seems more like support care—such as housework—than interactive care (for details, see the appendix to the book). Table 3.4 shows that participation in

TABLE 3.4 / Daily Time Devoted to Specific Adult Care Activities, by Age and Gender of Unpaid Care Worker, 2003 to 2008

	Caring	Helping	Travel
Engaged in specific activity, conditional on engaging in some adult care activity			
Ages fifteen to twenty-four			
Women	9%	61%	30%
Men	4	64	32
Ages twenty-five to sixty-four			
Women	16	56	27
Men	10	61	30
Ages sixty-five and over			
Women	21	50	28
Men	18	55	27
Average minutes spent on specific activities by those engaging in some adult care activity			
Ages fifteen to twenty-four			
Women	7	29	19
Men	4	33	18
Ages twenty-five to sixty-four			
Women	24	30	17
Men	11	45	21
Ages sixty-five and over			
Women	38	27	17
Men	30	39	19

Source: Authors' calculations from the American Time Use Survey (U.S. Bureau of Labor Statistics, various years).

that category was far higher for those who reported some adult care on their diary day than was participation in more narrowly defined caring activities. Not only do more people provide this type of help, but more minutes per day are devoted to helping by every age and gender category except women age sixty-five and over. Both the incidence and amount of time devoted to assisting with travel were also high—though not quite at the levels for child care. Both women (21 percent) and men (18 percent) age sixty-five and over were most likely to provide adult care other than helping or travel on the diary day, averaging thirty-eight and thirty minutes, respectively.

Finally, as shown in table 3.5, the ATUS provides an estimate of supervisory or "on-call" care for children under age thirteen. The percentages of men and women reporting some time devoted to supervisory child care were about the same as for those reporting some time in interactive child care, with the exception of those age sixty-five and over, who were less likely to provide this form of care (for details, compare table 3.5 with table 3.1). However, average amounts of time devoted to supervisory care were far higher—4.5 hours a day or more for all age categories of men and 5 hours a day or more for all women reporting any

TABLE 3.5 / Daily Time Devoted to Supervisory Child Care, by Age and Gender of Unpaid Care Worker, 2003 to 2008

	Engaged in Supervisory Care on Diary Day		Average Hours Spent by Those Providing Supervisory Care	
	Women	Men	Women	Men
Fifteen to twenty-four	35%	17%	6.0	4.7
Twenty-five to sixty-four	48	38	7.0	5.8
Sixty-five and over	6	5	5.0	4.5

Source: Authors' calculations from the American Time Use Survey (U.S. Bureau of Labor Statistics, various years).

supervisory care. Women between the ages of twenty-five and sixty-four providing supervisory care reported 7 hours on the diary day, while those who provided interactive care reported just 2.4 hours on average. It is unfortunate that neither the ATUS nor other time use surveys measure supervisory time devoted to adults suffering from mental or physical disabilities such as paralysis, dementia, or Alzheimer's disease. The need for such measures should rank high on any agenda for further research.

In chapter 5, we will return to a consideration of the number of hours of unpaid care provided nationwide, comparing it to the magnitude of time devoted to paid care (discussed in chapter 4) and calculating what it would cost to purchase a replacement for it.

COSTS, STRESSES, AND INEQUALITIES

Care provision requires time, physical effort, and emotional energy. Whatever its intrinsic rewards, it can also impose costs and stresses. However, it is often difficult to sort out cause and effect, since concern about a family member in need of care is often a source of stress whether or not it is met by specific efforts. Further, it can be difficult to determine why some individuals are motivated to take on care responsibilities and why others may avoid them. These decisions are complicated, involving rational calculations about who has time and who else might be available to provide care. But caregiving also has an emotional component that may make it difficult for individuals to clearly articulate why they are or are not providing care in a given situation.

For all these reasons, there has been little research documenting motivations for care work. A recent review (Quinn, Clare, and Woods 2010) found only four studies of dementia care providers published since 1960 that included quantitative analyses of care motivation; the motivations most often reported included personal attachments—that is, feelings of concern or love for the care recipient—

a sense of duty or obligation, and guilt. We are not aware of any research that attempts to analyze reasons why people are *not* engaged in care provision.

The Economic Costs of Providing Unpaid Care

The economic costs of unpaid care can take several forms: loss of employment or opportunities for advancement, restricted job choices, reduced current and future income, and loss of leisure. A large literature focuses on the costs of motherhood. Even a brief period of time withdrawn from full-time paid employment early in an adult career can have a significant negative effect on future earnings, and mothers are far more likely than fathers to withdraw from the labor force or reduce their hours of work to provide care to children. Mothers tend to earn less than other women even when they do not significantly reduce their hours of paid employment (Joshi 1998; Waldfogel 1997; Budig and England 2001; Phipps, Burton, and Lethbridge 2001). Differences in their preferences or behavior may help explain this gap. Mothers may put less effort than other women into their paid jobs, or they may turn down promotions that would interfere with family responsibilities. Audit studies suggest that employers may discriminate against mothers in hiring and promotion decisions (Correll, Benard, and Paik 2007).

The reduction in earnings of mothers, independent of hours worked, contributes to what has been termed the "family gap" and the "motherhood penalty." It adds up to a substantial sum of money above and beyond the costs incurred by simply going without a paycheck for a couple of years while taking care of an infant. In the United States, the relative importance of the motherhood penalty has been increasing over time, in part because other sources of difference in men's and women's earnings (such as overt discrimination) have declined (Waldfogel 1998). In 1991, by one estimate, motherhood accounted for more than 60 percent of the difference in men's and women's earnings (Waldfogel 1998; Sigle-Rushton and Waldfogel 2004).

The motherhood penalty is buffered to some extent by income pooling between married or cohabiting parents. While mothers tend to reduce their hours of market work, fathers tend to increase theirs. If mothers and fathers share income, they also share the costs of forgone earnings. But sharing may be influenced by relative bargaining power, and lower earnings leave mothers vulnerable to poverty in the event that income pooling comes to an end. Divorce often has adverse consequences for women, not only because it increases their reliance on their own (lower) earnings, but also because it reduces their eligibility for benefits, such as pensions, that are based on a husband's (higher) earnings (Folbre 2008a).

Care for adults tends to come later in the life cycle than care for children and therefore may have fewer consequences for lifetime earnings. Nonetheless, its negative economic impact on those individuals who curtail their employment can be substantial. Some estimates of the additional income that caregivers of adults could have earned if they had not reduced their paid work hours are startlingly high—ranging from about $660,000 to over $1 million (NAC/MMMI 2006; MMMI

2009). It is difficult to determine the net effects of caregiving on employment and earnings because the "counterfactual"—the labor force attachment, hours of work, and wage rates or earnings of those who are providing care, in the hypothetical alternative situation of not providing care—cannot be directly observed.

Some studies have found evidence of employment or earnings reductions among caregivers (McLanahan and Monson 1990), while others have not (Boaz 1996; Wolf and Soldo 1994). A comprehensive review of research produced over a twenty-year period concluded from the available evidence that, on the whole, caregivers are not less likely to be employed than non-caregivers, but that employed caregivers do tend to reduce their labor market hours on average (Lilly, Laporte, and Coyte 2007). These labor market reductions also depend on various aspects of the caring situation; those with more intensive care responsibilities and those who coreside with the care recipient tend to make larger labor market adjustments than others.

Stresses and Rewards of Caregiving

Since the early 1980s, research on the stressful aspects of being a caregiver, especially for those who provide care to an older spouse or parent, has figured prominently in social gerontology, psychology, and related fields. By 1989 a leading scholar could claim that "[the] point that caregiving is stressful is now well-established" (Zarit 1989, 147). Caregiver depression and other adverse mental health consequences of providing elder care are persistent themes.[9] Other negative effects studied include reduced immune system responses (Kiecolt-Glaser et al. 1996; Vedhara et al. 1999), elevated risk of coronary heart disease (Lee et al. 2003), an increase in the number of chronic conditions (Pinquart and Sörensen 2007), lower self-rated health (Pinquart and Sörensen 2007), health risk factors such as poorer nutrition and reduced exercise (Burton et al. 1997), and even excess mortality (Schulz and Beach 1999; Christakis and Allison 2009). Additional recent research focuses on caregiver populations defined by the care recipient's condition or disease—for example, stroke (White et al. 2004), multiple sclerosis (Pozzilli et al. 2004), or cancer (Kim and Given 2008)—rather than the care recipient's age. Some studies have demonstrated adverse physical health (Musil and Ahmad 2002) or mental health outcomes (Blustein, Chan, and Guanais 2004) among grandmothers who care for a grandchild compared to those who do not.

Although there seems to be overwhelming support for the proposition that caregiving is hazardous to caregivers' health, at least three counterarguments cast doubt on it. First, most research on caregiver consequences pays little or no attention to the positive or beneficial outcomes associated with the provision of care. Several studies have pointed out that caregivers often derive satisfaction from their caring, even in combination with the feeling of being burdened (Lawton et al. 1991). Others have noted that caregiving costs are accompanied by rewards (Raschick and Ingersoll-Dayton 2004; Reidel, Fredman, and Langenberg 1998), or that "hassles" are paired with "uplifts" (Kinney and Stephens 1989). These positive aspects of caregiving are often conceptualized as representing different underlying dimensions than the negative ones of stress and burden. In other words, it is possible for caregivers to experience both positive and negative consequences at the same time. Sarah Matthews (2002), reflecting on the more positive picture of family caregiving that emerges from her qualitative study of 149 family groups compared to the negative picture common in the literature, suggests that the widespread use of closed-ended survey questions to elicit caregivers' appraisals of their situation encourages the depiction of family care as burdensome and stressful.

Second, conclusions about the consequences of care provision often rest on the use of inappropriate comparison groups. In caregiver research, it is impossible to adopt the standards of experimental clinical trials, where random assignment is used to place some subjects in a treatment group and others in a control group. Many studies of caregiver stress use no comparison group at all; they simply compare average caregiver-group outcomes to those in the general population. But even when comparing a group of caregivers to a matched group of otherwise similar non-caregivers, there are two important differences between the two groups: the caregivers have a close family member with care needs *and* they are actively involved in providing that care, while the latter group—non-caregivers—generally share neither attribute. In such a situation, it can be misleading to attribute the entire difference in outcomes between the two groups to just one of these factors, the activity of caring.

Although the positive effects of caregiving can be experienced only by active caregivers, some of the stresses that caregivers often experience—including a breakdown of established family relationships and the experience of watching a loved one decline and approach eventual death—are often experienced by non-caregivers as well (Schulz, Visintainer, and Williamson 1990). These contrasts can perhaps be most easily studied in cases of parent care in which one or more siblings participate in caring for an older mother or father while other siblings do not. Yet only two published studies have contrasted "caregiver stress," manifested as heightened depressive symptoms among those actively providing hands-on help to an elderly parent, to "non-caregiver stress," a parallel increase in indicators of depression among adult children whose parents need help but who do not actively provide such help (Amirkhanyan and Wolf 2003, 2006). In both studies, depression levels were similar among caregivers and non-caregivers, the only significant difference being much higher levels among people whose parents had care needs than among comparable people whose parents did not. That research suggests that much of what has been interpreted as an adverse outcome of being a caregiver may actually be a consequence of having an older parent who *needs* care, irrespective of one's own care provision efforts.

A third problem is the failure in the great majority of caregiver-stress studies to recognize "selectivity"—the potential for unobserved differences between caregivers and non-caregivers (Vitaliano, Zhang, and Scanlan 2003). For example, within a group of siblings there may be one who is less attached to the labor force and therefore more likely to become a family caregiver. Preexisting differences—rather than the activity of caregiving itself—may explain higher levels of depression or poor health.

Class and Racial-Ethnic Differences

Individual, household, and community-level differences based on class, race, and ethnicity clearly shape unpaid care provision. The cost of taking time away from paid work to provide care for children or other family members is lower for those in low-paying jobs. On the other hand, their needs for income are greater. Low-income families rely more heavily on parental care and kin care than more affluent families, who can afford child care centers that offer children more early education (Williams and Boushey 2010). Relationships between mothers and fathers tend to be fragile at the bottom of the income distribution, where the likelihood of non-marital births is greater and there are complex, shifting patterns of coresidence between adult women and men. Grandparents and other kin may help compensate for this family instability, but we currently have limited information on these intergenerational ties of support.

Low-income families also are more likely to be providing care for elders, at least partly because they do not have the resources to pay someone else to do so. One study found that families with income under the poverty line were more than twice as likely as others to provide more than thirty hours of unpaid assistance each week to parents (Heymann 2005, 102). The burden of care is higher for other reasons as well. Low-income families typically report more health problems and a higher incidence of disability among both children and adults than other families.

Extended family, as well as friends and neighbors, may help unpaid caregivers meet the needs of their dependents. However, both legal immigrants and undocumented workers may live a long way from close family members. Proponents of the "superintegration" hypothesis (Stack 1974; Baca Zinn and Wells 2000) argue that African American and Latino families tend to have stronger care networks with extended kin, while proponents of the "disintegration" hypothesis hold the opposite view (Menjivar 2000). One recent study based on the National Survey of Families and Households (NSFH) finds that Mexican American women (but not men) are more likely than European American women to provide housework and care assistance to kin (Sarkisian, Gerena, and Gerstel 2006). Similarly, African Americans—particularly women—tend to provide more practical support for kin, while whites provide more financial assistance and emotional support (Sarkisian and Gerstel 2004b). Data from the 2009 National Alliance of Caregivers/American Association of Retired Persons survey shows that African American and Hispanic households were more likely to include a caregiver than either white or Asian households. (NAC/AARP 2009a, 12).

Low-income caregivers have less flexibility in their efforts to balance paid employment with family care, since they have few or no savings to fall back on if they reduce the time they spend working for pay. Although there are government programs aimed at easing the burden on impoverished parents, paid work requirements and lifetime caps limit parents' ability to reduce the time they spend at paying jobs in exchange for cash assistance through Temporary Assistance to Needy Families (TANF). And even though families with income below the poverty level theoretically have access to subsidized child care, the supply of such services does not meet the demand (see the discussion in chapter 7). In addition, many low-income mothers have difficulty finding adequate transportation to work and child care (Yoshikawa, Weisner, and Lowe 2006).

Racial-ethnic differences are often difficult to separate from differences in family income (Angel and Tienda 1982). However, nonmarital child-rearing and multiple-partner fertility tend to be higher among African Americans, even controlling for income. Perhaps as a result, spouses are less prominent and daughters are more prominent sources of informal care for elderly African Americans than is the case among other groups (Roth et al. 2007).

In general, coresidence of elderly parents with children is higher among blacks, Hispanics, and immigrants than among native-born whites (Burr and Mutchler 1999; Cohen and Casper 2002). Elderly Latinos are more likely than elderly non-Hispanic whites or African Americans to receive informal care and less likely to receive institutional care (Weiss et al. 2005; Herrera et al. 2008). Elderly African Americans living in rural areas typically experience a longer duration of care from family members than those living in urban areas (Chadiha, Feld, and Rafferty 2010). Extended kin ties are probably a source of greater support among African Americans and Latinos than among whites (Gerstel 2011). This suggests that the burden of unpaid care may be greater among these groups as well.

SUMMARY

A number of changes are altering the landscape for unpaid care, not the least of which is the aging of the baby boom generation. At least two factors have reduced the potential supply of unpaid care: the greater labor force participation of women and increased family instability. A variety of estimates, including those based on the nationally representative American Time Use Survey, show that Americans continue to devote a substantial amount of time to the care of both children and adults. However, it is difficult to assess past or future trends in family members' willingness to devote time to those who need it.

Those who provide unpaid care often derive important benefits, including a sense of purpose, love, support, and connection with others. But they also encounter significant economic costs and difficulties, particularly when care demands are great. Women bear a disproportionate burden, especially for the care of young children. Unpaid care needs loom large among low-income families because they are often characterized by a relatively high ratio of dependents to working-age adults.

APPENDIX: THE AMERICAN TIME USE SURVEY

The ATUS is a stratified random sample drawn from households that have completed their participation in the Current Population Survey (CPS), which is representative of the U.S. civilian non-institutional population ages fifteen and over. One individual from each household is surveyed by the ATUS between two and five months after the household's final CPS survey. Labor force information is included for each respondent, including whether they are unable to work for pay as a result of disability. No other questions regarding disability are asked.

The ATUS computer-assisted telephone interview asks respondents to sequentially report their activities during the twenty-four-hour period that began at 4:00 AM the preceding day and ended at 4:00 AM on the interview day. Respondents describe their activity episodes, including start and stop times and other information, such as who else was present and where they were. The data used in this chapter cover the period from January 2003 through December 2008. Interviews were conducted every day except on a few major holidays. The total sample of diary days comes to about 85,645. Overall response rates were 57.8 percent in 2003, 57.3 percent in 2004, 56.6 percent in 2005, 55.1 percent in 2006, 52.5 percent in 2007, and 54.6 percent in 2008. Analysis of nonresponse suggests that people who are only loosely connected to households do not respond. The weighting adjustments provided by the U.S. Bureau of Labor Statistics (BLS) do a good job of adjusting estimates for potential biases and lack of representativeness (See Abraham, Maitland, and Bianchi 2006).

NOTES

1. U.S. Census Bureau, "Table 1a: Childcare Arrangements of Preschoolers Living with Mother, by Employment Status of Mother and Selected Characteristics: Spring 2010." Available at: "Child Care: Who's Minding the Kids? Child Care Arrangements 2010," http://www.census. gov/hhes/childcare/data/sipp/2010/tables.html (accessed December 21, 2011).
2. U.S. Census Bureau, "Table C1: Household Relationship and Family Status of Children Under 18 Years, by Age and Sex: 2011," available at: http://www.census.gov/ population/www/socdemo/hh-fam/cps2011.html (accessed February 22, 2011).
3. Calculations based on the Child Development Supplement to the Panel Study of Income Dynamics (PSID). Available at: http://psidonline.isr.umich.edu/ (accessed February 27, 2012).
4. The characterization of "need" is different for parents and spouses. For parents, it is determined by the survey respondent's report that a parent "needs help" with basic personal needs (such as dressing, eating, or bathing), or cannot be left alone for even one hour, or has a diagnosed "memory-related disease." For spouses, the need variable reflects the spouse's own self-characterization as having a "difficulty . . . because of a physical, mental, emotional or memory problem" with any of six ADLs: dressing, walking, bathing, eating, getting into or out of bed, and using the toilet.
5. Additional HRS data not shown here indicate that nearly all surviving parents of people age sixty-five and older are judged to need care.
6. The survey asked the following question regarding adult care: "In the last 12 months, has anyone in your household provided unpaid care to a relative or friend 18 years or older to help them take care of themselves? Unpaid care may include help with personal needs or household chores. It might be managing a person's finances, arranging for outside services, or visiting regularly to see how they are doing. This person need not live

with you" (NAC/AARP 2009a, 2). Note that this report does not include unpaid care for a child without special needs under its rubric. For further discussion of these measurement issues, see the appendix.

7. For example, data from the 1994 HRS indicate that among active caregivers (that is, among those providing *any* hours of care) the average number of care hours per week was 19.4 (Amirkhanyan and Wolf 2003). This number reflects care provided to parents and parents-in-law exclusively. The 1996 Survey of Income and Program Participation (SIPP) panel (whose caregiving activities were surveyed in 1998), which records care provided to a broader group—relatives or friends of *all* ages—yields an estimate of 24.2 hours of care per week on average (Alecxih, Zeruld, and Olearczyk 2001). The 2009 NAC/AARP *Caregiving in the U.S.* survey finds that among those caring for someone age fifty or older, the average number of weekly hours spent in caring is 18.8 (NAC/AARP 2009a). These three estimates are very similar, despite their very different vintages and coverage. Moreover, both the HRS and NAC/AARP surveys ask about care provided over the twelve-month period prior to the survey, while the SIPP asks about only one month prior to the survey. In contrast, an analysis of 2002 HRS data found that caregivers spent an average of 11.2 hours per week providing care (Johnson and Schaner 2005). One reason for this comparatively low estimate may be that the 2002 HRS asked people to report the number of hours they had spent on caregiving over a two-year period rather than to estimate the hours spent in a "typical" or "average" week, as in the SIPP and NAC/AARP studies.

8. Space constraints limit our ability to disaggregate these data further. However, we note that differences in care provision by socioeconomic status have been documented. For example, Kenneth Couch, Mary Daly, and Douglas Wolf (1999) found that higher-wage and more-educated married men devoted less time to "helping" their parents—a category broader than interactive care—although no such differences were found among their wives, nor among unmarried men. Higher-wage unmarried women also spent less of their time helping their parents than did lower-wage unmarried women.

9. One review by Richard Schulz, Paul Visintainer, and Gail Williamson (1990) counts thirty-four studies on the psychiatric and physical morbidity effects of caregiving, twenty-two of which include depression as a key outcome—and often as the only outcome of interest. More recently, Martin Pinquart and Silvia Sörensen's 2005 meta-analysis synthesized ninety-three studies of depression and concluded that the differences in depression between caregivers and non-caregivers are large and statistically significant.

Chapter 4

Paid Care Work

Candace Howes, Carrie Leana, and Kristin Smith

T hat most people enter caring occupations in order to earn a living and help support their family members does not diminish the importance of the moral values, caring norms, and personal attachments that often infuse their performance on the job. In this chapter, we call attention to the motivational commitments and institutional similarities of care work across very different occupations because these are relevant to the development of political alliances and sectoral labor force development policies. However, we focus on two sets of care occupations that parallel the unpaid tasks described in the preceding chapter: child care and adult care.

The first section provides an overview of paid care work, reviewing the existing literature and providing empirical details based on analysis of the 2010 Current Population Survey. We highlight commonalities across care occupations but also focus on important differences between high- and low-wage interactive care jobs. The next two sections, focusing on child care and adult care jobs, explore the institutional features of these jobs and the economic and demographic characteristics of the workers who fill them. These jobs represent an important subset of all low-wage jobs because they provide earnings and potential economic mobility for workers in many African American, Latino, and immigrant communities. We also explore links between poor job quality and poor service quality and build a case for a sectoral high-road strategy, which we outline in the conclusion and return to in more detail in the final chapter.

EMPLOYMENT IN PAID CARE

Labor force statistics in the United States categorize workers according to the type of goods or services produced ("industry") and the type of work they do ("occupation"). Such categorizations are necessarily approximate, but nonetheless useful. A number of major care industries help produce, develop, and maintain the nation's human resources. Workers in interactive care occupations—where concern for the well-being of others is likely to affect the quality of the services provided—are primarily but not exclusively located in care industries. While these interactive occupations also share some common characteristics, they differ widely in skill requirements, pay, and unionization rates.

Care Industries

Our categorization of care industries encompasses several industrial categories, predominantly in health, education, and social assistance (see figure 4.1). Our categorization is based on minor revisions to previous research (Albelda, Duffy, and Folbre 2009).[1] Private household services, which include some child and adult care services provided in homes, amount to only about 2 percent of total employment but may not be fully captured by existing labor force surveys.

The previous chapter on unpaid care distinguished between interactive and support care. Making an analogous distinction here, we can characterize all workers in care industries as providing either interactive or support care. By this definition, employment in the paid care sector amounts to 24 percent of all employment (U.S. Bureau of Labor Statistics, Current Population Survey 2010b).

Employment in care industries depends heavily on public spending. More than 34 percent of all employees in these industries work in the public sector, a significantly higher percentage than any other grouping. Many public dollars are also spent to help pay for private-sector employees in hospitals, nursing homes, private homes, community settings, and schools. Only 6 percent are self-employed (see table 4.1).[2] Employment in care industries is also distinctively female. In 2010 women represented 47 percent of all employees, but 75 percent of all those in education and health services—a far higher percentage than in any other major sector. Employees in education and health services are also more likely to be African American (14 percent compared to 11 percent for all employees) and less likely to be Hispanic (10 percent compared to 14 percent for all employees; U.S. Bureau of Labor Statistics, Current Population Survey 2010c).

Care Occupations

Our categorization of interactive care occupations—those in which concern for the well-being of others is likely to affect the quality of services provided—also builds on previous research (Albelda, Duffy, and Folbre 2009) (see box A.4 in the appendix). Some of these interactive occupations, such as teachers, nurses, child care workers, and personal aides, clearly entail high levels of interactive personal care. Others, such as pharmacists and dieticians, may entail lower or more intermittent interactions. By the same token, some workers who provide interactive

FIGURE 4.1 / Employment in Care Industries in the United States, 2010

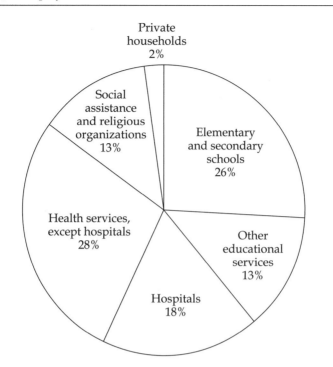

Source: Author's calculations of data from U.S. Bureau of Labor Statistics, Current Population Survey (2010c).

care may not be included on our list. However, our categorization yields a rough estimate: about 15 percent of all paid workers in 2010 were engaged in interactive care occupations (see table 4.1).

Care occupations are heterogeneous, ranging from one of the highest-paid major occupational groupings (professional and related occupations, which includes doctors, nurses, teachers, and college professors) to one of the lowest-paid (service occupations, in which child and adult care workers are classified) (see box A.4 in the appendix). Overall, interactive care occupations are tilted toward the top end of the occupational spectrum: professional and related occupations represent 77 percent of all interactive care jobs. By contrast, professional and related occupations represent only about 22 percent of jobs in the economy as a whole (U.S. Bureau of Labor Statistics, Current Population Survey 2010a). As a result, the occupational spread is greater among women in care jobs than in the economy as a whole.

Women and African American professionals are disproportionately located in interactive care occupations.[3] Women represent about 57 percent of all workers in professional and related occupations, but about 73 percent of all those in

TABLE 4.1 / Characteristics of Workers in Interactive Care Occupations, 2010

	All Workers	Interactive Care Workers	All Low-Wage Workers[a]	Child Care Workers	Adult Care Workers
Number (in thousands)	152,145	22,783	42,634	1,776	3,042
Percentage of all workers	100.0%	14.9%	28.0%	1.2%	2.0%
Percentage female	47.1	77.7	55.0	96.5	88.7
Economic characteristics					
Median family income	$64,030	$74,020	$33,000	$50,000	$34,500
In poverty	7.5	6.2	21.4	18.6	18.2
Median hourly wage[b]	$16.82	$18.26	$7.75	$9.17	$10.58
Average weekly hours worked	38.5	37.3	35.4	33.1	35.1
Overtime (more than forty hours per week)	20.9%	18.8%	13.5%	13.7%	9.0%
Full-time employment[c]	79.3	75.4	64.5	58.6	67.5
Year-round full-time employment[d]	65.0	62.2	46.0	41.8	53.4
Self-employed	9.5	5.9	10.0	20.7	3.7
Two or more jobs	9.8	13.2	9.4	12.4	12.1
Union membership[e]	12.0	23.2	4.6	3.1	13.2
Health insurance					
Public	12.6	12.8	18.8	18.6	24.4
Private	74.2	82.0	52.2	59.1	54.9
No health insurance	19.3	11.9	35.1	27.7	27.8
Demographic characteristics					
Average age	41.9	43.3	37.7	37.7	41.9
Education					
High school or less	38.3%	17.7%	55.5%	42.4%	54.3%
Some college, no degree	19.8	13.7	23.7	27.8	15.7
Associate's degree	9.8	12.6	7.8	9.4	11.4
Bachelor's degree	21.0	27.3	10.1	17.7	7.1
More than bachelor's degree	11.0	28.6	2.9	2.7	1.5
Race and ethnicity					
White, non-Hispanic	68.8	69.7	59.6	63.4	45.9
Black, non-Hispanic	10.6	13.9	12.9	15.1	30.8
Asian, non-Hispanic	4.6	5.0	3.9	3.5	4.6
Other, non-Hispanic	1.9	19.6	2.2	1.6	2.8
Hispanic	14.1	9.4	21.4	16.5	15.8
Foreign-born	15.4	12.9	19.9	16.6	22.8

TABLE 4.1 / *Continued*

	All Workers	Interactive Care Workers	All Low-Wage Workersᵃ	Child Care Workers	Adult Care Workers
Marital status		.			
Married	54.9	59.2	38.8	47.4	36.7
Previously married	16.7	17.5	18.0	18.0	29.0
Never married	28.3	23.3	43.2	34.6	34.4
Children under age eighteen	37.3	40.5	36.5	50.1	40.3
Single mothers	10.1	10.8	17.3	20.7	22.9

Source: U.S. Bureau of Labor Statistics, Current Population Survey (2010d), analyzed by Kristin Smith and Andrew Schaefer.

Notes: Percentages are based on weighted data for all workers age eighteen and older. Hourly wages, family income, poverty status, and work hours reflect 2009 employment; all other characteristics refer to 2010.

ᵃLow-wage workers are those making less than two-thirds of the gross median wage in 2009.
ᵇHourly wages are calculated using total annual earnings in 2009 divided by usual hours worked per week, multiplied by the number of weeks worked in 2009.
ᶜIncludes those working thirty-five or more hours per week.
ᵈIncludes those working thirty-five or more hours per week and fifty or more weeks annually.
ᵉThe union membership question is asked for one-quarter of the sample.

interactive care jobs in that occupational category. Similarly, African Americans, who make up 9 percent of all professionals, comprise 19 percent of community and social service professionals and are also disproportionately represented in some education and health services professions. Likewise, women in service jobs are disproportionately located in interactive care work. While they represent 57 percent of all those in service occupations, they represent about 90 percent of all those in interactive care service occupations (U.S. Bureau of Labor Statistics, Current Population Survey 2010a). Two of the largest occupational groups—nurses and teachers—typically require postsecondary education. Across all levels of education, teachers account for about 37 percent of all interactive care workers, and nurses account for 15 percent (U.S. Bureau of Labor Statistics, Current Population Survey 2010a).

In this chapter, we focus on two large occupational groups working in institutional environments that we believe pose problems for both job quality and service quality: child care workers, who account for about 8 percent of all interactive care workers, and adult care workers, who account for about 14 percent.[4] Adult care workers (nursing assistants, home health aides, and personal and home care aides), working in hospitals, nursing homes and other long-term care facilities, group homes for people with disabilities, and care recipients' own homes, represent the fastest-growing component of the paid care labor force.

THE GROWTH OF PAID CARE JOBS

Employment in care industries and occupations expanded faster than overall employment between 2000 and 2010 and is projected to continue to grow more rapidly in the near future (U.S. Bureau of Labor Statistics 2012). This rapid expansion helps explain why women now represent about one-half of all employees on nonagricultural payrolls, a historic benchmark (English, Hartmann, and Hayes 2010). Many factors help explain this growth. Increases in women's labor force participation increased the demand for services that were once provided free of charge by wives and mothers (see the discussion in chapter 5). The aging of the population associated with fertility decline and increased longevity has increased demand for adult care services. In recent years, the increased availability of low-wage and especially immigrant workers to provide child care and care for disabled working-age adults and the frail elderly has probably made it easier for highly educated women to combine family care with paid employment (Furtado and Hock 2010). In other words, the expansion of paid care services itself has increased both the demand for and the supply of women workers.

High relative rates of growth in paid care work may also reflect the fact that most care jobs are less vulnerable to international competition and less easily relocated overseas than manufacturing and other jobs, owing to the personal, often hands-on interaction that is central to interactive care work (Blinder 2006). The nature of care jobs also makes them resistant to automation, although the development of robot technology offers the opportunity to provide enhanced medical monitoring and also supervisory assistance through remote video (Horowitz 2010). "Carebots" may be on the way (Masi 2009).

Although the direction of future technological change remains unclear, the projected growth in care occupations seems to be tilted toward jobs at the bottom of the occupational distribution. Employment in health care practitioner occupations, including nursing, is expected to grow by just over 26 percent between 2010 and 2020, but employment is expected to grow by 69 percent for home health aides and by 70 percent for personal and home care aides (U.S. Bureau of Labor Statistics 2012). This shift seems consistent with a larger pattern of increased demand for low-wage compared to mid-wage workers in the United States (Autor 2010). It also highlights the need for close attention to the characteristics of low-wage care jobs.

CHARACTERISTICS OF INTERACTIVE CARE WORKERS

Analysis of the 2010 Current Population Survey provides an overview of similarities and differences between interactive care workers and all paid workers. We begin with a discussion of characteristics that differentiate care workers from all other workers.

The biggest difference lies in gender composition: about 78 percent of all paid care workers are women, compared to 47 percent of all paid workers (see table 4.1). Also common across categories of interactive care workers is that they spend fewer hours per week at their primary job, are less likely to be working full-time or year-round, and are more likely to hold multiple jobs than all workers. Although, overall, interactive care workers are less likely to be self-employed, child care workers are more than twice as likely to be self-employed. These differences in job characteristics suggest that, whether willingly or not, interactive care workers experience less regular—and possibly seek more flexible—employment.

Certain personal or demographic characteristics support speculation that interactive care workers may be motivated to find flexible work arrangements so that they can meet other family obligations. Interactive care workers are more likely to be married or to have been married than all workers. They are somewhat more likely to have children under age eighteen and to be single mothers.

Interactive care workers earn a median pay of $18.26 per hour, substantially higher than the median of $16.82 per hour for all workers. But pay comparisons that do not control for factors such as education, experience, and sector tell us little about the relative position of one group of workers. Interactive care jobs are disproportionately concentrated in professional occupations, and care workers have attained significantly higher levels of education. About 27 percent have a bachelor's degree, compared to 21 percent of all workers. Even more—29 percent compared to 11 percent of all workers—have more than a bachelor's degree.

Interactive care workers are also more likely to report belonging to a union (reflecting the relatively high unionization rates of teachers and nurses and some healthcare support workers). Almost twice as many interactive care workers (23 percent) compared to workers as a whole (12 percent) belong to unions.

Child care workers and adult care workers represent the low-wage component of the care workforce, earning far less than all interactive care workers, but more, on average, than all low-wage workers (defined as earning less than two-thirds of the gross median wage).[5] In 2009 low-wage workers earned a median hourly wage of $7.75, while child care workers and adult care workers earned $9.17 and $10.58 per hour, respectively. However, this simple comparison does not control for differences in age, education, or unionization.[6]

As table 4.1 indicates, child care workers are far more likely than low-wage workers in general to have a bachelor's degree (18 percent compared to 10 percent). Although adult care workers are less likely than child care workers to have a bachelor's degree, they are more likely than low-wage workers to have an associate's degree (11 percent compared to 8 percent). Adult care workers are older, on average, than low-wage workers and child care workers. While professionalization and higher education may explain child care workers' higher wages relative to all low-wage workers, the higher rates of unionization among adult care workers—13 percent compared to 5 percent among all low-wage workers—probably explain their apparent wage premium.

The Pay Penalty in Care Jobs

Although the median wage for interactive care workers may exceed the median wage for other workers, care workers are paid less than other workers with

FIGURE 4.2 / Median Hourly Wages for All Workers and Interactive Care Workers, by Education Level, 2009

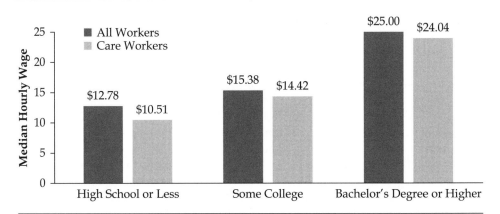

Source: U.S. Bureau of Labor Statistics, Current Population Survey (2010d), analyzed by Kristin Smith and Andrew Schaefer.
Notes: Percentages are based on weighted data for all workers age eighteen and older. Data refer to 2009 hourly wages. "Some college" includes those with an associate's degree and those who have not completed a degree.

similar characteristics. The higher-than-average wage reported in the previous section disappears once differences in education are taken into account, as indicated by figure 4.2. More detailed cross-sectional analyses of pay by occupation in the early 1990s show that interactive service jobs (a broader category than care work because it includes sales workers) impose a pay penalty even after controlling for worker education levels and unionization rates, how much cognitive skill and physical skill the jobs require, and the percentage of women in the occupation (England 1992). A more comprehensive analysis of earnings by occupation, controlling for differences among individuals, found that care workers pay a 5 to 6 percent hourly wage penalty, net of their education, experience, seniority, whether they work part-time, and a number of other job characteristics—including the amount of cognitive skill and physical strength required by the jobs and the percentage of female workers in the jobs (England, Budig, and Folbre 2002). The estimated penalty varied across occupations. For instance, a group of occupations dominated by nursing paid no penalty, perhaps because nurses are relatively likely to be union members and are often required to work overtime, for which they are paid a premium. More research is needed to determine how the care penalty varies by industry and occupation and also how it may be changing over time. Figure 4.2 indicates that the penalty, controlling only for education, is proportionally larger for low-wage than for high-wage interactive care workers. Controls for experience, job characteristics, and unionization might reveal an even greater penalty for low-wage care workers.

Many care workers may place a high priority on work flexibility, in part because they are providing unpaid care to family members such as children and parents. Approximately 39 percent of certified nursing assistants (CNAs) and 30 percent of home health aides, for example, reported that, in addition to their paid care job, they were caring for a child or a relative who had a disability or was ill at home (U.S. Department of Health and Human Services/ASPE/DALTCP 2011). Nurses typically bargain more heavily for control over their scheduling than firefighters, who are more likely to look for opportunities to earn supplemental income through overtime (Crocker 2010). Home care workers in California ranked flexibility in the job among the three most important reasons why they chose to work in the field; pay ranked in the top three only for a small percentage of respondents (Howes 2008).

Although the studies that quantify the care penalty control for the percentage of females in the job, revealing that female-dominated care jobs average lower pay than female-dominated noncare jobs at similar skill levels, gender bias may still be implicated (England, Budig, and Folbre 2002). It may be that care is more culturally devalued than other kinds of women's work precisely because it is strongly associated with women and unpaid work in the home.

Characteristics of Low-Wage Interactive Care Workers

All interactive care workers share some personal, motivational, and job characteristics that distinguish them from all workers. But low-wage interactive care workers experience difficulties related to low-wage work itself. Numerous structural changes in the U.S. economy and U.S. labor markets since the mid-1970s have increased competitive pressure on employers to cut costs (Appelbaum, Bernhardt, and Murnane 2003). Globalization, deregulation of financial and labor markets, falling unionization rates, and, recently, high unemployment rates have all weakened the bargaining position of the low-wage labor force (Noah 2010). Women have fared better than men, largely because it is difficult to offshore, outsource, or automate interactive care, but on average real wages for production and non-supervisory workers are only slightly above what they were in 1973 (Economic Policy Institute 2010).

In terms of race, ethnicity, and nativity, low-wage interactive care workers look more like the low-wage workforce than the interactive care workforce. Between all care occupations and all workers there is little difference in the percentage of white non-Hispanic workers. Black non-Hispanics are slightly overrepresented (14 percent compared to 11 percent for all workers), and Hispanics are underrepresented (9 percent compared to 14 percent for all workers). But underlying these averages, we find significant differences between low- and high-wage care jobs. Although blacks are well represented in the lower-paying professional care occupations, they are greatly overrepresented, along with Hispanics, in the very low-wage child care and adult care occupations (U.S. Bureau of Labor Statistics, Current Population Survey 2010a). Racial-ethnic differences between these two occupations are also significant: white non-Hispanic workers dominate child care jobs (representing 63 percent of the total), but not adult care jobs (representing only 46 percent). Almost one-third of adult care workers are black non-Hispanics, compared to only about 15 percent of child care workers.

Care workers are slightly less likely to be foreign-born—13 percent compared to 15 percent for all workers—but among low-wage care workers, the chance of being foreign-born is similar to the rate among all low-wage workers. Nearly one-quarter of the adult care workforce is foreign-born, a larger percentage than the child care workforce (17 percent). The foreign-born and native-born child care workforces differ in significant ways. Child care workers who are foreign-born are less likely to be black non-Hispanic and more likely to work full-time, to be Hispanic, and to have lower education levels. A larger proportion of foreign-born than native-born child care workers have no health insurance coverage (44 percent and 26 percent, respectively). Foreign-born adult care workers also work longer hours than their native-born counterparts, and in adult care both black non-Hispanics and Hispanics comprise a larger share of the foreign-born than the native-born workforce.

Very few child care workers belong to unions (about 3 percent). The unionization rate for adult care workers is about 13 percent, only slightly higher than the average for all workers, but lower than the average rate for the health care sector where many are employed. Child care workers and adult care workers, like all low-wage workers, work fewer hours per week, are less likely to work full-time or year-round, and are more likely to have a second job compared to all workers. Adult care workers are less likely to work overtime (defined as more than forty hours per week). Almost half of child care workers are married, a higher percentage than that of either generic low-wage workers as a whole (42 percent) or adult care workers (37 percent). Partly because a lower proportion of adult care workers are married, they tend to have lower family incomes even though they generally earn higher wages. Preliminary research suggests that this pattern may also reflect a tendency for female child care workers to marry men who are, like themselves, white, non-Hispanic, and college-educated; thus, their husbands tend to earn more than the husbands of female adult care workers (Smith and Churilla 2010).

Family poverty rates are high among child care and adult care workers. In 2009 about 18 percent of adult care and child care workers lived in families with incomes below the poverty line. Child care and adult care workers are more likely than low-wage workers in general, but less likely than care workers in general, to have health insurance coverage. Child care workers and adult care workers have similar private-sector coverage, but adult care workers have higher public-sector coverage, a side effect of lower family earnings among adult care workers (see table 4.1).

The official labor force statistics that we draw from do not fully include undocumented workers, who live in fear of deportation and enjoy no labor law protections. Child care and adult care workers employed by private households in the United States are particularly likely to fall into this category. Relatively few employers of household workers in the United States pay legally required Social Security taxes or contributions to unemployment insurance. In 2006 the American Community Survey tallied over 800,000 household workers, but the Internal Revenue Service (IRS) counted only 200,000 household employer tax returns, indicating a noncompliance rate of more than 74 percent (Haskins 2010). A recent survey of labor law violations in American cities found that more than 40 percent of household workers were paid less than the minimum wage (Bernhardt et al. 2009, 21).

PAID CHILD CARE

Paid child care includes a range of formal and informal jobs, some of which blur the lines between paid and unpaid care. Teachers and teacher's aides at school-based or center-based programs—including those employed by elementary schools, Head Start programs, prekindergarten, nursery schools, and community-based child care centers—clearly lie within the formal sector. Some of these workers may receive a discount or subsidy for the care of their own children in exchange for their work, but they are typically paid employees. The public sector directly subsidizes child care in a variety of ways—through direct provision of early childhood education on the state level, through vouchers to low-income parents, and through the federal Head Start program (for more detailed discussion of these policies, see chapter 6).

The informal sector adds another layer of complexity. Family day care providers who care for other people's children (sometimes in addition to their own) in their own homes are subject to state regulation (and eligible, in some cases, for state reimbursement for services to low-income families). However, an estimated three-quarters of children in family day care are in homes that are not regulated or registered, and fewer than half of unregulated providers report their income (Brown-Lyons, Robertson, and Layzer 2001). Recent efforts to assess the number of family day care workers have been hampered by inconsistent definitions: some studies count all nonrelatives who are paid to provide care, while others count only those who are registered or licensed (Morrissey and Banghart 2007). About 29 percent of grandparents providing child care receive some remuneration, often for providing care in their own homes, yet they are often lumped into the category of family/friend/neighbor care (Brown-Lyons, Robertson, and Layzer 2001, 15). Nannies who work in private homes are often paid under the table. By one estimate, the informal sector comprised almost half the total paid child care workforce in the late 1990s, with considerable variation across states (Burton et al. 2002). This sector is poorly measured by conventional labor force surveys.

Child Care Occupations

Institutional complexity contributes to considerable segmentation of the child care workforce. Paid workers in the public sector enjoy significantly higher pay and benefits than those in the private sector, and small differences in the ages of the children being cared for are associated with large differences in pay. Kindergarten teachers, who are primarily responsible for five-year-olds, earn considerably more than preschool teachers, who are primarily responsible for four-year-olds, despite the importance of high-quality care for young children and the advantages of institutional continuity between preschool and grade 3. As one preschool teacher put it: "People need to realize that preschool teachers are not just babysitters; I get so much more respect now that I have left and become an elementary school teacher, but I am still doing the same job" (Whitebook and Sakai 2004, 97).

As highly educated women have gained new opportunities in paid employment, they have moved up in the occupational hierarchy. As a result, average skill levels in interactive care of young children have declined. The share of early childhood education teachers and administrators with at least a four-year college degree averaged 43 percent in the period 1983 to 1985, but only 30 percent in 2002 to 2005 (Herzenberg, Price, and Bradley 2005). Older workers in this industry are more likely to have a college degree than younger workers, a pattern that suggests difficulty attracting younger workers.

Characteristics of Child Care Workers

Our analysis of the 2010 CPS examines the economic and demographic characteristics of workers in center-based child care and family day care centers as well as nannies working in private homes. In 2010 two-thirds of child care workers were employed in centers, roughly one-quarter were self-employed and working out of their own homes, and the remaining 10 percent were nannies (see table 4.2). Center-based child care workers and nannies earned $9.60 per hour, and family day care workers had the lowest hourly wages ($7.14). They also worked the longest hours, with 47 percent working more than forty hours per week. On the other hand, family day care workers had the highest levels of year-round, full-time employment. Their steadier flow of paychecks narrows the annual earnings gap between them and their peers.

Center-based care workers are more highly educated than workers in either of the two other categories, with almost one-quarter holding a bachelor's degree or higher in 2010. They are also more likely to be white, non-Hispanic, and native-born than family day care workers and nannies. Family day care workers are more likely to be married and are older than the other care workers (forty-three years old on average). About one in four nannies are Hispanic, and they are younger, tend to have never married, and are less likely to have children than other child care workers. Roughly one-fifth of all child care workers are covered by public health insurance, with public health insurance coverage more prominent among center-based child care providers than family day care workers.

Job Quality, Care Quality, and Turnover in Child Care

A growing emphasis on the value of center-based early childhood education has intensified concerns about the quality of jobs in that segment of the child care workforce. Licensing and regulation vary considerably from state to state, and most

TABLE 4.2 / Characteristics of Child Care Workers, 2010

	Total	Center-Based Care Provider	Family Day Care Provider	Nannies
Number (in thousands)	1,776	1,223	368	185
Percentage of all workers	1.2%	68.9%	20.7%	10.4%
Percentage female	96.5	96.2	97.8	96.1
Economic characteristics				
Median family income	$50,000	$50,200	$45,752	$54,100
In poverty	18.6%	17.3%	23.5%	17.4%
Median hourly wage	$9.17	$9.60	$7.14	$9.60
Average weekly hours worked	33.1	30.9	42.1	28.8
Overtime (more than forty hours per week)	13.7%	4.4%	47.0%	9.5%
Full-time employment[a]	58.6	54.0	78.7	49.3
Year-round full-time employment[b]	41.8	37.8	62.9	26.6
Self-employed	20.7	0.0	100.0	0.0
Two or more jobs	12.4	87.9	89.8	81.6
Union membership[c]	3.1	3.5	0.0	0.0
Health insurance				
Public	18.6	19.5	18.5	13.2
Private	59.1	60.7	49.7	67.1
No health insurance	27.7	25.8	34.3	27.1
Demographic characteristics				
Average age	37.7	36.7	43.5	32.2
Education				
High school or less	42.4%	40.5%	52.3%	35.6%
Some college, no degree	27.8	27.6	20.9	42.2
Associate's degree	9.4	9.6	10.4	6.1
Bachelor's degree	17.7	19.3	15.0	13.3
More than bachelor's degree	2.7	3.1	1.4	2.8
Race and ethnicity				
White, non-Hispanic	63.4	65.1	56.8	64.9
Black, non-Hispanic	15.1	16.3	16.9	4.1
Asian, non-Hispanic	3.5	3.6	3.0	3.4
Other, non-Hispanic	1.6	1.6	0.8	2.6
Hispanic	16.5	13.4	22.5	25.0
Foreign-born	16.6	12.9	23.0	28.1
Marital status				
Married	47.4	47.9	55.7	28.0
Previously married	18.0	15.4	28.2	14.7
Never married	34.6	36.8	16.1	57.3
Children under age eighteen	50.1	50.6	55.8	35.5
Single mothers	20.7	21.0	20.2	19.7

Source: U.S. Bureau of Labor Statistics, Current Population Survey (2010d), analyzed by Kristin Smith and Andrew Schaefer.

Notes: Percentages are based on weighted data for all workers age eighteen and older. Hourly wages, family income, poverty status, and work hours reflect 2009 employment; all other characteristics refer to 2010.

[a]Includes those working thirty-five or more hours per week.
[b]Includes those working thirty-five or more hours per week and fifty or more weeks annually.
[c]The union membership question is asked for one-quarter of the sample.

child care jobs have few entry requirements, licensing standards, or opportunities for career advancement (Helburn and Bergmann 2002).[7] Education and training enhance outcomes for children (Bowman, Donovan, and Burns 2000). However, it can be difficult to find convincing links between classroom quality and children's academic gains (Early et al. 2007), perhaps because of the confounding effects of family background. It is difficult to accurately measure the relationship between inputs and outputs in child development (Blau 2001). Teachers' credentials may be less important than less tangible characteristics such as energy, enthusiasm, and motivation (Blau 2001, 209). Such characteristics are likely to be affected by the workplace environment, including flexibility and the degree to which autonomy and collaboration are encouraged (Leana, Appelbaum, and Shevchuk 2009). Neither education nor experience has a very significant positive effect on what a child care worker earns. Parents are reluctant to pay more for quality, perhaps because of the difficulty of accurately assessing it (Blau 2001).

Collaboration among workers—and between workers and young children—is a central aspect of the labor process in child care centers. Classrooms are often staffed with two or more teachers and aides, who must coordinate their work as they share a physical space and responsibility for a group of children. Such coordination can take many forms, ranging from a clear division of labor (as when one adult always directs play activities for the children while the other organizes feeding and napping) to a more improvised sharing of mutual responsibilities (as when adults work together to collaboratively organize play and feeding activities each day). Child care teachers and those they care for know each other by name and often form warm relationships.

Children are not likely to thrive unless they trust and like their caregivers, who play an important role as "available, responsive adults who can help children build an internal image of the world as safe and of themselves as valuable persons" (Whitebook and Sakai 2004, 13). Children who form close relationships with teachers tend to show better language skills and more sociability and to demonstrate fewer behavior problems than those who do not (Moon and Burbank 2004), and close relationships require a certain minimum threshold of continuity of care. Yet about one-third of early childhood education teachers leave their jobs every year (Whitebook and Sakai 2004). Turnover rates have been particularly high in for-profit centers, averaging around 45 percent a year (Helburn and Bergmann 2002, 180). A detailed analysis of California centers found that turnover was also particularly high in publicly subsidized child care (Whitebook, Kipnis, and Bellm 2007). Turnover can be amplified over time as departures disrupt the working environment, leading to further departures.

Low wages and lack of "voice," or opportunity to participate in the organization of work, contribute to high turnover rates (Whitebook and Sakai 2004; Hatch 2009). Part-time employment reduces job attachment. The odds of remaining in the workforce increase by 2 percent with every additional hour worked per week. White non-Hispanic women, as well as those with a child under eighteen, are more likely than Hispanic women to remain in their job (Smith and Baughman 2007b). Collaborative work may not affect turnover intentions for all classroom staff, but it does have an encouraging impact on those teachers and aides who provide the highest-quality care, improving retention of high-performing teachers (Leana, Appelbaum, and Shevchuk 2009). Developmental and supportive supervisory actions for center directors and others in leadership positions can foster a culture that supports effective collaboration (Leana, Appelbaum, and Shevchuk 2009).

High turnover can have detrimental effects on both employees and care recipients because it tends to reduce the quality of services provided, compromise developmental outcomes for children, and contribute to program attrition (Whitebook and Sakai 2004). Low wages and inadequate professional development opportunities discourage new entrants (Kagan, Kauerz, and Tarrant 2008).

In recent years, both nonprofit organizations and unions have made concerted efforts to build alliances among child care workers and the families they serve in order to improve the quality of care provided. The spirit of this effort is captured in a popular slogan: "Parents can't afford to pay, teachers can't afford to stay, there's got to be a better way." The grassroots Worthy Wage Campaign effectively publicized problems of low job quality and high turnover in paid child care between 1991 and 1999.[8]

Advocates for unionization argue that unions could play a vital role in upgrading service quality and increasing public support by making it easier for committed workers to stick with a vocation that they love. Child care workers are difficult to organize because centers are typically small and workers are dispersed. Public support is also difficult to muster, as families are fearful of cost increases. However, the United Auto Workers (UAW) successfully organized some child care workers in the 1970s, and affiliates of two large international unions, the Service Employees International Union (SEIU) and the American Federation of State, County, and Municipal Employees (AFSCME), inspired in part by the Worthy Wage Campaign, have launched strategic child care organizing efforts in Seattle, Washington, and Philadelphia, Pennsylvania. AFSCME's national Union of Hospital and Health Care Employees (1199) partnered with child care advocates based in Philadelphia to charter a new child care union called the United Child Care Union.

Because family child care providers are self-employed, they are not covered by the National Labor Relations Act (NLRA). Efforts to organize these workers have required the development of a new bargaining model, one based on state-level executive orders or on enabling legislation that defines an "employer of record" for the purposes of collective bargaining (Smith 2009b). Campaigns have been targeted to family child care providers who care for the children of low-income working people, often partially funded by public monies. Efforts to build coalitions among families, providers, and advocacy groups to fight for greater access to public resources and to link quality care and quality jobs have proved strategically effective. Successful examples include the Family Care Providers Association of San Francisco and a new statewide union of home-based child care providers in Pennsylvania.[9] As of 2007, ten states had passed legislation that would create an employer of record for family child care providers (Smith 2009b).

Another innovative approach is exemplified by Childspace, a worker-owned child care cooperative in Philadelphia. In addition to promoting local economic development by providing families with high-quality care and workers with high-quality jobs, this organization aims to empower workers to help manage their workplaces, improve their compensation, and join efforts to advocate for better subsidy rates, health insurance coverage for low-income workers, and management of the state's subsidy programs.[10]

PAID ADULT CARE

Adult care, often described as long-term care, is assistance provided to people over the age of eighteen who need help performing some activities of daily living (such as bathing, dressing, eating, transferring from bed to chair) owing to physical or mental disability, chronic illness, or the effects of aging. Although adult care workers are not nurses or paramedics, they often administer medication, monitor vital signs, and provide medical oversight. They may also provide companionship and help with cooking, housework, and transportation (Institute of Medicine 2008). Job titles tend to vary between states and work sites, but the most common include nurse's aide, nursing assistant, personal care aide, home care aide, home health aide, certified nursing assistant, and direct support professional (National Direct Service Workforce Resource Center 2008).[11]

Adult care workers can be found in a variety of settings, from for-profit and not-for-profit nursing facilities, assisted living facilities, and continuing care retirement communities (CCRCs) to private households to group homes for people with psychological or developmental disabilities (National Direct Service Workforce Resource Center 2008). Some independent and self-employed providers work in very informal arrangements that are not included in standard labor force surveys. A little less than half of adult care workers in the United States currently report to a facility each workday in a traditional employer-employee arrangement (PHI 2010).

The Adult Care Industry

Adult care is stratified by client—adults with physical disabilities, elderly persons, persons with intellectual and developmental disabilities (ID/DD)—and by settings—nursing homes, residential care facilities for persons with ID/DD, community facilities, adult day care, and care in the home. Since adult care is expensive and public funding is available only for persons whose household income is at or close to the poverty line, the industry is also stratified by income level and payment source. Almost half of all financing for long-term care comes from Medicaid, and its rules and reimbursement policies substantially shape the industry (Kaye, Harrington, and LaPlante 2010). Over the past thirty years, program rules have gradually evolved to support more community-based and less institutional-based care (Harrington et al. 2009). Most people with intellectual or developmental disabilities receive personal care services in community settings or family homes. More recently, states have begun to move or redirect older persons and adults with disabilities to home- and community-based services. Consumer preference, state fiscal crises, and the Supreme Court's *Olmstead* decision in 1999 have all contributed to the shift away from nursing homes (Howes 2010).[12]

Assisted living facilities and continuing care retirement communities are rapidly growing; most of them are private, for-profit, private-pay establishments that cater to high-income elderly persons. As of 2006, about 700,000 people lived in assisted living and continuing care retirement communities (Spillman and Black 2008).

The Home Health Care and Home Care Industries

The fastest-growing segment of the long-term care sector is the home health and home care industries (Seavey and Marquand 2011). The formal sector includes Medicare- and Medicaid-certified home health care companies that supply services ranging from skilled nursing, home health care, and personal care to durable medical equipment. Some for-profit chains and smaller proprietary and non-proprietary firms limit their services to nonmedical, limited personal care and homemaking (Seavey and Marquand 2011).

Within the home-based care segment, consumer-directed, publicly funded home care is gaining ground in many states. Under this model, individuals hire providers of their own choice, supervising and paying them either directly using cash support from Medicaid or having the provider paid directly by the state or an intermediary, such as a "public authority." Under the public authority model, which originated in California, the consumer hires the provider, the state pays the provider directly, and the public authority maintains a registry of providers, offers training for consumers and providers, and serves as the employer of record. Whether the employer-of-record is a state or private sector entity, consumer-directed home care workers are reclassified from independent contractors to employees, which means they are covered either by state statutes that govern collective bargaining for public employees or the National Labor Relations Act that covers private sector employees. They can join unions, engage in collective bargaining, and access group benefits such as worker's compensation and health care benefits (Delp and Quan 2002; Boris and Klein 2008; Smith 2008).[13] Including California, where there are over 350,000 independent providers, eleven states now provide Medicaid personal care services under this model of "consumer-directed" care (Seavey and Marquand 2011).

Other home care providers work as independent contractors, either declaring self-employment or working under the table. As with child care workers, the true number may be considerably higher than reports based on the Current Population Survey owing to the high number of independent home care workers who provide care off the books.

States' rebalancing projects, combined with the demographic trends described in chapter 3, help account for the very high rate of projected job growth in the home health and home care industries. Between 1989 and 2004, the workforce providing non-institutional personal assistance and home health services tripled, while the workforce providing similar services in institutional settings remained relatively stable (Kaye et al. 2006). Home health care and services for the elderly and persons with disabilities ("home care") are now the industries with the first- and second-fastest rate of growth of employment in the United States (U.S. Bureau of Labor Statistics 2012). Together, adult or long-term care industries, which made up about 3 percent of all jobs in 2010, are projected to account for 10 percent of all expected new jobs between 2010 and 2020. Two-thirds of these jobs will be in home health and home care (U.S. Bureau of Labor Statistics 2012).[14]

Adult Care Occupations

Most research to date on adult care workers has focused on the institutional workforce, whose members are easier to identify and track than those who provide home-based care (Ochsner, Leana, and Appelbaum 2009). Nurse's aides, certified nursing assistants, and psychiatric aides work in hospitals, nursing homes, and residential care facilities under the supervision of nursing staff. They generally work in highly structured and hierarchical settings and provide assistance only with feeding, bathing, dressing, transferring, and other personal care services.

In contrast, home health aides work in care recipients' homes or residential facilities, in adult day programs and hospices, doing work similar to nurse's aides and CNAs.[15] Home health aides are employed mainly through Medicare-certified home health care agencies, Medicare rules specify that they must work under the supervision of a health care professional, usually a nurse, although supervision is intermittent and occasional. Their duties may range from light housekeeping, shopping, and food preparation to basic health-related services such as checking temperature, pulse rate, or respiration rate, occasionally changing bandages, and assisting in the administration of medications. Personal care aides perform the same nonmedical functions as home health aides but do not work under the supervision of a health care professional, receive little if any supervision from anyone, and are not supposed to provide health-related services. About one-third are employed by home health agencies and another third by home care companies. The remaining third work as independent providers in private households, where their only supervision comes from the client and family (U.S. Bureau of Labor Statistics 2010b).

Because home health aides and personal and home care aides are fast-growing occupations, policymakers in many states have expressed doubts about their state's ability to fill the new openings as they proliferate, concerned that low wages, poor working conditions, and a lack of affordable benefits will keep turnover rates high and that these occupations will fail to attract enough new workers.[16] The abrupt increase in unemployment associated with the Great Recession that began in 2007 may have allayed labor shortages, but the recession has also decreased the economic resources available to pay for such services. In general, today's labor market suffers from instabilities that make it difficult to promote sustainable and effective care.

Characteristics of Adult Care Workers

Our analysis of the 2010 Current Population Survey illustrates key components of the adult care workforce. More than 50 percent of adult care workers are employed in home and community settings, 22 percent as home health aides and 31 percent as personal and home care aides, while nursing homes employ 26 percent as nursing assistants. The remaining 21 percent work in hospitals as nursing assistants or orderlies (see table 4.3). A clear occupational hierarchy is evident: Hospital aides are the best paid, at $12.98 per hour. They work more hours than home health and personal and home care aides, are most likely to work full time and are far more likely to have private health insurance. In contrast, personal and home care aides earn a much lower median wage ($9.50 an hour), work fewer hours and are much less likely to work full time than hospital and nursing home aides. Nursing home aides fall somewhere in the middle.

Hospital aides are also more likely to be married and to have higher education levels than nursing aides and home health aides. They are younger, on average, than home health and personal and home care aides. Nursing home aides are more likely to be black and non-Hispanic, while home health aides are more likely to be foreign-born. Hospital aides and nursing aides who are foreign-born are older, on average, and are more likely to be married than their native-born colleagues.[17] Foreign-born home health aides are also older than native-born home health aides, and nearly three-quarters have a high school degree or less. Foreign-born personal and home care workers are more likely to work full-time compared to native-born personal care workers, and they are more likely to be married. Roughly one-third of home health aides and personal and home care aides have no health insurance, and another third are covered by public insurance. In contrast, three-fourths of hospital aides are covered by employer-sponsored health insurance.

Real wages fell for both home health and home care workers between 1999 and 2007 despite a steady increase in the demand for their labor (PHI/DCWA-NC 2009). By contrast, wages rose for nursing aides and orderlies and attendants, in part because they work in hospitals, where 20 percent are unionized and where their wages are linked to those of other unionized employees.

Job Quality, Care Quality, and Turnover in Adult Care

As with child care, the link between quality jobs and the quality of care provided is key. Job settings matter. Home health and personal care aides often enjoy more autonomy and discretion than adult care workers employed in institutional settings, but they earn lower pay and often experience more hazardous working conditions.

In contrast to child care, long-term care is moving in the direction of decentralized provision of care in homes and community settings. Because home-based aides tend to care for fewer clients, they have greater opportunity to build longer-lived and trusting relationships with those clients (Stacey 2011). However, they

TABLE 4.3 / Characteristics of Adult Care Workers, 2010

	Total	Hospital Aide	Nursing Home Aide	Home Health Aide	Personal Care Aide
Number (in thousands)	3,042	626	802	669	945
Percentage of all workers	2.0%	20.6%	26.4%	22.0%	31.1%
Percentage female	88.7	85.9	88.9	92.3	88.0
Economic characteristics					
Median family income	$34,500	$46,006	$32,976	$28,673	$30,800
In poverty	18.2%	8.7%	17.0%	23.1%	22.0%
Median hourly wage	$10.58	$12.98	$11.40	$10.00	$9.50
Average weekly hours worked	35.1	37.2	36.3	33.4	33.9
Overtime (more than forty hours per week)	9.0%	6.2%	6.7%	10.0%	12.1%
Full-time employment[a]	67.5	81.4	74.3	59.1	58.4
Year-round full-time employment[b]	53.4	69.3	60.8	45.1	42.4
Self-employed	3.7	0.1	0.6	5.7	7.2
Two or more jobs	12.1	10.3	11.6	11.7	14.1
Union membership[c]	13.2	20.1	16.3	11.5	8.2
Health insurance					
Public	24.4	14.6	18.2	28.5	33.3
Private	54.9	75.8	59.4	43.9	45.1
No health insurance	27.8	18.1	26.9	33.1	31.2
Demographic characteristics					
Average age	41.9	40.6	40.1	42.6	43.9
Education					
High school or less	54.3%	44.3%	57.4%	58.9%	55.2%
Some college, no degree	15.7	31.7	26.5	20.9	24.4
Associate's degree	11.4	14.8	10.0	14.2	8.4
Bachelor's degree	7.1	7.6	6.0	4.4	9.6
More than bachelor's degree	1.5	1.7	0.3	1.6	2.4
Race and ethnicity					
White, non-Hispanic	45.9	45.4	45.8	42.0	49.2
Black, non-Hispanic	30.8	31.7	39.0	31.1	23.2
Asian, non-Hispanic	4.6	5.7	3.9	2.1	2.1
Other, non-Hispanic	2.8	3.6	1.2	3.5	3.2
Hispanic	15.8	13.6	10.1	21.3	18.1
Foreign-born	22.8	20.3	21.5	27.1	22.7
Marital status					
Married	36.7	42.4	35.6	34.6	35.2
Previously married	29.0	23.1	30.3	29.8	31.2
Never married	34.4	34.5	34.2	35.6	35.6
Children under age eighteen	40.3	39.1	44.9	39.3	37.9
Single mothers	22.9	17.7	26.9	23.7	22.3

Source: U.S. Bureau of Labor Statistics, Current Population Survey (2010d), analyzed by Kristin Smith and Andrew Schaefer.
Notes: Percentages are based on weighted data for all workers age eighteen and older. Hourly wages, family income, poverty status, and work hours reflect 2009 employment; all other characteristics refer to 2010.
[a]Includes those working thirty-five or more hours per week.
[b]Includes those working thirty-five or more hours per week and fifty or more weeks annually.
[c]The union membership question is asked for one-quarter of the sample.

are more likely to work part-time and to work for more than one agency or family at a time. These workers are prone to social isolation, difficulty juggling multiple employers, and time-consuming (and often uncompensated) travel time between client homes. Despite the hazards of the job, there are no or limited training requirements for home health and personal care aides, there is little if any supervision, and wages and benefits are lower. These workers are currently not covered under the federal Fair Labor Standards Act (FLSA), which guarantees payment of a minimum wage and overtime pay, on the grounds that they are primarily providing "companionship" rather than compensable services (Smith 2009a; Forhan 2010). The Obama administration has recently proposed a rule change that would eliminate this exclusion (Smith 2012).[18]

Turnover is a generally accepted indicator of job quality. While many adult care workers find intrinsic satisfaction in their job, low pay and poor working conditions often prompt them to leave (Howes 2008). Turnover related to problems of low wages, low morale, absenteeism, and burnout is high across all sectors of the adult care industry (NDSWRC 2008). One recent study of three categories of female adult care workers found that hospital aides and nursing home aides had a higher propensity for remaining in their occupation than home health aides. Higher wages, being older, having children, and being Hispanic were other significant predictors of remaining in the adult care profession (Smith and Baughman 2007a). CNA turnover averages 71 percent a year in nursing homes nationwide, and it reaches even higher levels in many states (Decker et al. 2003). An estimated 40 to 60 percent of home health aides leave after less than one year on the job, and 80 to 90 percent leave within the first two years (Institute of Medicine 2008). There are no large-scale studies of turnover among home care workers, but small-scale studies have found that turnover rates are lower than those in home health care, and considerably lower than in nursing homes, suggesting the possibility that increased autonomy may offset some of the negative effects of low wages and benefits.[19]

Home health and home care aides may also be trading off their physical safety. Care of adults is physically demanding. In 2009, nursing home aides, orderlies, and attendants had the fourth-highest occupational injury rates of any workers in government or private industry. They followed EMTs and paramedics, but ranked higher than correctional officers, fire fighters, and construction workers. Home care workers have been studied less than other paid caregivers, but their reported injury rate is three times that of registered nurses; while their injury rate is lower than nursing home aides working in private industry, home care workers employed through state governments have an astronomically high incidence of injury. More than five out of every ten workers—almost fifty times the national average for all workers in government and private sector employment, which is 117 out of every 10,000—sustained a work-related injury that resulted in lost days at work (U.S. Bureau of Labor Statistics 2010a).

Unlike in nursing homes, where regulations require that a second person be present to assist, home health and home care workers are expected to lift a client on their own, usually without the aid of mechanical lifts, which are rarely found in private homes (Meyer and Muntaner 1999). The physical demands of the job contribute substantially to the risk of musculo-skeletal injury (Kim et al. 2010). Improved training and supervision tends to lower injury rates as well as reduce turnover (McCaughey et al. 2010).

Although the training and licensing of adult care workers varies from state to state, it is widely considered inadequate. As the Institute of Medicine (2008, 204) puts it, "The education and training of the direct-care workforce is insufficient to prepare these workers to provide quality care to older adults." Certified nursing assistants and certified home health aides (who work in Medicare- and Medicaid-certified nursing homes and home health agencies) must receive 75 hours of federally mandated training. Some states have extended these requirements up to 175 hours. There are no federal training requirements for personal care and home care aides. As of 2007, however, ten states reported having adopted entry-level training for personal and home care aides and direct support professionals (who provide care for persons with intellectual and developmental disabilities), and six states had adopted training requirements for workers in consumer-directed home care programs (PHI/DCWA-NC 2009; U.S. Department of Health and Human Services/ASPE/DALTCP 2006; NDSWRC 2008). Other state initiatives have focused on training supervisors and creating career ladders using training requirements. High turnover disrupts the collaborative process of care provision. While nursing home aides interact with residents throughout the workday, they also often coordinate their care with other aides who provide care to the same residents on earlier or later shifts. They may also coordinate with nurses who provide medical services and with other professionals, ranging from dietary aides and recreational specialists to housekeeping staff. Personal relationships among workers as well as between workers and care recipients can expedite the flow of information and contribute to emotional support. The disruption that comes from turnover is likely to lower the quality of care provided. When these personal relationships become temporary, workers have less incentive to invest in them.

Further, frequent turnover requires that existing care workers work overtime, which makes them "susceptible to exhaustion, increased mistakes and decreasing quality of performance" (Hewitt and Lakin 2001, 6). Turnover increases employer costs because of the need for continuous recruitment and training. The costs of adult care worker turnover on the national level have been estimated at $4.1 billion per year (Seavey 2004). State-level studies also yield high estimates (Leon, Marainen, and Marcotte 2001).

Turnover and retention seem to be driven by different forces. Workers in nursing homes report that they remain in these jobs because of their sense of satisfaction from doing the work and their interactions and relationships with care recipients and their families; they tend to leave these jobs because of extrinsic conditions like poor management, lack of respect, and the sheer physical and emotional difficulty of the work (Mittal, Rosen, and Leana 2009). Studies of home-based adult care workers show that turnover rates are elevated by low wages and benefits and mitigated by attachment to the consumer (Howes 2004, 2005; Stacey 2011). Consumers show a significant tendency to hire family members, friends, or individuals who share their ethnic background when given the opportunity (Howes 2004, 2005). This "dual-driver model" suggests that institutions must respect both intrinsic and extrinsic motivations, providing better wages and working conditions but also creating a supportive work environment that facilitates autonomy, discretion, and collaboration. The lesson is similar for home-based workers, but the challenges are different. Too much autonomy and discretion, little or no training, little or no supervision, and low wages and benefits all contribute to a lower quality of care.

A SECTORAL HIGH-ROAD STRATEGY

Even care that is motivated by concern for the care recipient can be crushed by work organizations that obstruct the caregiver's ability to care. The most effective forms of work organization mimic the organization of high-quality care provision in the home when the care provider is motivated by a deep commitment to the care recipient, has sufficient autonomy and discretion to respond to the specific needs of the care recipient, and is able to collaborate effectively with other care providers. Whether in schools, hospitals, nursing homes, or the family home, the organization of work has a huge impact on the quality of care. In some ways, managers in care industries are confronting problems similar to those confronted by managers in manufacturing firms during an earlier stage. Men moving out of autonomous craft jobs into monotonous factory work had little incentive to work harder than necessary to hold on to their jobs (Lewchuk 2003). Similar problems are becoming apparent in many service jobs.

Poor job quality in child care and adult care leads to poor care quality. A growing literature describes the economic benefits of a positive work environment and opportunities for employee advancement (Appelbaum et al. 2000; Appelbaum, Gittell, and Leana 2008). This high-road strategy offers a particularly high payoff in the care sector of the economy, especially in relatively poorly paid child care and adult care jobs. The labor process in these jobs is typically improved by the development of long-term relationships between workers and between workers and care recipients. Better pay, benefits, and working conditions could help strengthen the intrinsic motivation that brings many into this field of employment, reducing turnover and mitigating worker burnout. Consumers and care recipients would benefit from the resulting enhancements in care quality.

All high-quality care jobs include a significant degree of worker control or autonomy, good collaboration with the others involved in the recipients' care, and compensation that inspires job commitment. While the factors that make a job good are consistent across jobs and settings, what makes them bad differs from setting to setting. Settings in both child care and adult care vary in their organizational formality, from child care centers and nursing homes to home-based child care and nannies and home health and personal care in homes. In some settings more autonomy and cooperation is needed, and in others more external support, such as training, access to group health benefits, and time off, is needed.

At this point in time, about two-thirds of child care workers (among those officially counted) work in child care centers. In long-term care, in contrast, two-thirds of care providers work in home-based or community-based settings, not in large institutions. The trend in long-term care is toward increased use of home-based care, whereas child care is headed in the opposite direction. So while policies and work practices that enhance the quality of jobs in institutions are important, so too are policies that improve job quality in home-based work.

Child care and long-term care policies, which are discussed in detail in chapters 6 and 7, can have an important impact on the quality of the job as well. In both home-based child care and home care, for example, some institutional arrangements are better for simultaneously protecting the caring relationship between the worker and recipient and the labor rights of workers.

Care relationships appear to be stronger if there is no direct cash exchange between the adult care recipient and the worker (Ungerson 1997, 2004). Independent contractor status makes it difficult for workers to bargain or form unions. With third-party intermediaries as the "employer of record," workers are far more likely to see their rights enforced, including their entitlement to contributions to the Social Security fund and to overtime and minimum wage payments. The public authority model, in which government serves as the employer of record, has improved working conditions for consumer-directed home care (Howes 2011). Higher-than-average wages, higher levels of employer-provided health insurance, and much lower-than-average turnover rates have resulted.

Similarly, a vision of workforce development, especially if tied to other labor market policies designed to raise the floor on wages, could inform efforts to improve training opportunities and develop career ladders for low-wage care workers (Holzer et al. 2011). Many states have already experimented with such initiatives, although they have tended to be small-scale efforts with precarious funding sources (Moon and Burbank 2004). Examples in child care include programs in North Carolina to raise the earnings of center staff and family child care providers and the California CARES (Compensation and Recognition Enhances Stability) program (Helburn and Bergmann 2002). Adult care examples include the Massachusetts Extended Care Ladder Initiative, which coordinated the efforts of fifteen community colleges and 150 nursing homes to offer career ladders to nursing assistants, and Cooperative Home Care Associates, a worker-owned home care business in the Bronx that provides new workers with free training that is considerably more extensive than the minimum required by the federal government (Holzer 2009, 316). Living wage ordinances in many locales, for example, have had a direct impact on the living standards of low-wage care workers because they are paid from public funds. We return to this issue in chapter 8 after a closer consideration of the social value of both unpaid and paid care services and an analysis of existing care policies.

SUMMARY

One of the ironies of care work in the United States is that it has created opportunities for women and blacks to advance in professional care occupations where they can earn high wages. But this has been possible in large part because weak labor market regulations and open immigration policies have helped create an extremely low-wage labor market in which many women have found the care jobs that release other women from performing household labor.

This chapter has explored the common characteristics of care jobs at the high and low end of the labor market while also highlighting what is different about low-wage workers. It has raised questions about why women in care work pay a wage penalty and whether that penalty is greater in the low-wage market. It has suggested the importance of turning our focus to the quality of low-wage jobs, in part because of the link between quality jobs and quality care. We have shown that quality jobs have common features across care occupations, including autonomy, discretion, flexibility, the opportunity to collaborate, and decent wages and benefits. Among the many remaining challenges is to find a path that allows women to participate fully in the labor force without having to rely on extremely low-wage care labor to substitute for household labor. We return to these challenges in the conclusion.

NOTES

1. Our measure differs in that we include all educational services (not just primary and secondary schools) and exclude pharmacies and drugstores. For a specific listing, see boxes A.3 and A.4 in the appendix.
2. Unpaid family workers represent another "class of worker" but are not included in the table because they represent less than 1 percent of the total in every industry grouping.
3. Although managers are not included in our interactive care occupations, women managers are disproportionately concentrated at the helm of care industries—38 percent of managers are women, but 68 percent of managers in human resources, education, medical and health services, and social and community services are women (U.S. Bureau of Labor Statistics, Current Population Survey 2010a).
4. Empirical details about child care and adult care jobs also come from our analysis of the 2010 Current Population Survey (CPS), using the following methodology: The direct care and child care workforce is identified based on both occupation and industry variables in the CPS for the longest job held in the previous year, or in 2010. By including both occupation and industry in the definition we can exclude occupations or industries that are not generally considered part of the direct care or child care workforce (such as health aides that work in manufacturing plants), and assign more distinct classifications of care workers than the occupational grouping alone allows. Specifically, the direct care occupation codes included are personal and home care aides (3600) and nursing, psychiatric, and home health aides (4610). Direct care industries include employment services (7580), offices of physicians (7970), dentists (7980), chiropractors (7990), optometrists (8070), other health practitioners (8080), outpatient care centers (8090), home health care services (8170), other health care services (8180), hospitals (8190), nursing care facilities (8270), residential care facilities without nursing (8290), individual and family services (8370), private households (9290), and executive offices and legislative bodies (9370). Our classification yields a sample size of 2,154 direct care workers: 462 hospital aides, 594 nursing home aides, 448 home health aides, and 650 personal care aides.

With regard to the child care workforce, the child care occupation codes included are preschool teachers (2300), teacher assistants (2540), and child care workers (4600), and child care industries include child day care services (8470), religious organizations (9160), and private households (9290). We also use self-employment to differentiate between child care worker classifications. Our methodology yields a sample size of 1,297 child care workers: 783 center care providers, 387 home-based family day care providers, and 127 nannies.

5. We follow the definition used by Gautié and Schmitt (2010, 3) in the introduction and overview to their edited volume on low-wage work.

6. Further, although the general category of low-wage workers is defined as those earning less than two-thirds of the gross median wage, the low-wage care occupations include some workers whose earnings exceed the low-wage threshold.

7. For a comprehensive list of state regulations, see National Resource Center for Health and Safety in Child Care and Early Education (n.d.).

8. For more information on the Worthy Wage Campaign, see Center for the Childcare Workforce (n.d.).

9. For more information on the Pennsylvania union, see Keystone Research Center (2007).

10. For more information on Childspace, see Childspace Cooperative Development, Inc., http://www.childspacecdi.org/.

11. The plethora of job titles makes it difficult to collect consistent and reliable data on this workforce. People attempting to analyze or organize these workers, in search of an umbrella term, often use the phrase "direct care workers." This term is misleading for our purposes, however, since child care workers also provide direct interactive care.

12. In its 1999 Olmstead v. L.C. decision, the Supreme Court ruled that states must do a better job of funding noninstitutional long-term care. The court found that Georgia's failure to provide sufficient home- and community-based long-term care violated the Americans with Disabilities Act's "integration mandate." The court indicated that states should make reasonable accommodations to their long-term care systems, and intent could be demonstrated by comprehensive, effective working plans to increase community-based services and reduce institutionalization (see http://www.law.cornell.edu/supct/html/98-536.ZS.html).

13. By state statute, the public authority is usually given the authority to set wage rates and benefits through collective bargaining with a union, but it is constrained by state policies regarding Medicaid reimbursement rates for services.

14. Under the North American Industrial Classification System (NAICS), the following industries comprise the institutional/residential sector of adult care: (1) home health care services (621600), and (2) services for the elderly and persons with disabilities (624120, as part of the social assistance subsector), which "comprises establishments primarily engaged in providing nonresidential social assistance services to improve the quality of life for the elderly, persons diagnosed with mental retardation, or persons with disabilities. These establishments provide for the welfare of these individuals in such areas as day care, nonmedical home care or homemaker services, social activities, group support, and companionship." See NAICS (2010) at http:://www.census.gov/cgi-bin/sssd/naics/naicsrch?code=624120&search=2007%20NAICS%20Search (accessed February 27, 2012).

15. Under the Standard Industrial Classification (SIC, distinct from the classification used by the U.S. Census, the Current Population Survey, and the American Community Survey), adult care workers include nursing aides, orderlies and attendants, psychiatric aides, and home health aides (SIC 31-1011: home health aides; 31-1013: psychiatric aides; 31-1014: nurse's assistants; 39-9021: personal care aides). Orderlies and attendants (31-1015) are not included in this analysis because their job definition does not include hands-on, or interactive, care other than to transport patients.

16. In a 2007 survey of states, thirty-three of the thirty-four respondents ranked "direct care" vacancies and/or turnover as a "serious" or "very serious" issue—a substantial increase from 2005, when only 76 percent of respondents indicated that this was a serious issue (PHI/DCWA-NC 2009).

17. Data are not shown for comparisons between foreign and native-born but are available upon request.

18. Smith (2012) finds that overtime is relatively uncommon among home care workers, but that a substantial proportion work part-time hours for involuntary or economic reasons, indicating an unmet need for more work hours. Some of the increased costs projected to arise from requiring overtime pay for home care aides could be avoided by redistributing work hours to those who indicate a desire for more work hours.

19. A survey of home care agency staff in Pennsylvania found a turnover rate of 44 percent (University of Pittsburgh 2006). A review of thirteen state and two national studies of in-home care for persons with intellectual and developmental disabilities found an average turnover rate of 65 percent (Hewitt and Larson 2007). A study of agency-employed home care workers in Maine found a turnover rate of 46 percent (Morris 2009). A study of consumer-directed home care workers in one county in California found a turnover rate of 24 percent—and for the entire state a turnover rate of 27 percent—in 2003 (Howes 2004, 2005). One intent-to-leave study showed that 37 percent of home care workers intended to leave their job in the following year (Brannon et al. 2007). One statewide study conducted over a two-year period found that 47 percent of home care workers intended to leave over a two-year period and that 46 percent actually did (Morris 2009). Another statewide study of consumer-directed home care workers found a turnover rate of 27 percent in 2003 (Howes 2004). Staff turnover rates in assisted living range from 21 percent to 135 percent, with an average of 42 percent (Maas and Buckwalter 2006). In contrast to job turnover, occupational turnover may be lower among workers in institutions.

Chapter 5

Valuing Care

Nancy Folbre

Both unpaid and paid care work represent important contributions to economic and social well-being, but how should we assign a value to them? Measuring both in terms of some common denominator can help us assess their relative importance and understand their joint outcomes, and estimates of the time devoted to care activities provide one such common denominator. Estimates of time use can be valued in monetary terms by reference to some market equivalent, such as an hourly wage rate. Although efforts to provide accurate monetary valuation of nonmarket work yield only approximate results, they shine a bright light on otherwise hidden dimensions of care provision.

They also help illustrate the conceptual difficulties of defining the final product of care work, which may have a value far greater than its market price. Whether paid or unpaid, care work helps develop human capabilities in many ways; the benefits of investment in human and social capital spill over to taxpayers and to future generations. The costs and benefits of care services influence living standards both among and within families. Accurate assessment of their value can contribute to expanded measures of economic well-being relevant to the definition of poverty and inequality and to a better understanding of economic development.

This chapter explores ways of assigning an economic value to care that encompass both unpaid and paid work. The first section shows how conventional industrial and occupational categories can be modified to provide a more unified picture of changes in care provision over time in the United States. It culminates with a measure of the relative significance of unpaid and paid care based on labor hours, drawing from the estimates of the two preceding chapters.

The second section delves more deeply into monetary valuation of care time, emphasizing the difficulty of measuring the total output of care activities. It reviews empirical studies relevant to the valuation of unpaid care, both in the aggregate and within individual households, demonstrating their relevance to the measurement of economic well-being. The third section builds on the discussion of care valuation by emphasizing the public benefits of care provision—benefits that are not necessarily captured by market prices but that exert a significant impact on economic productivity, economic inequality, and public-sector finance.

THE CARE SECTOR

The line that traditional national accounting systems draw between unpaid and paid work—enumerating only the latter—creates a misleading picture of economic development and change. When identical activities are shifted over the payment boundary from unpaid to paid, they are counted as a net addition to economic activity even though nothing has changed except the form of payment. When an increase in paid work leads to a decrease in unpaid work, only the increase is counted, overstating the actual gain in goods or services provided. For these reasons, the shift from the unpaid to the paid realm of care services for children and for adults needing personal assistance may overstate actual economic growth.

On the other hand, care services provided in the market may differ substantially in quality and intensity from care services provided free of charge. Paid care work is often provided in environments where there are economies of scale, such as child care centers or nursing homes. While a mother typically tends to no more than three children at a time, a child care worker often tends more. Similarly, an unpaid adult caregiver generally focuses her energy on one or two needy family members, while a paid adult care worker often has several clients—going from room to room in a nursing home or traveling to several clients' homes in the course of a week. Paid care sometimes requires training and certification that unpaid care work does not, and it often entails more specialization and a greater emphasis on interactive than supervisory care.

Home-provided care may be less focused and less intense than paid care, and it more often involves activities combined with self-care and routine household tasks (Wolf 2004). Unpaid care often draws on long-term relationships, person-specific skills, and strong personal attachments that can increase its value to recipients—but strong positive relationships often develop between paid caregivers and care recipients as well. Quality issues are key. If, for instance, an increase in the number of people cared for leads to a proportionate decline in the quality of care each person receives, any apparent gain in productivity is illusory. Issues of privacy, personal affinity, and cultural appropriateness complicate the quality and value of both unpaid and paid care, suggesting that their similarities are at least as important as their differences.

Most families in the United States combine unpaid and paid care services over their life cycle. Parents put in plenty of hours of child care, but also rely on child care workers and teachers. Family members and friends tend to those who need their help, but also make use of paid assistance. Although many people try to find a good balance between unpaid and paid care, their ability to do so is often constrained by a shortage of both financial resources and reliable information.

Likewise, policymakers often lack the knowledge required to encourage and support appropriate care provision.

Public policies aimed at improving the supply of care can take the form of subsidizing either unpaid family members (through such means as dependent care exemptions, child tax credits, and elder care tax credits) or paid care workers (through such means as child care or elder care expenditure deductions or direct subsidies of child care, early childhood education, nursing homes, or home- and community-based services). Which form of subsidy is best? It is difficult to answer this question without a clear picture of the relative dimensions of unpaid and paid care.

One way to gain perspective on this issue is to modify traditional occupational/industry statistics to include a category for individuals who devote most of their energies to unpaid family care. From this perspective, the labor force must be redefined to include not just those who are working for pay or seeking paid employment but also those who are providing interactive or support care services free of charge. If we count all individuals who care for family members without working for pay as a specific "occupation," how have their numbers changed over time, and how important are they in today's labor force? The answer to this question provides a new way of measuring occupational change. However, it still assumes that an individual can only be assigned one occupation, despite the fact that many people both provide care in the home and work for pay in a "standard" occupation in the market.

Therefore, another question provides a useful framework: if all unpaid care services were withdrawn, how many paid workers would be required to replace them? The answer reveals the quantitative significance of unpaid care. If family members went "on strike," the increased demand for purchased replacement services would dramatically increase the number of paid care jobs. Although this standard of comparison, like the earlier one, is rather simplistic, it vividly illustrates how a relatively large supply of unpaid care, largely motivated by concern for the well-being of family members, reduces the demand for paid care workers.

The Occupation of Housewife

The notion that a housewife is employed in a gainful occupation, even though she or he is not paid a wage or salary, may sound odd to the modern ear. Yet this notion has a long history in economic theory and has inspired considerable historical research (Folbre 2009; Folbre and Nelson 2002). For instance, the 1875 census of Massachusetts categorized married women who neither worked for pay, engaged in housework, nor superintended household work as "wives, merely ornamental." (These amounted to fewer than 2 percent of all married women.) Obviously, no such category is enumerated today—although in principle one could use time use data to ask whether some married women engage in neither paid nor unpaid work. No category of "husbands, merely ornamental" appeared in the 1875 census, but it did enumerate a small number of men who primarily cared for other family members as "houseworkers" (Folbre 1991, 57).

TABLE 5.1 / Full-Time Homemaking As an Occupation in the United States, 1870 to 2000

	Housewives and Homemakers As a Percentage of All Women Workers	Women in Paid Employment As a Percentage of All Women Workers	Housewives and Homemakers As a Percentage of All Workers
1870	70.2%	29.8%	40.1%
1900	64.4	35.6	35.6
1930	59.7	40.3	34.1
1960	56.0	44.0	34.1
1990	32.7	67.3	22.0
2000	29.5	70.5	19.4

Source: For discussion of data for 1870 to 1930, see Wagman and Folbre (1996). Data for 1960 from U.S. Census Bureau (1975); for 1990 and 2000, from U.S. Census Bureau (1997).

To trace long-run changes in the provision of care services, it is useful to define the total labor force broadly to include both paid and unpaid workers, excluding only adults who are likely to be unable to work. In 1870 about 85 percent of all men age sixteen and over reported a paid occupation. Assuming this means that about 15 percent of men sixteen and over were unable or unwilling to work in either paid or unpaid activities, and extending the same assumption to women, yields a measure of the total labor force.[1]

We can then estimate the number of homemakers by subtracting the number of women engaged in paid employment from the number in the total labor force.[2] Note that a homemaker is not simply a person who performs unpaid care work, since most adult women (and many men) perform such work. Rather, a homemaker is defined as a woman who specializes in unpaid care provision. By this measure, about 70 percent of all women workers—and about 40 percent of all workers in general—were homemakers in 1870 (see table 5.1).

This percentage declined steadily over time as the number of women in paid employment increased, but it remains substantial. In the year 2000, "housewives and homemakers" still represented about 30 percent of all women in the total labor force, and about 19 percent of all women and men (Folbre and Nelson 2002, 126).[3] Indeed, the number of housewives and homemakers in the United States in that year exceeded the number of paid workers in manufacturing.

Many of the women who entered the paid labor force took jobs in care industries such as education and health and social services, whose growth largely represented the marketization of services once provided in the home. The expansion of these jobs provided a means for women to enter paid employment and diversify their skills while remaining specialists in care provision. Meanwhile, household spending on substitutes for services once produced in the home—such as restaurant meals, takeout, and frozen dinners—helped fuel the growth of other sectors.

Another vantage point on this alternative way of defining occupation and industry is provided by analysis of the Current Population Survey between 1972 and 1993, when it allowed respondents to describe "keeping house" as a category of "major activity" in its classification system. This definition of homemakers yields numerical estimates for this time period similar to those reported earlier and offers a new perspective on gender job segregation. Treating "keeping house" as an occupation implies that women make choices to specialize in that activity, subject to constraints and opportunities, much as they choose paid occupations such as teaching or nursing.

As with standard measures of occupational segregation, we cannot ascertain whether choices to specialize in "keeping house" reflect individual preferences, social norms, institutional barriers, direct discrimination, or some combination of these factors. However, we get a more complete picture of gender segregation by looking at a larger segment of economic activities than just paid occupations. Not surprisingly, treating "keeping house" as an occupation increases estimates of the extent of occupational segregation by gender. The decline in occupational segregation over the period is significantly steeper than if segregation is measured only in terms of paid occupations (Cohen 2004).

It is also interesting to note that many jobs are less gender-segregated in paid employment than in unpaid work. In 1995, for instance, women provided 74 percent of all time devoted to cooking at home but represented only 45 percent of all employed cooks. Similarly, women provided 80 percent of time devoted to unpaid housecleaning but represented only 35 percent of janitors and cleaners (Cohen 2004, 241). Perhaps men are simply more willing to undertake such jobs if pay is involved. Direct interactive care jobs, on the other hand, tend to be more female-dominated than other jobs, as indicated in the previous chapter.

The designation "keeping house" has disappeared from the Current Population Survey and been replaced by the new terminology of "family responsibilities." But while family responsibilities can be listed as a reason for not working (along with categories such as "ill or disabled" and "unable to find work"), it cannot be listed as a "major activity" in the classification scheme. In 2009 relatively few women who were not part of the paid labor force (fewer than 1 percent) said that they wanted to work for pay but were unable to as a result of family responsibilities.[4] Respondents were not allowed to designate "family care work responsibilities" as a reason why they were not seeking paid employment, only as a constraint on their ability to find a paying job if they wanted one. Yet the lack of affordable, high-quality alternatives to maternal care directly influences the preference that many mothers express to stay home with their young children.

If Paid Caregivers Were Hired to Perform Unpaid Care

Rather than simply recategorizing workers in ways that cross the boundaries between unpaid and paid work, another way to measure the contributions of

TABLE 5.2 / Full-Time Job Equivalents Required to Replace All Unpaid Care, Average for 2003 to 2008

Age Group of Care Providers	Population Size of Care Providers (in Thousands)		Average Hours per Day		Total Hours per Year (in Millions)		Full-Time Job Equivalents (in Millions)		
	Women	Men	Women	Men	Women	Men	Women	Men	Total
15 to 24	20,387	21,541	2.4	0.9	17,859	14,939	8.9	0.5	6.4
25 to 64	79,003	78,170	3.8	0.6	109,577	74,183	54.8	7.1	1.9
65 and over	21,431	15,749	4.3	0.5	33,636	20,120	16.8	0.1	6.9
Total	120,821	115,460	3.7	0.6	161,072	109,242	80.5	4.6	35.2

Source: Population estimates based on U.S. Census Bureau (2010a).
Notes: Average hours per day is based on estimates reported in figure 3.3. Total hours is average hours per person per day multiplied by 365 days per year multiplied by the number in the group providing unpaid care.

unpaid caregivers is to ask how many paid workers would need to be employed to replace them (Albelda, Duffy, and Folbre 2009). The American Time Use Survey (ATUS) tallies the number of hours devoted to the interactive care of children and adults on a representative day, as reported in chapter 3, making it possible to estimate the total number of hours of support and interactive care provided per year by specific age and gender groups. Analysis of pooled data from 2003 to 2008 shows that women provided, on average, about 161 billion hours of support and interactive care per year and men about 109 billion hours (see table 5.2). These numbers would be far higher if supervisory care were included.

A full-time paid job typically requires about forty hours per week, fifty weeks per year, for an average of two thousand hours per year. Dividing the total hours per year of unpaid work by this measure yields an estimate of the number of paid employees that would be required to substitute for unpaid care, assuming that the paid workers could simply take the place of the unpaid ones, with no changes in productivity or in the ratio of care providers to care recipients. Under these assumptions, the total number of full-time employees required would amount to 135.2 million (see table 5.2), or about the number of workers employed in all occupations in 2010 (138.9 million).[5] In other words, the size of the paid labor force would double if all unpaid caregivers were paid for their work.

The same exercise can be performed for the more narrowly defined tasks of interactive child care and adult care. The average amount of time devoted per day to these activities is small because care demands vary greatly over the life cycle and many adults are not providing care at a particular point in time. Still, women provide 0.9 hour of child care per day and men about 0.5 hour, while both men and women average 0.2 hour of adult care (see table 5.3). Because

TABLE 5.3 / Full-Time Job Equivalents Required to Replace Unpaid Interactive Child Care and Adult Care Per Year, Average for 2003 to 2008

Age Group of Care Providers	Population Size of Care Providers (in Thousands)		Average Hours per Day		Total Hours per Year (in Millions)		Full-Time Job Equivalents (in Millions)		
	Women	Men	Women	Men	Women	Men	Women	Men	Total
Interactive care of children									
15 to 24	20,387	21,541	0.7	0.2	13.6	0.9	2.5	0.9	3.4
25 to 64	79,003	78,170	1.2	0.6	92.3	7.3	16.9	0.6	25.5
65 and over	21,431	15,749	0.2	0.2	4.6	0.7	0.8	0.5	1.3
Total	120,821	115,460	0.9	0.5	110.5	4.8	20.2	0.0	30.2
Interactive care of adults									
15 to 24	20,387	21,541	0.1	0.1	2.7	0.8	0.5	0.5	1.0
25 to 64	79,003	78,170	0.2	0.2	13.6	2.9	2.5	0.4	4.8
65 and over	21,431	15,749	0.2	0.2	3.7	0.3	0.7	0.6	1.3
Total	120,821	115,460	0.2	0.2	20.0	8.9	3.6	0.5	7.1

Source: Population estimates based on U.S. Census Bureau (2010b).
Notes: Average hours per day is the product of percentage engaged and mean time conditional on engagement, based on table 3.2. Total hours is average hours per person per day multiplied by 365 days per year multiplied by the number in the group providing unpaid care. Total number of full-time job equivalents is total hours divided by 2,000 hours (assuming a forty-hour workweek, fifty weeks per year).

the size of the population is large, so too are the total hours of care provided. Women devote about 110.5 million hours a year, and men about 54.8 million hours, to unpaid interactive child care. Gender differences are smaller in interactive adult care: women devote about 20 million hours a year and men about 18.9 million hours.

About 30.2 million full-time child care workers and 7.1 million full-time adult care workers would be required to provide substitutes for this unpaid interactive care. By way of comparison, the number of paid child care workers, preschool and kindergarten teachers, elementary and middle school teachers, and secondary school teachers combined in 2010 amounted to about 6 million, or only about 20 percent that many. About 0.9 million personal and home care aides, or about 13 percent as many, provided care for adults.[6] Clearly, the supply of unpaid work to these activities is extremely large, and reduction of that supply would increase demand for paid substitutes.

This quantitative exercise does not imply that unpaid caregivers should be paid a wage or salary. Nor does it imply that unpaid caregivers are currently providing exactly the right amount of care. Some families may be devoting more time to care activities than is actually needed, for instance, doting on their children or providing attention or instruction that could more effectively be provided in a group care setting. Other families, because of time constraints or geographical or other barriers, may not be providing the care for children, aging parents and grandparents, or disabled members that is either desired or needed.

This exercise does, however, make it possible to compare the gender division of labor in paid and unpaid care work. In certain occupations, the level of gender segregation is higher in paid than in unpaid interactive care. About 95 percent of paid child care workers and 82 percent of elementary and middle school teachers are women, for instance, while women provide only about 67 percent of all unpaid interactive child care labor hours. Similarly, close to 90 percent of nursing assistants, home health aides, and personal and home care aides are women, but women provide only a little more than half (51 percent) of all unpaid interactive adult care labor hours. As pointed out earlier, women's movement from unpaid work into paid support care jobs may reduce gender segregation, but their movement into many care occupations increases it.

We chose not to include an analysis of the total amount of time devoted to supervisory care here because it is often combined with other activities and it goes unmeasured in the ATUS, except for people supervising children under the age of twelve. However, it is worth noting that an important study of Australian time use data that defined child care more broadly estimated that the amount of time spent on caring for children in that country in 1997 was equivalent to almost two-thirds of the entire labor time absorbed by the market economy (Ironmonger 2004).

ASSIGNING A MONETARY VALUE TO UNPAID CARE

Moving beyond comparisons of labor hours to estimates of dollar value is important for several reasons. Labor hours can vary in terms of intensity, skill, quality, and productivity, and differences in wages and prices can capture at least part of this variation. Estimates of the dollar value of work also make it possible to assess the relative importance of labor costs relative to other costs of providing care. The costs of raising children, for instance, are far greater when the costs of the labor required, as well as the costs of food, clothing, and shelter, are taken into account.

However, efforts to impute a value to nonmarket work are based on strong—and not necessarily accurate—assumptions regarding market equivalents, so a careful analysis of these assumptions is needed in order to interpret those estimates and explain why the market value of care work may understate its value to society. The "output" of care work has at least three dimensions relevant to its valuation:

- Benefits to the care recipient in the form of increases in their well-being, which presumably influence their willingness to pay for services
- Process benefits received by the care provider, such as intrinsic satisfaction or pleasure from increasing the well-being of the care recipient
- Externalities, or spillover effects, on others, which can be characterized as public benefits (or costs)

Furthermore, care services often represent an investment in the development of human capabilities, or what is often termed "human capital." The valuation of an investment good, unlike a consumption good, requires the calculation of a flow of costs and benefits over time. These factors all bear heavily on the valuation of both paid and unpaid care.

Methods of Valuation

Efforts to assign a monetary value to nonmarket work have intensified in recent years, with particular attention to the care of dependents. A recent National Research Council (NRC) study, entitled *Beyond the Market*, calls for major revisions to the U.S. national income accounts and highlights the role of family work in the creation of human capital (Abraham and Mackie 2005). The international Commission on the Measurement of Economic Performance and Social Progress (2009) appointed by President Sarkozy of France has also called for the valuation of unpaid work performed on behalf of family, friends, and community members. At least two recent empirical studies have estimated the monetary value of care work across European households in recent years, with important implications for both the level and distribution of economic well-being (Giannelli, Mangiavacchi, and Piccoli 2010; Folbre et al. 2010).

Standard approaches to the valuation of unpaid work typically emphasize the logic of individual choice, assuming that individuals know what they want and how best to get it. As emphasized in chapter 1, this assumption often does not hold for care work. Still, it provides a framework for gaining at least some empirical traction. In deciding whether to provide a service or to purchase it, rational individuals should consider both the replacement cost of their time (the cost of purchasing the service) and the opportunity cost (the benefits they forgo by devoting time to providing the service). If the opportunity cost is lower than the replacement cost, a rational individual would choose to provide the service directly rather than to purchase it if money were the only relevant consideration, so wages are often used as an estimate of opportunity cost.

However, care work often entails nonpecuniary costs and benefits, and rational individuals compare the utility or happiness they will gain from alternative activities, as well as the pecuniary costs and benefits, when calculating opportunity costs.[7] As a result, opportunity cost is a distinctly individual measure, and it reflects only the valuation that the caregiver places on his or her time, not its value to the care recipient or to society at large. For instance, a lawyer who takes a day off work to care for a sick child faces a much higher opportunity cost than a clerical assistant in terms of forgone earnings per hour. However, the benefits may be the same from the child's point of view, since the lawyer is not necessarily any better at making soup, taking a temperature, administering aspirin, reading aloud, or sitting by the child's bedside.

Many decisions to provide care are based on prosocial preferences, but some individuals are more altruistic than others, and as explained in chapter 2, women often feel greater obligations toward family members than men do. The value that individuals place on their time may differ from the assessments of other family members. Parents may not invest enough in their children's education to maximize their children's earnings unless they are "rich enough and altruistic enough" (Behrman, Pollak, and Taubman 1995). Similarly, their decisions about how to provide child care are influenced by their own preferences and constraints, not purely by consideration of what is best for the children.

Many factors make it difficult for people to assess the consequences of their decisions. Noncustodial parents, for instance, may fear that their contributions to care will crowd out those of custodial parents—if every dollar they add is met by the reduction of a dollar from the other parent, the child will not benefit (Weiss and Willis 1985). The risk of divorce or some other form of disruption of implicit family contracts can also make it difficult to judge potential risks and rewards. For instance, a married woman might be more willing to leave paid employment to care for an infant child if she is confident that her marriage will remain secure or that her husband will later take a turn at staying home with the children, allowing her to focus on her career. Similarly, a daughter might be more willing to leave paid employment to care for an elderly parent if she is confident that a bequest will help defray her losses of income, or that her siblings will help her out. In both cases, uncertainty about opportunity costs might discourage family members from making commitments to provide unpaid care (Lundberg and Pollak 2003).

Individuals may find it difficult to accurately estimate opportunity costs, but they can use their expected hourly wage rate to approximate what they give up when they reallocate time to unpaid work. Researchers can go further, moving beyond reliance on a simple measure of expected hourly wage rates to compare the lifetime income of individuals who provide care with that of those who do not, as discussed in chapter 3. Similarly, researchers can estimate the "pay penalty" for entering a care occupation by looking at the financial impact of changing from a care occupation to a noncare occupation requiring similar skills and education levels or vice versa, as discussed in chapter 4.

Replacement costs also affect individual decisions, but valuations based on replacement cost—unlike those based on opportunity cost—do not reflect differences in individual preferences.[8] They simply ask what the cost of a market substitute for a nonmarket good or service would be. This question, therefore, can only be answered with an "all else equal" caveat.[9] Even calculating the cost of replacement care is not as straightforward as one might think, since increased demand might drive up the price of paid care if enough people opt to purchase replacements for the unpaid care they are providing.

Choosing the appropriate wage rates for determining replacement costs is also a challenge. Market care at both ends of the age spectrum includes both low-paid workers, such as home care aides and family day care providers, and better-paid workers, such as nurses and teachers. A "specialist" approach to valuing household production applies specific wage rates to various tasks. For instance, time spent preparing meals would be valued at a cook's wage, and time spent engaging in complex medical procedures at a nurse's wage. A "generalist" approach uses a single wage—for instance, the wage of a housekeeper—to value time spent in a range of activities. One early study by the National Bureau of Economic Research (NBER) simply multiplied the number of women primarily engaged in housework by an estimate of an annual wage for women employed in "domestic and personal service" (in other words, maids) (King et al. 1921). A few years later, economists Hazel Kyrk (1929) and Margaret Reid (1934) estimated the number of homemakers in the United States and suggested that higher wage rates might be appropriate. Many recent approaches to the valuation of child care activities adopt a specialist approach, using different wage rates for interactive and supervisory care (Albelda, Duffy, and Folbre 2009) or distinguishing "developmental" child care, such as teaching or reading aloud, from other activities (Bittman, Craig, and Folbre 2004; Folbre and Yoon 2007a).

Both opportunity-cost and replacement-cost valuations are based on input valuation, multiplying the number of hours devoted to different tasks (ideally quality-adjusted) by some vector of wage rates. An alternative method, output valuation, estimates the total cost of a market substitute for a nonmarket good or service, subtracts the cost of capital, raw materials, and other nonlabor costs, and takes the remainder as an indicator of the value of the labor. For instance, the value of preparing a hamburger at home can be calculated by asking what it would cost to purchase a comparable hamburger to go at a fast-food restaurant, including the cost of transportation to the restaurant and back home. The value of the time devoted to preparing a hamburger at home can then be set as this output price minus the costs of the hamburger meat, bun, condiments, and other inputs, such as the cost of the gas or electricity used to cook it.

Rather than multiplying the number of hours a parent spends by an hourly wage rate, one could ask what it would cost to send a child to a day care center for that many hours and subtract the nonlabor costs associated with providing child care at home (such as extra space in the home or milk and cookies) to arrive at an output valuation of the unpaid labor time. A similar method can be applied to adult care using the costs of adult care centers or nursing homes. The Office of National Statistics of the United Kingdom has experimented with applying this methodology to its national income accounts (Holloway, Short, and Tamplin 2002). The cost of market-provided services (for example, the cost of sending a child or adult to a day care center) can also be used as an estimate of the total value (rather than the value of labor inputs alone) of the nonmarket service. It is important to note, however, that market services can typically take greater advantage of economies of scale (particularly in supervision) than is possible in individual households (Fitzgerald and Wicks 1990; Dalenberg, Fitzgerald, and Wicks 2004).

Opportunity cost, replacement cost, and output valuation all represent important tools for the valuation of nonmarket work, and each has its own strengths and weaknesses. Opportunity cost is especially helpful in assessing the causes and consequences of individual decisions, but can be as much the result of those decisions as the cause.[10] Replacement cost provides a sound accounting perspective consistent with national income accounts, but it can be difficult to assess the quality and intensity of the paid and unpaid work being measured to ensure that they are comparable. Output valuation provides a means of cross-checking input valuation, but raises difficult questions about correct definition of output (see the following section for further discussion). In an ideal world of survey data, both input and output valuations of the market value of non-market care could be made and cross-checked with one another (Abraham and Mackie 2005).

Intrinsic Rewards, Intensity, and Density of Care

All these methods of quantifying unpaid care work should be qualified by consideration of their limitations, especially those that can be overcome by careful empirical research. For instance, one might argue that the subjective experience of unpaid work differs significantly from that of paid work because it tends to be more discretionary. Perhaps unpaid care offers so much greater satisfaction that it should not even be termed "work." On the other hand, most people derive considerable process benefits from paid as well as unpaid work (Juster and Stafford 1985). Consistent measurement of subjective well-being is not an easy task, but efforts to develop instruments that can be used in conjunction with time use surveys are well under way (Kahneman et al. 2004).

A second issue, related to but distinct from measures of subjective satisfaction, concerns the intensity of work. Unpaid work may be conducted at a more leisurely pace or in conjunction with other more pleasurable activities than paid work (for a more detailed discussion of joint production, see the appendix). On the other hand, pressure to complete unpaid care tasks in the time available may lead to high levels of multitasking, as reflected in reports of participation in what are called secondary activities. Multitasking often increases work intensity. For instance, a mother watching a small child may be preparing dinner at the same time. Evidence suggests that multitasking is widespread in unpaid work, particularly among women (Floro 1995).

A related issue concerns care density, or the ratio of care providers to recipients. An adult who reports spending an hour of time engaged in child care may be the only person in charge of three children or one of three adults engaged in caring for one child. An input-oriented adult-centric survey that simply tallies hours supplied would show the same result in either case: one hour of care time supplied. But a survey of the care received—based on a child-centric survey such as the Child Development Supplement of the Panel Study of Income Dynamics (PSID)—will show three hours of child care consumed in the first case and only one in the second.

Like other household public goods, care is not perfectly rivalrous in consumption. In other words, when one adult cares for two children, the care each receives is surely more than half what they would receive if cared for alone. Yet care quality is almost certainly diluted as the ratio of children to adults increases, and economies of scale—improvements in efficiency achieved by caring for more than one child at a time—are limited. Many time use surveys, including the ATUS and the PSID Child Development Supplement, include questions about who else was present that make it possible to calculate the ratio of adults to children, also known as the density of care (Folbre et al. 2005). The implications of density, however, are difficult for economists to interpret.[11] Developmental psychologists need to tell us more about the effects of the ratio of care providers to recipients on the value of care, in both unpaid and paid care.

Estimating the Value of Unpaid Care

The best way to estimate the aggregate value of care provided in terms consistent with our national income accounts is a quality-adjusted replacement-cost approach (Abraham and Mackie 2005). Many historical precedents adopted this methodology, including the early studies already cited (King et al. 1921; Kyrk 1929; Reid 1934). Current estimates of the value of unpaid work—most of which falls into our categories of support care and interactive care—range from about 20 percent to 40 percent of gross domestic product (GDP), depending on the method applied (Landefeld and McCulla 2000; Abraham and Mackie 2005; Giannelli, Mangiavacchi, and Piccoli 2010). A recent study based on the ATUS disaggregated child care activities in 2003 into seven categories of supervisory and interactive care activities, applying a vector of wage rates ranging from the then-minimum hourly wage of $5.15 for supervisory care to $25 (close to the median wage for kindergarten teachers) for developmental care such as reading aloud and teaching (Folbre and Yoon 2007a). Focusing on households that included only children under the age of twelve in order to fully consider the impact of supervisory time, this study found that the value of child care services provided by women in these households totaled about $33,000 a year, and the value provided by men about $17,100. By comparison, the annual wages for a nanny who did not live with her employer averaged about $30,680 that year (Folbre and Yoon 2007a).

Estimates of the value of adult care have typically been based on surveys of that population, such as the National Long-Term Care Survey (NLTCS) or the National

Health Interview Survey on Disability (NHIS-D). As a result of differences in definition and measurement across these surveys, researchers often take an average or offer a range when estimating the hours of care provided (see the appendix for details). One early study estimated the value of unpaid personal assistance to adults with disabilities at $168 billion in 1996, compared to $32 billion spent on paid personal assistance (LaPlante, Harrington, and Kang 2002). This study also found that the elderly were more likely than working-age adults with disabilities to rely on paid care.

A recent study offering state-by-state estimates of the value of family caregiving in 2004 uses a replacement-cost approach, applying an average of the minimum wage at the time ($5.15 an hour) and the average national wage rate for home health aides and other workers in the home health industry ($14.68), which comes to $9.92 per hour (Arno, Levine, and Memmnott 1999; NFCA/FCA 2006). A review of five different estimates that projected these to the U.S. population in 2006 found that the annual economic value of unpaid caregiving for adults was about $354 billion, more than total public spending on Medicaid and far higher than total spending on nursing home and home health care (Gibson and Houser 2007). A recent estimate published by the American Association of Retired Persons (AARP) based on 2009 data put the total value of unpaid care for adults at $450 billion, more than twice the total of paid long-term care services from all sources (Feinberg et al. 2011).

Measuring Living Standards

The valuation of care work has important implications for measuring household living standards. Comparisons of household income are typically adjusted by some measure of household composition to allow for differences in family need through the use of equivalence scales, but standard equivalence scales place a smaller weight on children than on working adults in calculating household needs, since they cost less to feed and clothe. Taking the time cost of raising children into account would lead to a very different calculation, altering estimates of the relative well-being of households with and without children (Folbre 2008a). Similarly, the time cost of caring for adults who need assistance as a result of age-related or other disabilities should be factored into equivalence scales.

Our standard economic measuring stick—market income—ignores both the value of unpaid work in households and the value of government services such as subsidized child care and elder care (Esping-Anderson 2009a; Folbre et al. 2010). Adding in the value of these services to calculate the value of extended income would obviously increase estimates of family income. But changes in the level of household income based on alternative measures are perhaps less significant than changes in its distribution. The valuation of unpaid work alters the picture of changes in poverty and inequality over time. As women enter paid employment, the market income of their family goes up. Yet a substantial portion of that market income must be devoted to the purchase of substitutes for the unpaid care services that are reduced as a result. The increase in the family's market income overstates the gain in their standard of living.

In particular, our current method of measuring income overstates the well-being of employed single parents with dependent children, since many of them incur significant child care and babysitting costs. Even middle-class and upper-class households have been affected by the rising cost of substitute care for dependents, which has been increasing at a significantly higher rate than wages and which is not accurately measured by aggregate cost-of-living measures. The U.S. Census Bureau recently announced plans to develop a new supplemental poverty measure (SPM) that will subtract some work-related costs, such as the child care expenditures of employed parents, to better capture real disposable income.[12]

Most estimates suggest that extended income is distributed more equally than market income because there is less variation in the value of unpaid work than in household market income (Frazis and Stewart 2006). But for this very reason, the use of extended income as a measure of household well-being leads to different conclusions about trends in household well-being over time than the use of market income alone. Many studies have found that increases in women's employment and earnings have lowered household income inequality in the United States and other countries over the past forty years (Cancian, Danziger, and Gottschalk 1993; Cancian and Schoeni 1992; Harkness 2010). These studies focus entirely, however, on increased market income, ignoring the corresponding declines in the value of households' extended income as unpaid care was replaced by paid care. Comparisons of the inequality of extended and market income suggest that extended income is distributed more equally; therefore, an increase in the relative importance of market income has probably increased overall inequality in living standards (Folbre et al. 2010).

The valuation of unpaid work has significant implications for income inequality across households. Consider two households with the same level of market income and the same household composition. If one household includes an adult who specializes in the provision of family care and the other does not, the former household clearly enjoys a higher living standard (Folbre 2008a). Similarly, households that enjoy a significant quantity of unpaid care from nonresident family members—say, grandparents willing to provide child care while parents are working—enjoy a higher living standard than households with similar incomes that lack such assistance.

Proper valuation of unpaid care also puts public support for unpaid care into perspective. Tax subsidies provided in the United States in 2000, including the dependent tax exemption and child tax credit, amounted to between 10 and 26 percent of the average annual parental expenditures on a child under eighteen in a middle-income, two-parent family (Folbre 2008a). If the lower-bound replacement value of parental time is taken into account, the relative public contribution appears much smaller, amounting to between only 4 and 9 percent of average costs. Comparable figures for adult care are not available, but the ratio of public to private expenditure would clearly drop considerably if the value of unpaid time was taken into account.

THE PUBLIC BENEFITS OF CARE PROVISION

Market valuation of nonmarket care work provides a useful metric for comparing the relative importance of paid and unpaid work, but it distracts attention from an even more fundamental issue: the undervaluation of both types of work. Unlike sovereign consumers, care recipients often do not choose how much should be spent on them. The decisions made by third parties to spend on care are often determined by norms or altruistic preferences rather than by consideration of the gain to either the recipient or society as a whole. Yet the benefits of successful care typically spill over to other beneficiaries who do not participate in the private care transactions. In other words, the private costs and benefits of care decisions often diverge from the social costs and benefits. As a result, decentralized individual decisions may not lead to efficient outcomes.

Care work is not unique in this respect. Indeed, it is difficult to describe any private market transaction that does not create spillovers or externalities, especially given the growing sensitivity of global climate to carbon emissions. However, the public benefits of successful care are particularly large relative to the private costs because care work contributes to the development of human capabilities that influence the quality of virtually all social transactions. Furthermore—and perhaps as a result of that fact—our social contract specifies a basic level of provision for dependents who need assistance through no fault of their own and provides taxpayer-funded care to people who cannot get the care they need from either their family or the market. Another feature of our social contract provides citizens with a means of partially capturing the benefits of care provision that enhance productivity: we impose taxes on future workers in order to finance current expenditures. Public liabilities represent, in essence, a claim on the income of the next generation.

Economists often emphasize the benefits of investment in human capital. Too often, however, they restrict this emphasis to investing in young children, although investing in the elderly also yields future benefits. The investments that we promise working adults will reap benefits for them in their old age strengthen the social contract that ensures their contributions to investments in the young. But improved health and well-being in old age has offered important gains in economic efficiency as well as intrinsic benefits. Elderly individuals make important contributions to our collective standard of living, even when they have retired from paid employment, by providing family care and engaging in volunteer work.

Investments in Young Children

The emergence of social cost-benefit analyses of investments in early childhood education offers a fascinating prototype for efforts to estimate social spillovers.

The HighScope Perry Preschool Program followed a group of children enrolled in an intensive preschool program over time, comparing a series of outcomes for those children who participated with outcomes for those who did not. These outcomes included the incidence of crime, earnings and economic status, educational attainment, and marriage versus single parenthood. By assigning estimates of social cost to the adverse outcomes, one widely cited study found that by age twenty-seven the cumulative benefits of the program had far exceeded the costs. Stated in terms of a social rate of return, they found that every public dollar spent on the program saved $7.16 in tax dollars.[13]

Nobel Prize winner James Heckman has collaborated on the development of many detailed estimates of the potential for well-designed early childhood education investments to counter the effects of growing up in a disadvantaged environment (Heckman and Masterov 2007). Rob Grunewald and Art Rolnick of the Federal Reserve Bank of Minneapolis have published a number of reports using social rates of return as a rationale for greater public investment in early childhood education.[14] A recent meta-analysis of the effects of 123 early childhood education interventions confirms large positive effects (Camilli et al. 2010). Such investments are increasingly being framed as a strategy for community economic development whose impact on jobs and earnings will far exceed that of state tax subsidies designed to attract industry.[15] Paid child care can also provide valuable complements to family care. A recent study of New York mothers found that some child care centers were particularly effective in helping to develop informal social networks that the mothers could draw on for support and assistance (Small 2009).

Child education and health are coproduced by families, communities, and public programs, and the long-run economic impact of unpaid care also deserves consideration. Longitudinal studies tracking family members over a long period of time suggest that acute and prolonged poverty in early childhood has harmful effects (Duncan and Brooks Gunn 1999). The effect of family income is mediated by other factors, including parental efficacy (Mayer 1998). On the other hand, many adult behavioral problems may be rooted in poorly understood effects of economic inequality and stress. Improved care provision could help mitigate the negative effects of poverty, improve parental efficacy, and improve outcomes for adults.

Randomized experiments provide a way for researchers to assess the effects of public policy packages on outcomes for children. For instance, the New Hope experiment conducted in Milwaukee, Wisconsin, between 1994 and 1998 provided a wage supplement, health insurance, child care, and after-school programs for parents and other adults who worked full-time (Duncan, Huston, and Weisner 2007). Children of families randomly selected to receive this economic treatment fared better over time in school than children in the families who did not. Boys in particular earned higher grades, were less likely to get in trouble, and developed higher aspirations for the future. In addition to measuring the quantitative dimensions of the gains that children enjoyed, New Hope researchers highlighted gains that were more difficult to measure, including improvements in the quality of family life such as parents and their children feeling less stressed out.

Family Care and Health Costs

Increased pressure to cut costs in the formal health care system has generated pressures to offload more care responsibilities onto people who need care and their families. Medicare beneficiaries who receive informal care use significantly less Medicare-funded care (van Houtven and Norton 2004). The same apparently applies to Medicaid beneficiaries, since elderly women without surviving children are far more likely to live in Medicaid-financed nursing homes than elders with adult children (Wolf 1999). Causality can also run the other way. Payment caps specific to the Medicare home health care benefit have been shown to increase the amount of informal care provided by low-income families (Golberstein et al. 2009).

However, the apparent savings realized by the system when care is offloaded to unpaid family members (some units save money simply by shifting costs elsewhere, off their own books) can prove illusory for two reasons. First, poor continuity of care can lead to adverse outcomes, as when care recipients or their unpaid caregivers fail to correctly administer medication, resulting in expensive hospital stays or other medical care. Second, the mere transfer of costs from the formal accounting system to family and community support systems does not necessarily lead to greater efficiency. As indicated in chapter 3, caregiving can impose significant costs on caregivers in reduced market income, reduced leisure, and physical and mental stress.

The Net Value of Child-Rearing

Part of the monetary value of unpaid care comes from the future tax revenues likely to be generated as a result of improvements in human capabilities. A growing literature on fiscal externalities estimates the net value to society of a birth, taking into account the tax revenues and expenditures associated with that child and its descendants. One study estimates that net value to be between $92,000 and $245,000 (in 1996 dollars), depending on the education level of the newborn's parents (Lee and Edwards 2001).

In a more recent study, Douglas Wolf and his colleagues (2010) use longitudinal data along with simulations to compare average net taxes (individual taxes paid minus individual government benefits received) paid over a lifetime by parents and nonparents. They define parents in economic rather than biological terms as people who devote uncompensated time or monetary resources to, or coreside with, either biological, adoptive, or stepchildren under the age of eighteen. In other words, a deadbeat who has never paid child support, cared for, or lived with his children is not counted as a parent.

Parental status affects individual earnings, the taxes people pay (as a result of tax deductions and tax credits) and the benefits they receive. Even taking earnings differences into account, parents tend to pay lower income taxes than nonparents when young, but more once they have grown older and their children have left home (because their income goes up and their tax deductions decline). Overall, parents pay less in net taxes than nonparents do—until the future net tax contributions of their children are taken into account. These more than offset the difference, leading the authors to conclude that the average parent contributes about $200,000 more (in 2009 dollars) than the average nonparent to net taxes (discounting future contributions at an annual rate of 3 percent). This disparity in contributions helps explain why greater public support for child-rearing may be justified.

SUMMARY

An accurate measure of the market value of unpaid care work would improve our economic accounting systems and contribute to a better understanding of economic growth. Most major developed countries now regularly administer time use surveys like the ATUS, and many are now being launched in developing countries, including China. Unfortunately, they do not always include clear or consistent measures of interactive care, support care, and supervisory care.

Further, relatively little effort has been devoted to improving methods of assigning a monetary value to unpaid care. Standard methods of valuation suffer from a bias induced by circular causality. Wage rates for paid caregivers are often relatively low, in part because a large supply of unpaid care reduces market demand for paid care and in part because paid caregivers often cycle in and out of the labor market in order to meet their own family's care demands. Applying these wage rates to unpaid labor allows us to assign it a market value that approximates its current replacement cost, but it does not tell us much about the long-run cost of a possible decline in the supply of unpaid labor, since that decline would probably increase the price of paid care by increasing demand.

These problems contribute to persistent tendencies to take unpaid care for granted and to implement policies that may increase rather than ease the burdens borne by unpaid caregivers. Unpaid care work represents an important contribution to a kind of social commons, a process of reproducing ourselves and our social values. We know that declines in family stability pose some serious problems for the effective care and nurturance of dependents. We should also be concerned about possible declines in the supply of unpaid care that may take place independently of demographic trends. Serious consideration of the value of care work needs to move beyond direct measures of time use and wage rates to consider the complex spillovers and synergies that are not easily captured by a market-based metric.

NOTES

1. Many children under the age of sixteen also engaged in productive activities in 1875, but for the purpose of simplicity—and for comparability with later periods when school became mandatory—we ignore them here.

2. We use the term "homemakers" rather than "housewives" because not all these women were married; some were daughters, sisters, aunts, or widows.

3. Note that the figure on the percentage of the total labor force who were homemakers in 2000 represents a correction from Folbre and Nelson (2002), based on Nelson (2011).

4. See U.S. Bureau of Labor Statistics, Current Population Survey, Household Data Annual Averages, "Table 35: Persons Not in the Labor Force by Desire and Availability for Work, Age, and Sex," available at: http://www.bls.gov/cps/cpsaat35.pdf (accessed April 30, 2012).

5. Based on U.S. Bureau of Labor Statistics, Current Population Survey, Household Data Annual Averages, 2009, "Table 11: Employed Persons by Detailed Occupation, Sex, Race, and Hispanic or Latino Ethnicity," available at http://www.bls.gov/cps/cpsaat11.pdf (accessed April 30, 2012).

6. Based on U.S. Bureau of Labor Statistics, Current Population Survey, Household Data Annual Averages, 2009, "Table 11: Employed Persons by Detailed Occupation, Sex, Race, and Hispanic or Latino Ethnicity," available at: http://www.bls.gov/cps/cpsaat11.pdf (accessed April 30, 2012).

7. In this sense, calculations made on the basis of opportunity cost include a measure of what economists call "consumer surplus."

8. In this respect, replacement cost estimates are like the market prices used in national income accounts, including imputations for the value of owner-occupied housing: what the homeowner is likely to have paid in rent had he or she been renting.

9. In more technical terms, it represents a partial equilibrium rather than a general equilibrium approach.

10. That is, opportunity cost may be endogenous, determined by the prior effect of norms or preferences.

11. A nonlinear transformation of the density of care, such as the square root of the child-adult ratio, could provide a reasonable way of weighting inputs of time, paralleling the economies-of-scale parameters applied in household equivalence scales. But the relationship between density and care inputs probably varies with social context and age of children.

12. For an announcement of the Census Bureau plans, see Sam Robert, "U.S. Plans New Measure for Poverty," New York Times, March 2, 2010, available at: http://www.nytimes.com/2010/03/03/us/03poverty.html (accessed April 30, 2012). For a discussion of the supplemental poverty measure, see U.S. Census Bureau, "Poverty: Experimental Measures," available at: http://www.census.gov/hhes/www/povmeas/SPM_TWGObservations.pdf (accessed April 30, 2012).

13. See studies summarized at Schweinhart (2002).

14. These studies are available at the website of the Federal Reserve Bank of Minneapolis, http://www.minneapolisfed.org/publications_papers/studies/earlychild/index.cfm.

15. See Partnership for America's Economic Success, "Long-Term Economic Benefits of Investing in Early Childhood Programs" (issue brief 5), available at: http://partnershipforsuccess.org/docs/researchproject_dickens_bartik_200802_brief.pdf (accessed April 30, 2012).

Chapter 6

The Care Policy Landscape

Janet Gornick, Candace Howes, and Laura Braslow

"Care policy" is not a common category in American social policy research, which often organizes social policies simply by the characteristics of recipients. The widely referenced congressional publication *Compilation of the Social Security Laws* (the "Green Book"), for example, categorizes U.S. social policies primarily according to the groups served: the elderly, survivors of deceased workers, people with disabilities, the blind, the unemployed, veterans, mothers, and children. Academic social policy typically disaggregates policies into broad domains such as income support, employment, housing, and health policy (Blau and Abramovitz 2010). In the political arena, public initiatives with budgetary components are often separate from those that do not require direct fiscal outlays. That has the effect of decoupling, for example, child care policies (which generally require public spending) from family leave policies (which often grant leave rights but not wage replacement and thus do not require direct governmental expenditures).

Before we can give care policy the sustained and systematic attention that it deserves, we must develop a clear definition of its content and boundaries. As several contributors to this volume have argued, defining "care" presents an ongoing conceptual challenge; the same is true, of course, with respect to "care policy." Identifying and assessing care policies is especially challenging in the United States because of the complex, often overlapping divisions of labor between national and state governments. In many aspects of care policy, both federal and state levels of government are key actors in revenue generation, spending, and direct provision of care, as well as in various aspects of rule setting and regulation, from determining eligibility to quality assurance.

We begin this chapter by defining the universe and boundaries of care policy, limiting ourselves to policies that directly shape the provision or receipt of care for children or for adults who need personal assistance. The next section provides an overview of early childhood education and care policy, family leave policy, foster care policy, and services and special education for children with disabilities. The third section provides a parallel description of care for adults, focused on long-term care services and supports. For each of the policy categories, we clarify, in general terms, the nature of the policy, its intended purpose, the size of the population potentially and actually served, and its key components at both the national and state levels. We close each policy section with a discussion of current estimated national and state expenditure levels. We conclude the chapter with some remarks about the care policy landscape as a whole.

DEFINING CARE POLICY

A large system of policies, regulations, and institutions indirectly affects the nature and adequacy of care provided in the United States. This system includes an array of income transfers and tax expenditures (such as Social Security and the Earned Income Tax Credit [EITC]); near-cash and non-cash supports (such as food stamps, subsidized school lunches, and housing assistance); regulations that shape working conditions (such as minimum wages and overtime thresholds); public education (including investments in primary, secondary, and tertiary education); and institutions of social control (including the juvenile and adult criminal justice systems).

These government policies and institutions transfer crucial goods and services and shape the private acquisition of resources in ways that affect individuals' and families' access to care and to resources to be used for care. Under this wide umbrella are a number of policies that more *directly* shape care provision and receipt for children and adults needing personal assistance. We divide these two overarching categories of care recipients—children and adults—into seven subcategories and map them onto the main care policies that typically or potentially serve them and their caregivers, as shown in table 6.1. Our research suggests that the policies listed there are the largest and most substantial public initiatives related to the direct provision of care, as measured by the number of care recipients (or potential recipients), the level of expenditures, or both. Included are policies that operate through a diversity of mechanisms, such as direct provision, demand- or supply-side subsidies, and employment regulation. Also included are diverse governmental structures, from purely national programs to federal-state matching programs, federally funded block grants, state programs that extend eligibility for or benefits from national programs, and autonomous state programs.

The first two groups served are children in the early developmental stages who live with their families (a small subset of whom have disabilities). Children are often cared for in programs that supplement or substitute for parental child care or provide early educational opportunities on a daily basis. For the children of employed parents, crucial support is also granted through public family leave policies. These policies grant rights—and in some cases cash benefits—that enable parents to take temporary breaks from employment to care for their own children. They sometimes also cover care for other family members.

The third group is made up of children whose parents or guardians cannot care for them at home. These children are often cared for in the foster care system, sometimes being placed with extended kin but frequently with entirely new families.

TABLE 6.1 / Care Recipients and Care Policies

Groups That Need or Benefit from Care Policies	Policy Components				
	Early Childhood Education and Care (ECEC)	Family Leave[a]	Foster Care	Early Intervention and Special Education	Long-Term Services and Supports
Children					
Children with primary parent or caregiver who is not employed	X				
Children with primary parent or caregiver who is employed	X	X			
Children who need residential care[b]	x	x	X		
Children with disabilities	x	x	X	X	X
Adults					
Adults with intellectual and developmental disabilities (ID/DD)[c]		x	X		X
Adults with disabilities other than ID/DD		x	X		X
Frail elderly adults		x	X		X

Source: Authors' summary.
Notes: A large "X" signifies the policy arena(s) most central to providing care to this group or support for their caregivers. A small "x" denotes policies that affect access to and receipt of care but are arguably less crucial to responding to the need for care.
[a]Leaves granted to employees to care for infants or seriously ill family members.
[b]Because their parents are judged unable to care for them at home.
[c]Disabilities that have manifested at birth or prior to age twenty-two and are expected to continue indefinitely.

(There is also overlap between this group and the first two, since foster parents may place their foster children in early childhood education and care [ECEC] programs or draw on family leave options.)

The fourth group is children with disabilities. They receive an array of services and supports, including special education, whose goal is to help them achieve maximum possible social integration in adulthood. Some also receive long-term services and supports.

The three groups of adult recipients include individuals with a diverse range of physical and mental conditions that limit their capacity for social integration, work, or self-care. They are served by institutional and home- and community-based long-term care and support services that assist them with basic activities and help them live safely. Ideally, these services also maximize care recipients' independence and foster their integration into the community. These adults may also receive support in the form of short-term family leaves granted to their employed family caregivers if their caregivers need to take time off from work to help them during a temporary but serious illness.

POLICIES THAT SUPPORT THE CARE OF CHILDREN

Public policies that support children and their caregivers are directed at one of four areas: early childhood education and care, family leave, foster care, and disability services and supports.

Early Childhood Education and Care

Early childhood education and care is an essential form of support for families with children, especially those with children below primary school age.[1] We use the term "early childhood education and care" to encompass two types of programs: child care programs that are primarily intended to provide substitutes for parental care, and early education programs, such as Head Start and prekindergarten programs, that have an explicit educational purpose.

ECEC policies are crucial for children without a stay-at-home parent: they allow parents to commit to working outside the home secure in the knowledge that they can find reliable care for their children. But children whose primary caregivers do not work for pay also benefit from publicly supported ECEC programs, especially those with an educational focus.

RECIPIENTS AND POTENTIAL RECIPIENTS   While most nonparental care in the United States is arranged, provided, and financed privately, a substantial minority of the children who receive early childhood education and care are in programs that get most or all of their financing from public funds. In 2006 about 2.5 million children received care financed by the major means-tested assistance programs described here, while another 1.9 million were enrolled in state- or federally funded early education programs. In addition, 4.4 million families claimed federal Child and Dependent Care Tax Credits (CDCTC) in 2006, which subsidized some of their out-of-pocket expenditures, although an unknown (but most likely relatively small) number of these claims supported the care of adult dependents rather than children. An additional unknown number also benefited from tax benefits for dependent care through employer-provided Dependent Care Assistance Programs (DCAPs) (McKenna 2010).

According to the U.S. Census Bureau's *Who's Minding the Kids* report, in 2010, of the 8.7 million families with children under age five and mothers who were employed, nearly half (4.0 million) made payments for ECEC services. Of all children under age five with working mothers, nearly half were primarily cared for in institutional settings or by non-relatives, types of ECEC that typically require either public funding or private payment (U.S. Census Bureau 2011a). Another 12.6 million families with working mothers had children older than five but younger than fifteen. Nearly one-quarter (2.8 million) of these families used paid ECEC services (U.S. Census Bureau 2008c). The 21.2 million families with working mothers and children under age fifteen represented about two-thirds of the roughly 34 million U.S. families with children (U.S. Census Bureau 2011b). In the context of the utilization levels reported here for publicly-funded ECEC programs, this suggests that a substantial minority of families with children receive some type of publicly funded, non-parental ECEC.

THE POLICY LANDSCAPE   In this chapter, our focus is the publicly funded care provided to the substantial minority that received public support. As summarized in table 6.2, ECEC policy in the United States has four core components: (1) public early education policies, (2) means-tested programs that provide child care assistance, (3) tax benefits for parents, and (4) regulation of quality.

PUBLIC EARLY EDUCATION PROGRAMS   Although some early education programs, such as prekindergarten, serve children regardless of income, others are designed to enhance the social and intellectual development of low-income children and to reduce disparities in school-readiness between more and less affluent children. The single largest compensatory early education effort is the federal Head Start program, which provides part-day educational services funded through federal grants to state and local providers. About three-quarters of the states provide additional funding for Head Start or operate parallel state programs. Head Start provides high-quality, developmentally oriented education (and health) services to children. It also offers educational, social, and mental health services to their parents. Recent federal initiatives have extended Head Start services in some locations both downward (to serve younger children) and outward (to provide full-day services).

In recent years, states have also taken the lead in expanding early education programs. These programs are designed to increase the school-readiness of all children, with particular benefits for children with impoverished home environments or other forms of disadvantage. (In our later discussion of programs for children with disabilities, we describe programs with similar goals targeted to children with disabilities.) Well over half (thirty-eight) states currently operate state-funded prekindergarten programs. In 2008–2009, more than 1.5 million three- and four-year-olds were served by these programs—more than double the number served by Head Start programs (Barnett et al. 2009). In addition, all states provide kindergarten, which is attended by nearly all the nation's five-year-olds. However, there is evidence that state-funded prekindergarten programs may be facing substantial cuts in many states over the next several years as a result of the recession, leaving their future uncertain (Epstein and Barnett 2010).

MEANS-TESTED ASSISTANCE   Means-tested assistance is designed to reduce the cost of substitute care for low-income employed parents, either by subsidizing child care provision (supply subsidies) or by increasing the purchasing power of low-income families in the private child care market (demand subsidies). Means-tested

TABLE 6.2 / Early Childhood Education and Care Policies

	Early Education	Means-Tested Child Care Assistance	Tax Benefits	Quality Regulation
Federal-state	Head Start: Provides means-tested compensatory education for children primarily ages three and four	Child Care and Development Fund (CCDF): Provides means-tested subsidies for employed parents with children up to age thirteen Temporary Assistance to Needy Families (TANF): Provides means-tested subsidies for employed parents receiving or transitioning from public assistance Social Services Block Grant (SSBG): Provides means-tested subsidies for employed parents	Child and Dependent Care Tax Credit (CDCTC): Nonrefundable tax credit for out-of-pocket expenses Dependent Care Assistance Program (DCAP): Provides employer-sponsored "flexible spending accounts" exempting out-of-pocket expenses from payroll and income taxes	
State-local	Prekindergarten and kindergarten programs provide universal or targeted educationally oriented care to children ages three to five		State-based tax credits provide tax relief for out-of-pocket expenses	Licensing and regulatory mechanisms establish and enforce health, safety, and quality standards

Source: Authors' summary.

child care assistance has grown sharply in recent years as an element of welfare reform policies designed to require and support employment among welfare recipients (Meyers et al. 2011).

Since 1996, the federal government has provided the bulk of funding for means-tested child care assistance, through three block grants to the states. The single largest source of federal funding for means-tested subsidies is the Child Care and Development Fund (CCDF), a federal block grant to the states. States may use CCDF funds to provide child care assistance to working families with incomes up to 85 percent of the state median, although many choose to set the threshold lower. Federal guidelines require states to offer parents a choice of care types and providers, but states are free to set other CCDF policies, including standards for eligibility, levels of parental copayment, and provider reimbursement.

The second major funding stream for means-tested assistance is the Temporary Assistance for Needy Families (TANF) block grant, which replaced the Aid to Families with Dependent Children (AFDC) program in 1996. States are authorized to transfer up to 30 percent of their TANF funds to the CCDF program, and virtually all states transfer some of their TANF resources to child care expenditures. In some states, dedicated CCDF spending makes up almost 100 percent of state child care spending, while in others the majority is funded by TANF dollars allocated to child care (Meyers et al. 2011). States also use TANF funds directly to provide child care (largely through vouchers) for welfare-reliant families who are preparing for work and for current and former welfare recipients who are employed.

The Social Services Block Grant (SSBG) provides the third and smallest source of federal child care assistance for poor families. The SSBG provides federal funds for a wide range of services to the poor, and states have almost complete discretion in deciding how to allocate them, including whether to spend any on child care. As of 2007, an estimated 13 percent of all SSBG funds were used for child care services or vouchers (U.S. Department of Health and Human Services/OCS 2007).

TAX BENEFITS   Tax deductions and credits constitute the third-largest form of assistance. The federal Child and Dependent Care Tax Credit (CDCTC) allows parents to deduct 20 to 35 percent of their out-of-pocket expenses from their taxable earnings. Lower-earning parents deduct higher percentages, but because the federal CDCTC is a nonrefundable tax credit, it does not benefit families whose incomes are too low for them to pay income tax. Benefits under the federal tax credit are capped and decline in value for higher-income families, ranging from $600 to $1,050 for one child and from $1,200 to $2,100 for two or more. The lowest-income families (below $15,000 per year in adjusted gross income) can deduct 35 percent of child care expenses up to $3,000 for one child or $6,000 for two or more children—the percentage of expenses that can be deducted decreases incrementally, down to 20 percent for families making $43,000 or more annually (Internal Revenue Service 2009).

Families working for participating employers may elect to use a Dependent Care Assistance Program (DCAP) instead of the CDCTC to deduct their care expenses by diverting a portion of their salary into a tax-free account that can be used to pay for services. DCAP functions like a tax deduction, allowing families to deduct up to $5,000 in care expenses from their taxable income; the program may yield somewhat higher benefits than CDCTC for some families, depending on how many children they have and their income tax bracket. As with CDCTC, DCAP primarily benefits higher-income families who owe taxes, but the benefits are even greater for the highest-income families, as the net benefit of the program depends on the tax bracket of the participating family. DCAP deductions also benefit employers, who save their portion of payroll tax on the funds that their employees divert into the account. Despite this fact, DCAP is offered to only about one-third of all private-sector workers. Workers with higher income, those in certain industries, those in the public sector, and those in large firms are much more likely to work for employers that offer DCAP, while those who earn too little to owe income taxes are unlikely to have access to the program, nor would they gain any benefit from it (McKenna 2010).

Tax credits for care such as CDCTC and DCAP can provide substantial benefit to middle-income and higher-income families—these credits are potentially worth marginally more than the subsidies available to low-income families through CCDF. However, typically CCDF beneficiaries who do collect subsidies collect more through these programs than those with higher incomes who claim tax subsidies. In the final tally, what is most notable is that programs that provide support for child care are available across the income spectrum, at roughly equivalent (low) levels of subsidy—as such, they are broad-based, relatively flat in their redistributive impact by income, and, unfortunately, inadequate to cover the costs of quality child care (McKenna 2010).

In addition to the federal tax benefits outlined earlier, over half of all states now provide additional child care tax credits. Many are based in part on the federal credit (the CDCTC), but some diverge from the federal structure to target low-income families more directly, either by enacting refundable tax credits (which can be used even by families with income too low to owe income tax) or by limiting the credits to families at lower income levels (Maag 2005).

QUALITY REGULATION The effects of substitute care on children's safety, health, and intellectual and emotional development depend largely on the quality of care received. Quality is a product of several factors: basic health and safety characteristics (such as the cleanliness and safety of the setting), structural factors (such as the number of children cared for and the number of adults providing supervision), and characteristics of the providers (especially education and training, job experience, and level of investment or engagement in their work, all of which may have an impact on the type and quality of their interactions with children).

In the highly privatized U.S. system, the government provides largely post hoc control over the quality of care, through licensing requirements and enforcement. The licensing of ECEC services is left to state governments; outside of the federal Head Start program, there are no national standards for staffing, health and safety, or teaching curricula. State licensing requirements, standards, and rigor vary enormously from state to state. Many states exempt some forms of care from regulation (for example, small family day care homes or centers in religious institutions). For those they do not exempt, all states regulate basic health and safety standards and set maximums for group size and for numbers of children per adult provider. Few go beyond these basics, however, to address other issues such as provider education and training standards.

TOTAL ECEC EXPENDITURES   Public expenditures on child care via CCDF, TANF, and SSBG totaled $13.6 billion in 2006, the most recent year for which figures are available. CCDF spending accounted for $9.2 billion of that total, TANF funds allocated to child care totaled $4.3 billion (Meyers et al. 2011), and SSBG allocations were just under $100 million (net of TANF transfer) (U.S. Department of Health and Human Services/ACF/OCS 2008). In addition, nonrefundable tax credits granted through the federal CDCTC totaled $3.2 billion, and benefits provided via DCAPs amounted to $600 million (Maag 2007). Twenty-seven states contributed additional subsidies in the form of state-level tax dependent care credits, but total state-level expenditures for child care–related tax benefits are not available (National Women's Law Center 2006).

Public expenditures on early education are also substantial, amounting to nearly $10 billion in 2006. Of that total, federal and state expenditures on Head Start amounted to $5.8 billion and $123 million, respectively. State and federal expenditures on public prekindergarten programs added up to $3.6 billion and $154 million, respectively (Meyers et al. 2011). Although these programs do serve a large number of children at a significant cost, they are dwarfed by the cost of primary and secondary education in the United States—in the 2005–2006 school year, total spending on public elementary and secondary education totaled $528 billion (U.S. Department of Education/NCES 2011).

Family Leave

Family leave policy refers to a set of publicly secured rights and benefits that allow employees to take time off from paid work to temporarily care for family members. Family leaves, which exist at both federal and state levels and may be paid or unpaid, are typically granted to parents to care for infants (either born to the family or newly adopted) or to care for seriously ill family members. In addition to family leave laws, some public provisions grant medical leave, allowing workers to take time off when they themselves are incapacitated or ill. Because this volume focuses mainly on care for people other than oneself, we focus our attention here on family leave.

Family leave policies have diverse and overlapping goals: to provide new parents with time for recovery and bonding, to secure care for those in need, to increase and strengthen women's employment, to prevent employee turnover or raise labor force productivity, to protect families from economic insecurity during periods of caregiving, and, in some cases, to encourage men and women to share caregiving work more equally.

As with ECEC, in the United States family leave provisions are mainly provided through the market, with relatively limited public intervention. ECEC is primar-

TABLE 6.3 / Family Leave Policies

	Leaves for Mothers Due to Pregnancy or to Care for Infants	Leaves for Mothers and Fathers to Care for Infants	Leaves to Care for Ill Family Members
Federal	Pregnancy Discrimination Act (PDA): Requires that providers of disability benefits (employers, states) cover maternity	Family and Medical Leave Act (FMLA): Grants mothers and fathers the right to unpaid leave during first year of child's life	Family and Medical Leave Act (FMLA): Grants the right to unpaid leave to attend to serious illness of child, spouse, or parent
State	Temporary Disability Insurance (TDI): Provides limited paid maternity leaves to pregnant or new mothers (in California, Hawaii, New Jersey, New York, and Rhode Island only)	Various laws expand unpaid FMLA, mainly by reducing the minimum enterprise size threshold, increasing the benefit duration, extending the definition of family members (who can be cared for), and relaxing eligibility conditions. California and New Jersey provide paid leaves for infant and relative care. Washington passed a law providing paid infant care leaves, but it remains unfunded.	

Source: Authors' summary.

ily provided via consumer markets, while family leave rights and benefits—particularly the full or partial wage replacement that is granted to some employees while on leave—are, to a significant extent, left to the labor market.

The public component of family leave provisions summarized in table 6.3 has three core elements: leaves granted to birth mothers due to pregnancy or to care for infants (usually referred to as "maternity leave"), leaves granted to mothers and fathers to care for infants (often called "parental leave" or "bonding leave"), and leaves granted to care for seriously ill family members ("caring leave"). On the federal level, public family leave benefits pertain only to employees' right to take *unpaid* time off from work. Currently there are two states that provide *paid* parental and caring leaves; these two states, California and New Jersey, and three additional ones—Hawaii, New York, and Rhode Island—provide paid maternity leave benefits through state temporary disability insurance (TDI) programs.

RECIPIENTS AND POTENTIAL RECIPIENTS   Family leave rights and benefits affect an enormous number of Americans. Although it is difficult to estimate the number of workers who need or take family leave in a given year, some information is available related to the Family and Medical Leave Act (FMLA), the national law that grants unpaid leaves to qualified employees. Information is also available about the numbers served in the two states that have paid family leave programs up and running, California and New Jersey. Hawaii, New York, and Rhode Island also provide paid maternity leave as part of their state TDI programs, but it is impossible to distinguish maternity leaves from the larger universe of medical leaves that workers take to care for themselves. The FMLA and state paid family leave programs are described in detail later in this chapter.

Regarding unpaid leave, a 2007 Department of Labor study found that 76 million workers (about half of the U.S. workforce) were eligible to take unpaid leaves in 2005 under the provisions of the FMLA. Of those 76 million workers, between 6 million and 13 million took qualified leaves during 2005 (U.S. Department of Labor 2007). An earlier report (U.S. Department of Labor 2000) found that slightly over half of FMLA leaves are taken due to pregnancy or the need to care for family members, including caring for a new child or recovering from a maternity disability (26 percent), caring for a seriously ill parent (13 percent), caring for a seriously ill child (12 percent), or caring for a seriously ill spouse (6 percent). Medical leaves, taken due to an employee's own serious illness, constitute the other half of FMLA leaves. (As noted earlier, we largely omit consideration of medical leave in this volume.)

With respect to paid leave, the flagship paid-leave states—California and New Jersey—grant some wage replacement to substantial numbers of workers and their families. In California in 2009–2010, paid family leave benefits were granted to 181,000 women and men; in addition, California's TDI program paid pregnancy- or childbirth-related claims to about 170,000 women (State of California/EDD 2010b). Also in 2009–2010, the nation's newest paid family leave program, in New Jersey, awarded benefits to 28,000 men and women; in addition, New Jersey's TDI program granted pregnancy- or childbirth-related benefits to nearly 26,000 women (State of New Jersey/DOLWD 2010c). It is important to note that in both states, women may be eligible for both paid family leave and pregnancy-childbirth benefits under state TDI programs. Unfortunately, data that provide unduplicated counts of beneficiaries across these two programs are not available.

THE POLICY LANDSCAPE—UNPAID LEAVE   Rights to unpaid family leaves were established nationally in 1993 with the passage of the Family and Medical Leave Act (FMLA), the first piece of legislation signed by President Clinton and the culmination of an eight-year political battle. The FMLA applies to all public employers and to private employers with fifty or more employees—which includes only 4 percent of firms but more than 70 percent of workers (U.S. Small Business Administration 2010). Within the establishments it covers, eligibility is extended only to workers who have been employed for at least twelve months and have worked a minimum of 1,250 hours in the prior year. The law does not address wage replacement, although it requires employers to continue contributions to workers' health insurance during covered leaves.

Employees who meet FMLA eligibility standards have the right to up to twelve weeks of unpaid, job-protected leave to care for a child after birth or following placement for adoption or foster care. The FMLA also provides eligible workers up to twelve weeks a year to care for seriously ill family members—including sons, daughters, spouses, and parents. Nearly one-third of FMLA leaves are taken to care for family members other than infants (U.S. Department of Labor 2000).[2] The FMLA defines a son or daughter as a "biological, adopted, or foster child, a stepchild, a legal ward, or a child of a person standing in loco parentis" (U.S. Department of Labor 2010). It defines serious illness as a medical condition requiring hospitalization or continuing treatment by a health care provider. The FMLA allows workers to take these leaves in "chunks" when necessary—a few hours, a day, or a week at a time.

Several U.S. states supplement the FMLA with laws that expand the pool of workers who are eligible or increase the maximum time granted per leave. A variety of state provisions have been implemented that expand FMLA eligibility to more workers or more circumstances. Some states require private employers with fewer than fifty workers to provide leaves, some relax worker eligibility conditions related to tenure or hours worked, and some extend the range of family members who may be cared for (including, for example, grandparents, grandchildren, and in-laws). Several states have also increased the duration of job-protected leave benefits to grant more than twelve weeks of leave per year.

THE POLICY LANDSCAPE—PAID LEAVE   Two government mechanisms shape American mothers' access to paid maternity leave, both operating within the framework of disability policy. One is the national Pregnancy Discrimination Act (PDA) of 1978, an amendment to Title VII of the 1964 Civil Rights Act. The PDA mandates that public and private employers that offer disability benefits must extend them to employees for pregnancy, childbirth, and pregnancy-related medical conditions. Importantly, while the PDA mandates that employers that provide disability benefits must include maternity, it does not require employers to offer disability benefits.

In addition, five U.S. states—California, Hawaii, New Jersey, New York, and Rhode Island—provide paid maternity leaves to insured workers. These leaves are paid through state TDI programs,[3] which provide some wage replacement in the event of short-term disability—and thanks to the PDA, short-term disability must cover pregnancy and a postbirth period for new mothers. Weekly TDI benefits range from about $170 to $959, and the average duration of a claim is six to eight weeks (Fass 2009).

Three states have enacted paid family leave programs that serve both men and women. Two of the three are TDI states (California and New Jersey), and the third is Washington. California became the first state to extend what it calls paid "bonding leave" to fathers (in addition to mothers), in a 2002 law that grants six weeks of paid infant-care leave to parents of both genders, in addition to the TDI-covered maternity period granted to mothers. Benefits are set at approximately 55 percent of wages up to a maximum level of earnings. Washington's 2007 law will provide five-week leaves for both mothers and fathers, but it has yet to be funded. New Jersey's 2008 law provides for up to six weeks of paid leave in addition to TDI-based maternity benefits. The California and New Jersey laws also grant paid leaves to care for other family members during periods of serious illness, while Washington covers infant care only (Economic Opportunity Institute 2007).

EXPENDITURES   There are no estimates of total expenditures on maternity leave as distinct from other medical and disability leaves across the five TDI states. However, some expenditure data are available for both California and New Jersey. Those data include spending on these states' new paid family leave programs, as well as on pregnancy- and childbirth-related leaves in their long-standing TDI programs.

California operates the largest paid family leave program in the United States. The state spent $469 million on paid family leave benefits in 2009–2010. California also spent $4.4 billion on its TDI program overall, with maternity claims totaling $708 million (16 percent) of that total. Pregnant women and new mothers in California took an average of 10.5 weeks of leave, collecting an average benefit of $397 per week (State of California/EDD 2010b).

New Jersey spent $35 million on paid family leave benefits, from July 2009 through July 2010. During calendar year 2009, New Jersey also spent $437.4 million on its TDI program, with 25 percent of claims being paid to women for time taken off from work during pregnancy or after childbirth. Unlike in California's temporary disability program, the average weekly benefit for TDI maternity claims in New Jersey was virtually identical to the overall average weekly benefit in the program—about ten weeks. Assuming that the average weekly benefit for TDI maternity claimants and overall TDI claimants have the same relationship to each other in New Jersey as in California, then TDI maternity claims in New Jersey totaled roughly $92 million in 2009 (State of New Jersey/DOLWD 2010).

Foster Care

In foster care—also referred to as "out-of-home care"—minor children whose parents or guardians are unable to ensure their well-being, either temporarily or permanently, are placed in the homes of adults other than their parents or guardians or in institutional settings. Parents or guardians sometimes place children in foster care voluntarily. In other cases, children who have been found to face the risk or actual occurrence of physical or psychological harm at home are placed in foster care by the state without the participation of the parent or guardian.

Foster care may be short-term or long-term; in either case, it is intended to be temporary. The goal of the child welfare system is to find a safe and stable permanent home for children by either returning them to their original home, if possible, or placing them permanently with another family. A primary purpose of foster care, as part of the child welfare system, is to develop and achieve a plan for permanent placement. Foster care allows for a range of outcomes, from family reunification to adoption to emancipation, which happens when a foster child reaches the age at which they become legally independent.[4]

RECIPIENTS AND POTENTIAL RECIPIENTS   Nearly half a million children—an estimated 463,000—were in the foster care system in the United States in September 2008. As mentioned in chapter 1, this represents roughly one-half of 1 percent of all children under age eighteen nationwide. Seventy-one percent of children in foster care are placed with foster families, with the bulk of these placed in nonrelative homes (47 percent) and the remainder with relatives other than their parents or guardians (24 percent). Sixteen percent are placed in group homes or institutional care, with the remainder placed in preadoptive (4 percent) or trial homes (5 percent); a small share (2 percent) are unaccounted for—runaways, for example (U.S. Department of Health and Human Services/ACF/ACYF/CB 2008).

In addition, many children are in ad hoc out-of-home care arrangements that are not mediated by the foster care system, as when a relative or family friend takes in a child informally when the parents are unable to care for the child. According to findings from the National Survey of America's Families (NSAF), only 10 percent of children living with relatives other than their parents are in formal kinship foster care arrangements; over 2 million children have been placed in informal kin care or voluntary kinship care (where kin care arrangements are mediated by child welfare agencies but children are not in the custody of the state) rather than foster placements with family members per se (Urban Institute 2003; Geen 2004). Children in these informal kin care arrangements do not receive the services or financial support that would accrue to children in official foster care.

THE POLICY LANDSCAPE   The U.S. foster care policy system, as summarized in table 6.4, includes four main components: federal and state child welfare regulations; federal, state, and local foster care and adoption regulations; dedicated federal and state funding for foster care and adoption services; and federal block grant funding.

FEDERAL POLICIES   The primary responsibility for foster care—and for child welfare in general—has traditionally rested with state and local government agencies and, to some extent, with nonprofit child welfare organizations and foundations, which provide services both independently and as contractors to and collaborators with government agencies. However, the role of the federal government in the child welfare system has grown as the federal government has increased its targeted funding to states. This funding is tied to new requirements emphasizing greater state accountability in achieving positive outcomes for children. Several major pieces of federal legislation—including the Child Abuse Prevention and Treatment Act (CAPTA) and the Keeping Children and Families Safe Act (KCFSA)—have played a significant role in structuring the modern child welfare system, through a combination of financing provided to states and regulatory policy.

Federal funds, from more than thirty different programs, account for roughly half of states' total reported spending on child welfare services. The major federal funding source for foster care services, established in 1980, is the Title IV-E program (Federal Payments for Foster Care and Adoption Assistance); this funding stream shares the cost of foster care services with the states. The 1997 Adoption and Safe Families Act (ASFA) amended Title IV-E, shifting the emphasis to increasing the number of adoptions and encouraging states to emphasize permanency planning. Additional federal financing for foster care services comes through the Social Services Block Grants (SSBG) and Temporary Assistance for Needy Families (TANF) funding streams, which, as in the case of means-tested child care benefits, states may direct toward their foster care programs (Murray 2004).

Additional support to increase incentives for adoption among low-income families is provided through the Adoption Tax Credit, which became a permanent part of the

TABLE 6.4 / Foster Care Policies

	Regulatory Policy		Funding Streams	
	Child Welfare Policy Framework	Specific Foster Care and Adoption Regulatory Policies	Dedicated Foster Care and Adoption Funding	Nondedicated Funding Streams Used for Foster Care and Adoption
Federal-state	Child Abuse Prevention and Treatment Act (CAPTA) and Keeping Children and Families Safe Act (KCFSA): Help states improve practices in preventing and treating child abuse and neglect	Adoption and Safe Families Act (ASFA): Aims to accelerate permanent placements for children in foster care	Title IV-E (Federal Payments for Foster Care and Adoption Assistance): Provides funds to the states to cover a share of the cost of foster care Adoption Incentive Payments (established in ASFA) and the Adoption Tax Credit: Provide financial support to adoptive families	Social Services Block Grant (SSBG) Temporary Assistance for Needy Families (TANF): Provides additional funding for foster care
State-local	State and local agencies regulate and administer a wide array of child welfare programs.			

Source: Authors' summary.

tax code in 2001. In 2010, following expansion of the credit as part of the Health Care and Education Reconciliation Act (HCERA), adoptive families may claim refundable tax credits of more than $13,000 per eligible child, as long as family income does not exceed the average $22,000 phase-out cap (Internal Revenue Service 2009; Commission for Children at Risk 2010).

STATE AND LOCAL POLICIES   Beyond these national regulatory guidelines and funding structures, all other details of foster care policy are the responsibility of states and local agencies. States vary markedly with respect to the standards and procedures by which children are removed from their families, placed in foster care, and transitioned out of the system; the requirements imposed on foster parents and facilities and their remuneration; the procedures for determining permanency goals; family unification and visitation policies and rights; the training, support services, and other resources provided to families working toward reunification; and the legal processes governing adoption, which present a complex set of policy issues. In spite of this significant variation between states, some of the central policy issues have been addressed in the Interstate Compact on the Placement of Children, an agreement among the states regarding best practices for the placement of children and the sustainability of adoptive families.

EXPENDITURES   In 2006 estimated total spending on foster care, both federal and state, was $10 billion, of which approximately 40 percent ($4 billion) came from federal Title IV-E funds. Of that $4 billion in Title IV-E funding, about 43 percent was spent on payments to foster care providers (known as maintenance payments); the remainder was allocated to administration, child placement services, training, and child welfare information systems (Child Trends 2010). Unfortunately, similar data detailing the distribution of the state portion of foster care spending are unavailable.

Services for Children with Disabilities

Children with chronic illnesses or physical, mental, intellectual, or developmental disabilities or delays need a range of special medical, therapeutic, educational, and personal assistance services. A small number of children receive the long-term care services discussed in the next section on adults, but most of these children live in their own homes and are cared for by their parents. They receive services until the age of eighteen and twenty-two through two programs specifically targeted to children—Early and Periodic Screening, Diagnosis, and Treatment (EPSDT), which is a mandatory Medicaid benefit for low-income children, and programs under parts B and C of the Individuals with Disabilities Education Act (IDEA), a non-means-tested program that provides early intervention services for children from birth to age three and special education from age three to age twenty-two.

Both programs use a much broader definition of disability than that for adult programs. For children, the definition is based on a developmental model, which is meant to identify not just children who already have disabilities but also those at risk of developing chronic conditions or limitations if they do not receive medical treatment and educational remediation. Most children with disabilities enrolled in EPSDT and special education programs are not considered disabled by the time they reach adulthood. Those who continue to meet a Social Security Act definition of disabled for adults become eligible for the adult programs discussed later in this chapter (Institute of Medicine 2007).

Many states have also adopted Medicaid waiver programs—so-called because the state is allowed to waive some Medicaid rules, including with respect to income eligibility—which have expanded eligibility for children with disabilities. Many states and localities provide additional support services for the families of children with disabilities, and localities manage and partially finance special education programs through their school systems. Policies for children with disabilities are summarized in table 6.5.

RECIPIENTS AND POTENTIAL RECIPIENTS   In 2008 there were 74 million children below the age of nineteen in the United States, of whom roughly 4 million had a disability in the form of an activity-limiting health care need. That number included 3.5 million school-age children and another 500,000 under the age of six, about half in families whose incomes fell below 200 percent of the poverty level.[5] Two million children with disabilities were insured by the means-tested, Medicaid-financed EPSDT programs or by Children's Health Insurance Programs (CHIP), according to the 2007 National Survey of Children's Health (NSCH). Most low-income children with special health care needs get comprehensive health care services, including long-term medical and therapeutic treatments, personal assistance, or even institutional services, through EPSDT (Rosenbaum, Wilensky, and Allen 2008).

Estimates extrapolated from the 1994–1995 National Health Interview Survey on Disability reveal that approximately 1 million children age five and younger and another 1.5 million school-age children had intellectual and developmental disabilities (Larson et al. 2000).[6] Many low-income children with ID/DD are covered by EPSDT. Some whose families earn too much to qualify receive services through Medicaid waivers. In addition, twenty states had Medicaid waiver programs designed for medically fragile or technology-dependent children. Just over 20,000 children were enrolled in those programs in 2006, but almost as many— 19,000—were on waiting lists (Harrington, Ng, and Watts 2009).

Despite the many services available through Medicaid for children with disabilities, only about 15 percent of low-income children with disabilities and chronic care needs enter Medicaid through disability services (Rosenbaum, Wilensky, and Allen 2008). Medicaid's programs for people with disabilities, which are discussed later in more detail in the section on adults with disabilities, become important mainly when children age out of EPSDT at the age of twenty-one or nineteen.

Because early intervention and special education are not means-tested, public special education services are available to most children with ID/DD. Of the 1.5 million school-age children with ID/DD, an estimated 1.36 million received special education services (Larson et al. 2000). Overall, 6.6 million children age three through twenty-one received special education services, and another 280,000 children under age three were enrolled in early intervention services through the Individuals with Disabilities and Education Act in 2008 (U.S. Department of Education/ NCES/IES 2009).

HEALTH CARE (EPSDT AND CHIP)   Because of its broad range of services and flexible eligibility criteria, EPSDT is the primary source of acute and preventive medical care and long-term support for disabled children (Rosenbaum, Wilensky, and Allen 2008; Johnson 2010).[7] All children age five and younger living in families whose incomes fall below 133 percent of the federal poverty level are eligible

TABLE 6.5 / Children with Disabilities Policy Schematic

	Comprehensive Health Care	Long-Term Services and Supports	Early Intervention and Special Education	
Federal-state	Medicaid Early and Periodic Screening, Diagnosis, and Treatment (EPSDT): Requires that the states provide comprehensive means-tested health care for children under the age of twenty-two, including screening, diagnosis, and treatment	Medicaid long-term care provisions: Require that the states provide means-tested institutional care	Medicaid means-tested waivers and state plan personal care services option: Finance and deliver means-tested non-institutional care and family support services	Individuals with Disabilities Education Act (IDEA)—Part C: Provides in-home early intervention services for children below age three who show signs of developmental delay	Individuals with Disabilities Education Act (IDEA)—Part B: Provides special education for children age three to twenty-one
State-local			Some states provide additional family support services.		States and localities provide and fund special education programs.

Source: Authors' summary.

for comprehensive health care insurance under EPSDT. After age five, the federally mandated income eligibility requirement drops to 100 percent of the poverty level. However, states have the authority to expand Medicaid eligibility beyond these minimum standards—up to a maximum of 300 percent of the federal poverty level. Most states also have insurance programs for children whose incomes exceed the maximum allowable level for EPSDT eligibility. These programs are funded under the joint federal-state Children's Health Insurance Program; created in 1997, CHIP covers about 6 million children (Kaiser Family Foundation 2010).[8] Children enrolled in EPSDT are entitled to any service covered in the state's Medicaid plan.[9] Treatment under EPSDT may include a range of long-term services and supports, including personal care services (Rosenbaum 2008).

OTHER MEDICAID LONG-TERM SERVICES AND SUPPORTS   In most states, children qualify for Medicaid long-term supports and services if they have a disability or chronic illness and have qualified for Supplemental Security Income (SSI). Eligibility for SSI depends on the child's household satisfying a means test (Social Security Administration 2011).[10] The cost of institutional care or equivalent services in the home can have catastrophic financial implications for families whose incomes exceed the Medicaid threshold for eligibility. Prior to 1982, parents' income and assets were deemed part of their children's income and assets only if the children lived at home. Qualified children could get care free of charge as long as they lived in an institution, creating a perverse incentive for families to institutionalize children with severe disabilities. In 1982 Congress mandated that Medicaid-eligible children with disabilities who required an institutional level of services could get personal care and medical services in the home as long as care in the home was appropriate and the cost of providing services in the home did not exceed the cost of institutional care (U.S. Department of Health and Human Services/ASPE/DALTCP 2000). Twenty states have since adopted the TEFRA option (so-called because it was enacted as part of the Tax Equity and Fiscal Responsibility Act).

EARLY INTERVENTION AND SPECIAL EDUCATION   Many children with disabilities, especially those with ID/DD, receive services and special education under the auspices of the Individuals with Disabilities and Education Act, which entitles children with disabilities or developmental delays to a free appropriate public education (FAPE) from birth to the age of twenty-two or until they complete high school (U.S. Department of Education/OSERS/OSEP 2009).[11] The Infants and Toddlers with Disabilities component (IDEA: Part C—also known as "early intervention") provides services and supports to children who have (or are suspected of having) disabilities or developmental delays between their birth and their third birthday. The Assistance for Education of All Children with Disabilities component (Part B, commonly known as "special education") helps states provide special education and related services to children from ages three through twenty-one.

Any child who, upon evaluation, is found to have at least one of thirteen identified disabilities—autism, deafness, deaf-blindness, emotional disturbance, hearing impairment, mental retardation, multiple disabilities, orthopedic impairment, other health impairment, specific learning disability, speech or language impairment, traumatic brain injury, or visual impairment—is eligible for services. A school-based team collaborates with the child's family to develop a written individualized education program (IEP). The plan identifies educational goals and the necessary services and supports, which can include preventative medical care, therapeutic services, and long-term care services (Child Welfare League of America 2005; Rosenbaum 2008). In 1998 and 1999 at least eight states—Illinois, Maryland, Massachusetts, New York, Rhode Island, Vermont, West Virginia, and Wisconsin—financed the medical, therapeutic, and long-term care components of special education through EPSDT, which provided a total of between 10 and 34 percent of each state's share of special education funding (Parrish et al. 2004).

In 2008, 21 percent of all Medicaid payments—$63 billion—were spent on children through EPSDT. (An additional $10.3 billion was spent on CHIP-funded programs, including Medicaid expansions and stand-alone CHIP programs.) Genevieve Kenney, Joel Ruhter, and Thomas Seldon (2009) estimate that children in the top spending decile (which includes a high proportion of children with disabilities) accounted for 72 percent of all EPSDT spending (more than 14 percent of all Medicaid spending) during the period 2002 to 2005. Per capita spending for full-year enrollees in the top spending decile was almost $8,000 for that period, compared to $1,106 for all full-year enrollees. Although it is difficult to estimate precisely how much is spent through EPSDT and CHIP on children with special health care needs or disabilities, as distinct from children in the top decile of spending, $30 billion would represent a conservative estimate of these costs based on these data.

States and localities have primary responsibility for funding special education programs, with states paying an estimated 46 percent of the cost, localities another 46 percent, and the federal IDEA program about 9 percent. In total, states, localities, and the federal government combined spent an estimated $115 billion in 2008 to educate special education students—or $54 billion more than they would have spent to provide these students with a standard education (Parrish et al. 2004).[12]

POLICIES THAT SUPPORT THE CARE OF ADULTS WITH DISABILITIES AND THE FRAIL ELDERLY

Many adults living with impairments that limit their independence and ability to perform necessary activities of daily living without assistance require long-term services and supports. Impairments range from intellectual and developmental disabilities, which people are either born with or develop in childhood, to physical disabilities and chronic illnesses, which may occur at any age, to the frailty associated with old age.

Institutional and in-home services and supports for elders and for younger adults with disabilities—both ID/DD and non-ID/DD—consist mainly of nonmedical care, such as homemaker services and personal assistance. These include assistance with ADLs (bathing, dressing, eating, transferring, toileting, and mobility inside the home), with IADLs (which include housework, meal preparation, and bill paying), and with some health-related tasks. As described in chapter 4, these tasks are primarily performed by paid adult care workers.

People with ID/DD need a "combination and sequence of special, interdisciplinary, or generic care, treatment, or other services which are of lifelong or extended duration and are individually planned and coordinated" (Larson et al. 2000, 5). In addition to assistance with ADLs, adults with ID/DD often require case management, habilitation, supported employment, transportation, and therapies designed to help integrate them into the community. Assistance for people with ID/DD who live with their families comes in the form of services such as respite care, employment support, and adult day care. In addition, a very small number of family caregivers receive cash payments for their service from family support programs (Rizzolo 2009).

As noted in table 6.6, long-term services and supports are provided by a complex system that includes institutional long-term care and home- and community-based personal care and homemaker services, as well as an array of other community and rehabilitation support services. Most publicly funded long-term care is paid for through Medicaid. Several other laws, including the Older Americans Act (OAA) and the Rehabilitation Act, mandate and partially fund the coordination and provision of services for working-age and older adults with disabilities. The OAA funds nutrition and transportation services and provides some personal care for people who are not eligible for Medicaid-funded services. The Rehabilitation Services Administration (RSA) manages a set of programs designed to integrate working-age adults into the mainstream through employment and to support independent living in the community.

Recipients and Potential Recipients

According to an analysis of the American Community Survey of 2008, 18.3 million working-age (ages twenty-one to sixty-four) people and 14.2 million older adults (age sixty-five and over) living in the community had a disability. Among working-age people with disabilities, 6.2 million had what is called an independent living disability, meaning that they could not do errands without assistance. Among people over sixty-five living in the community, 6.3 million had independent living disabilities (Erickson, Lee, and von Schrader 2010). In addition, 1.8 million people lived in nursing facilities, of whom 1.5 million were sixty-five or older and 290,000, or about 16 percent, were under age sixty-five (U.S. Census Bureau 2010a).

Most of the 1.8 million people living in nursing homes, and another 1.4 million in community settings, received publicly supported services that were paid for mainly by Medicaid. Medicaid personal care services and Medicaid home- and community-based waivers supported personal care and homemaker services in the homes of eligible people with disabilities (Kaye, Harrington, and LaPlante 2010; Harrington et al. 2009).

TABLE 6.6 / Adults with Disabilities and the Frail Elderly Policies

	Long-Term Care, Institutional	Long-Term Services and Supports, Home- and Community-Based	Other Community-Based Services	Rehabilitation Services
Federal-state	Medicaid: Long-term care provisions require that states finance means-tested care in nursing homes, state hospitals, or intermediate care facilities for people with qualifying disability, chronic illness, or age-related infirmity	Medicaid Personal Care Services (PCS): Option to finance personal care services in the home and community for people meeting state eligibility requirements Medicaid Home- and Community-Based Services (HCBS) waivers: Finance long-term services and supports for people with an institutional level of need or less, including home health, homemaker, personal care, and adult day health services Social Services Block Grant (SSBG): Finances a range of means-tested, community-based services for low-income elderly	Administration on Aging: Provides nutrition services (congregate and home-delivered meals), family caregiver support, supportive services (personal care, homemaker, chore, adult day care), transportation, case management, outreach, disease prevention, and health promotion	Rehabilitation Services Administration: Provides vocational rehabilitation services, supported employment, and independent living programs
State-local			State aging agencies and local area agencies on aging (AAAs) provide an array of community-based services.	States sponsor additional vocational rehabilitation services, supported employment, and independent living programs.

Source: Authors' compilation.

Care and Support Services Received

In 2007 just under 1 million of the roughly 1.5 million adults with ID/DD received publicly supported care, either in residential facilities, community-based residences, or the home of a family member. About 38,000 received their services in state hospitals, 24,000 in larger congregate care facilities with more than sixteen residents, and 376,000 in a supervised residence such as a smaller congregate care facility, group home, foster/host home, or the care recipient's own home. Another 1 million lived with a family member. Of those, only about half—550,000—received publicly funded assistance in addition to the unpaid care provided by relatives (Prouty, Alba, amd Lakin 2008).

In 2005, 1.39 million adults with disabilities also received employment and training services through state and local vocational rehabilitation services, and over 200,000 people with disabilities who were living in the community received training, transportation, housing, personal care, and homemaking services through centers for independent living (U.S. Department of Education/OSERS/RSA 2009).

Services were provided under Title III Part B or C of the Older Americans Act (OAA) to 2.9 million older adults in 2008. Only 9 percent of eligible adults—persons age sixty and older whose incomes fell below 185 percent of the poverty threshold—received assistance with meals. An estimated 22 percent of eligible adults who needed help with transportation got it through these programs (U.S. General Accountability Office 2011).

Federal and State Policies That Support Care for Adults with Disabilities and the Frail Elderly

Medicaid, a means-tested aid program, is a jointly funded venture between federal and state governments that provides medical assistance to low-income people. Since its inception in 1965, Medicaid has been the primary source of public funding for long-term care services and supports for adults with disabilities and frail older persons.

People who meet the financial eligibility requirements for SSI and the Social Security Administration definition of disability—which covers people with physical and mental disabilities and with chronic illnesses—are automatically entitled to receive Medicaid-funded long-term services and supports. (For a discussion of how disability is defined, see the appendix).

Medicaid was the primary payer for 65 percent of nursing home residents in 2004, and for 34 percent of people receiving any long-term care services (personal assistance and home health services) at home in 2005–2006 (Kaye, Harrington, and LaPlante 2010). Medicare, the national health insurance program for everyone sixty-five and over, as well as for younger adults with disabilities, was the primary payer for 18 percent of nursing home residents and for 35 percent of people receiving long-term care services in the community during this period.[13] Assuming that these rates carried through to 2007, about 2.8 million receiving long-term care that year were funded primarily by either Medicaid (1.8 million) or Medicare (1.0 million). Over half of people with ID/DD are supported by state programs alone and the other half by Medicaid waiver programs, which we discuss later (Prouty, Alba, and Lakin 2008).

MEDICAID LONG-TERM CARE: INSTITUTIONAL AND HOME- AND COMMUNITY-BASED CARE   State Medicaid plans must provide institutional long-term care and home health care (as well as the EPSDT program) in order to be eligible for federal matching funds. In 1975 states were given the option to include in-home personal care services (the PCS option) as part of their Medicaid plans. As a condition of getting federal matching funds, states must offer any benefit provided to any beneficiaries in their state Medicaid plan to all Medicaid beneficiaries with comparable conditions. (These are known as the statewideness and comparability rules.) In other words, if a state wanted to make less expensive in-home personal care services available to elderly persons who were qualified for or already living in nursing homes, they would also have to offer the personal care services to nursing home–eligible working-age adults who were living independently in the community. Many states chose not to adopt the PCS option out of concern that it would stimulate demand and raise the overall cost of providing long-term care.

The Medicaid waiver authority—passed in 1981—allows states to waive statewideness and comparability rules, targeting specific services to particular populations. In 2009 there were 286 separate waivers operating in the fifty states and the District of Columbia, with a total of 1.346 million waiver slots. Another 365,000 people were on waiting lists for oversubscribed waiver services. Thirty-one percent of the waivers and 41 percent of the waiver slots were for people with ID/DD, who also represented 61 percent of those on waiting lists. Forty percent of waiver programs and 47 percent of slots were for people over age sixty-five or for people under sixty-five with disabilities. Waivers for people with physical disabilities, children, people with HIV/AIDS, and people with traumatic brain or spinal cord injuries made up the remaining slots (Harrington, Ng, and Watts 2011a). In 2008 there were 1.362 million waiver slots, and a total of 1.241 million participated in the waiver programs (Harrington, Ng, and Watts 2011b).[14]

Prior to passage of the Medicaid waiver authority, most publicly supported long-term care was delivered in state hospitals, other large institutions, and nursing homes. Between 1967 and 2007, the number of people with ID/DD living in state institutions fell from 195,000 to 36,650. As of 2007, only 9 percent of people with ID/DD still lived in facilities that had more than sixteen residents, while only 21 percent of adults with developmental disabilities were living in any kind of institution (Prouty, Alba, and Lakin 2008). In contrast, 68 percent of older adults receiving long-term care were still living in nursing homes in 2008 (Kaye, Harrington, and LaPlante 2010; Harrington, Carrillo, and Blank 2009).

OTHER COMMUNITY-BASED SERVICES AND SUPPORTS   Congress passed the Older Americans Act in 1965 in response to a concern that there were insufficient community social services for elderly people. Today the OAA is considered the principal vehicle for the delivery of nutritional and social services to older Americans. Title III of the OAA—Grants for State and Community Programs on Aging—authorizes the appropriation of funds for formula grants to states. These funds are used to provide supportive assistive services (transportation, personal care, homemaker services, case management, adult day health) and nutrition programs (congregate and home-delivered). A 2000 amendment to Title III added caregiver supports (training, counseling, support groups, and access assistance to local services and respite care) (U.S. General Accountability Office 2010a). All people over sixty years of age are eligible for OAA services, but the services are not entitlements, and lack of funding constrains the delivery of direct services. The OAA requires providers to target those with the greatest economic and social need: low-income people, minorities, people lacking proficiency in English, and rural residents.

State and local aging agencies may administer programs that are funded with a combination of OAA funds, other federal funds from Medicaid or social services block grants, state and local funds, and donations and income-based cost-sharing from participants (Rabiner et al. 2006; O'Shaughnessy 2009).

EXPENDITURES   Using an estimate of the daily cost of long-term care services delivered in nursing homes and in private homes, along with a range of estimates of the number of people receiving care in each setting in 2004–2005, Stephen Kaye, Charlene Harrington, and Mitchell LaPlante (2010) estimate that the total annual spending on paid long-term care services was between $147 million and $181 billion (in 2009 dollars), including both public and private expenditures but not including the economic value of unpaid care.[15] Medicaid expenditures of $106 billion in 2008 accounted for between 56 and 66 percent of estimated spending, and past estimates attribute about 20 percent of long-term care spending to Medicare (Georgetown University 2007). States spend 21 percent of their total budgets (including federal matching funds) on Medicaid, one-third of which pays for long-term care services (Burke, Feder, and van de Water 2005).

Disaggregating long-term care expenditures another way, between $113 billion and $136 billion (depending on the data source) is spent on nursing home care. Just $33 billion is spent on home- and community-based services, most of which is supplied through home health care agencies and paid for by Medicaid and Medicare (Kaye, Harrington, and LaPlante 2010). Only a small amount of home care is so-called consumer-directed care, given by independent providers under the direction of the care recipient, with most of that paid for directly by the person receiving services. However, as noted in the appendix, the number of people working as consumer-directed independent providers is seriously undercounted in government statistics. The growing significance of consumer-directed personal care services does not show up in official data either. It is also important to remember, as emphasized earlier in this volume, that most long-term care is provided by unpaid family caregivers.

SUMMARY

This large and complex package of public policies constitutes the core of the care policy landscape in the United States. The components of this package—ECEC, family leave, foster care, policies for children with disabilities, and policies that serve adults with disabilities and the frail elderly—operate across multiple levels of government. They take a variety of forms, providing direct services, granting cash payments, and regulating workplaces and service providers.

We began this chapter with the claim that the policies described here comprise the largest public care initiatives in the United States in terms of number of recipients, level of expenditures, or both. Indeed, as we have demonstrated, these policies serve millions of children and adults. About 4 million children are enrolled in the major means-tested child care programs or in publicly funded early education programs, and children in 3.7 million families receive services subsidized by the federal child care tax credit. In one recent year, between 6 million and 13 million U.S. workers took FMLA-qualified family leaves, about half of which were taken by workers to cope with a serious illness of their own, while the other half were taken to care for newborn children, aging parents, or other family members. Nearly half a million children are served in the public foster care system, nearly 7 million children receive federally funded special education services, and 4 million to 5 million children with special health care needs are enrolled in publicly funded EPSDT services. Furthermore, an estimated 2.8 million adults receive long-term care for which the primary payer is either Medicaid or Medicare, about 3 million elderly people receive services annually from programs authorized under the Older Americans Act, and another 1.8 million working-age adults receive employment assistance services and independent living services from the vocational rehabilitation centers funded by the Rehabilitation Services Administration.

These publicly supported care policies come with a substantial price tag. In one recent year, government expenditures on child care via the two main means-tested programs totaled nearly $11 billion, while public expenditures on early education amounted to nearly $10 billion. State and federal expenditures on public prekindergarten programs total another $3.8 billion, and tax credits granted through the federal dependent care credit total $3.2 billion each year. One state alone—California—spends about $1.4 billion a year on pregnancy benefits and family leave. An estimated $28 billion in public dollars is spent each year on health care and services for children with special health care needs. In addition, federal, state, and local governments spend about $115 billion a year on special education.

Turning to long-term care services for adults with disabilities and the frail elderly, recent estimates put combined Medicaid and Medicare spending on long-term care services in 2008 at close to $140 billion. And $1.44 billion in federal funding from the Older Americans Act is spent each year on supportive and nutrition services for the elderly and support services for caregivers, supplemented by the local area agencies on aging (AAAs) with between $3 billion and $4.4 billion from other public and private sources.

In short, our current care policy package clearly serves large numbers of recipients and requires substantial public funding. But how well is this complex set of policies working? Are needs being met? Are they being met equitably? In the next chapter, we assess how well these policies are working for people in need of care and for their families, with a focus on disparities by income and by geography.

NOTES

1. For more detail on the ECEC services and programs described in this chapter, see Gornick and Meyers (2003). We gratefully acknowledge Marcia Meyers, who constructed the ECEC typology we use here.
2. A comprehensive evaluation of the FMLA was completed and published in 2000. Later national data on FMLA coverage, eligibility, and usage are not yet available. In the spring of 2011, the U.S. Department of Labor, Wage and Hour Division, began conducting a replication of the 2000 study; to date, the results of this study have not yet been released.
3. Rhode Island enacted its TDI program in 1942; California enacted its state disability insurance program in 1946; New Jersey's TDI program dates to 1948; New York created its disability benefits law in 1949; and Hawaii launched its TDI program in 1969. After the passage of the PDA in 1978, these programs were required to cover maternity.
4. Typically, the age of emancipation has been eighteen. However as a result of the Fostering Connections to Success and Increasing Adoptions Act of 2008, federal Title IV-E foster care payments may be available for foster youth up to age twenty-one under certain conditions.
5. In the National Children's Health Survey 2007, the Maternal and Children's Health Bureau (MCHB) estimated that there were 14.1 million children under age eighteen with "special health care needs," ranging from the regular use of prescription drugs to health and functional limitations that limited participation in age-appropriate activities. "Children with special health care needs" are defined as those who are at increased risk for chronic physical, developmental, behavioral, or emotional conditions and who require services beyond those required by children generally. Prevalence estimates vary depending on whether special needs are narrowly defined as tied to limitations in specific types of activities or more broadly defined as in the MCHB definition (Rosenbaum 2008). An estimated 4 million of these children have an activity-limiting impairment that would be considered a disability. In all, 4 million to 5 million children with special health care needs were enrolled in EPSDT, including 2 million with activity-limiting impairments. The American Community Survey 2008 estimated that 3.5 million children between the ages of five and seventeen were disabled (U.S. Census Bureau 2009a).
6. Unfortunately, the disability supplement to the NHIS was conducted only in 1994–1995, so there are no more recent data.
7. Medicaid is a jointly funded federal-state program that finances health care for low-income people. EPSDT, which is best thought of as the pediatric component of Medicaid, is a mandatory Medicaid benefit, meaning that all states must offer it as a condition for receiving federal matching funds. Enacted as an amendment to the Social Security Act in 1967, EPSDT was designed to provide baseline preventive health care for all low-income children (not just children with disabilities) and to identify and treat chil-

dren who have, or are at risk of developing, physical and mental health conditions that could affect their development and growth.

8. States have the option to structure their CHIP programs so that they provide comprehensive medical services, comparable to EPSDT, or to provide a less comprehensive benefit that does not address the above-average needs of children with disabilities. State CHIP programs do not have to cover the comprehensive range of services mandated under EPSDT and therefore do not provide the full range of services required by children with "special health care needs" (Rosenbaum, Wilensky, and Allen 2008). CHIP funds can be used to set up separate CHIP programs or to expand Medicaid coverage. If used to expand Medicaid coverage, then all Medicaid rules and regulations, including cost sharing and benefits, apply, which means that the CHIP-funded Medicaid expansion program provides comprehensive services equivalent to EPSDT. States have much greater flexibility to set eligibility and benefit levels if the CHIP funds are used to set up separate CHIP programs. In 2008, of the 7.3 million children in CHIP-funded programs, only 2 million were in CHIP-funded Medicaid expansions (Ryan 2009).

9. Unlike other Medicaid benefits, and unlike CHIP and private insurance plans, EPSDT uses a developmental standard for assessment. Preventive and corrective services are defined as "medically necessary treatment," as they must be to qualify for Medicaid reimbursement.

10. Disabled children age eighteen or older may also be eligible for SSDI (Social Security Disability Insurance) if their parents have the required contributory history. Once eligible for SSDI, they will be eligible for Medicare after two years. The Social Security Administration refers to this as a "child's benefit" because it is paid on the parent's Social Security earnings record (Social Security Administration 2011).

11. This was first enacted in 1975 as the Education for All Handicapped Children Act and amended in 1990 with the new name, Individuals with Disabilities and Education Act.

12. There have been no reliable and comprehensive data on what public schools spend on special education since the Office of Special Education stopped requiring its collection in 1987 (Chambers et al. 1998). One recent estimate suggests that it costs 1.9 times as much to educate a special education student as to educate a regular education student (Parrish et al. 2003). Using the ratio of spending per special education student to spending per regular student estimated by Thomas Parrish and his colleagues (2004), and assuming that this ratio remained constant over the last ten years (Parrish 2010), we estimate that the total amount spent to educate special education students in 2008 was $115 billion and that the marginal cost was $54 billion, a number that Parrish himself found reasonable (personal communication, October 30–November 3, 2010).

13. Although Medicare does not pay for long-term care services, it does provide partial payment for up to one hundred days of rehabilitation in a nursing home following an acute medical episode that requires a hospital stay. Medicare also pays for home health care that involves some medical services in addition to personal care services.

14. The most recent data available on number of participants are from 2008.

15. This estimate is probably too low, given that it is based on their calculation of the number of people receiving assistance in institutions and home- and community-based services from the Survey of Income and Program Participation (SIPP), the National Health Interview Survey (NHIS), and the American Community Survey (ACS).

Chapter 7

The Disparate Impacts of Care Policy

Janet Gornick, Candace Howes, and Laura Braslow

Ational, state, and local governments provide a complex array of services, benefits, and regulations that support children and adults in need of care and their caregivers. In this chapter, we assess how well the current system is working—and for whom. Assessing the adequacy of U.S. care policy provisions requires identifying a set of standards against which to evaluate these provisions. Yet, as decades of policy analysis scholarship have established, there is no single framework to use in assessing the adequacy of policy provisions. In our case, one approach would be to focus on the efficiency or effectiveness of existing care supports—that is, to assess outputs or outcomes relative to expenditures and other inputs across several areas of care policy. Another would call for surveying care recipients and caregivers to assess the degree to which they judge their needs to be met. Yet another would require establishing some absolute standards—one or more floors below which access to (or receipt of) care supports should not fall—and assessing the extent to which those in need of care and their caregivers have access and supports consistent with those standards. All of these approaches would, of course, require tackling challenging normative questions, especially about who needs and deserves care supports, how much and what kind of care is optimal or acceptable, and what the balance should be between public and private provisions.

A comprehensive evaluation of this large package of care policies, using any of these frameworks, is outside the scope of this project. Instead, we focus on the adequacy of the current system from the vantage point of disparities in the receipt of care. Two axes strike us as particularly consequential: disparities by income and disparities by geography. In the first half of this chapter, we review relevant research to assess the interaction between household income and receipt of care, looking at families with high, low, and middle incomes. In the second half, we draw on policy data gathered for this project to assess the variations in the receipt of care across the U.S. states.

DISPARITIES BY INCOME

Income matters in at least two crucial ways. First, public supports for care are provided against the backdrop of an extensive system of private, market-based options, which only higher-income families and individuals can afford without substantial public support and which are often of superior quality or provide a greater range of choice or control relative to their publicly funded counterparts. For early childhood and care, private options include nannies, babysitters, family day care services, child care centers, and educational programs. Public family (and medical) leave programs supplement those provided by individual employers, which may be part of a standard employee-benefit package or individually negotiated. In adult care, publicly funded long-term care services and supports supplement an enormous and complex assortment of private services, including personal and home care aides, assisted living facilities, and retirement communities that offer a long menu of services for a substantial fee.

Second, some publicly provided care supports are means-tested—that is, they are available only to people with low household incomes. Other services—such as foster care services, early intervention and special education for children with learning disabilities, and maternity-related disability pay provided by state temporary disability insurance programs (see chapter 6 for details)—are available to recipients regardless of income. In other policy arenas, including several early childhood education and care services and long-term care programs, eligibility is conditioned on low income. When recipients are separated by income level, a frequent result is income-related disparities in the quantity and quality of the care and support received. In some policy areas, the use of nonrefundable tax credits leads to further disparities by benefiting only families with incomes high enough to pay income taxes.

These intertwined features of the U.S. care system lead to important and complex disparities. Many high-income families have the financial resources to purchase private services, often with the option of choosing among a range of care options, for example, between in-home and various types of institutional care. In addition, people in high-income households are more likely than their lower-earning counterparts to have access to employer-provided benefits.

Low-income families have fewer options, but they do have access to various means-tested public programs—although being low-income hardly guarantees actual access, let alone satisfactory services. In some cases, means-testing thresholds are set so low that they exclude all but the most impoverished families. Even those who qualify may remain without services because many means-tested programs lack entitlement status, allowing states to control costs by rationing access to care. Moreover, the available level of public support may be insufficient to enable recipients to obtain needed care. Many eligible individuals lack services simply because they (or their family caregivers) are not aware that they are entitled to them. Approximately half of uninsured children, for example, are eligible for public health insurance, but their parents or guardians do not apply for it. And finally, those who do access publicly funded services often find that they are of poor quality.

Not wealthy enough to afford private care and not poor enough for means-tested services, families in the middle of the income distribution often face the most limited options. Their employer-provided benefits are patchy at best, and they are ineligible for many public programs, yet they lack the resources to purchase adequate private care. They cannot afford to take unpaid time off work, but paying for ECEC or long-term care services is likely to cause them substantial financial hardship.

Early Childhood Education and Care

Families face remarkably different levels of support for and access to ECEC services depending on their income levels, yet families at all income levels face challenges in arranging ECEC (Williams and Boushey 2010).[1] As other researchers have reported, low-income families face specific ECEC challenges and inadequacies (Meyers et al. 2004). Most notably, they report the highest ECEC cost burden, yet their children receive the least amount of formal care. Low-income parents are more likely than their affluent counterparts to use informal arrangements, largely because they are less expensive.

In their analysis of 2008 national data sets, Joan Williams and Heather Boushey (2010) define low-income families as those in the bottom third of the income distribution, with income falling below 200 percent of the federal poverty level for a family of three. They define professional families as the 13 percent of families with incomes in the top 20 percent in which at least one adult is a college graduate. The remaining 53 percent represent the middle.

The typical low-income family using center-based care for young children spends 14 percent of its total monthly income on that care—about the same as those using in-home care spend, and much higher than the share of family income paid by middle- and upper-income families (Williams and Boushey 2010). When public support is unavailable or insufficient, many low-income families are forced to rely on a patchwork of unpaid child care. One study of poor working families with children found that 60 percent did not pay for ECEC at all (Meyers et al. 2004).

Family income imposes serious constraints on ECEC decisions. Children in low-income families are less likely than their more affluent counterparts to be enrolled in formal care and/or pre-primary school programs (Matthews 2009; U.S. Department of Health and Human Services/ACF/CCB 2008). One study found that three- and four-year-olds from families with incomes in the top quartile are 23 percent more likely to be enrolled in pre-primary school programs than those in the bottom quartile. Even after controlling for several covariates (such as race, ethnicity, and mother's education, employment, and marital status), more affluent children were still 15 to 16 percent more likely to be enrolled in pre-primary school. Because formal care for young children is associated with better cognitive and school-readiness outcomes, disparities in care during early childhood may exacerbate income inequality later in life (Meyers et al. 2004).

While a number of publicly available, means-tested, publicly supported ECEC programs are available to low-income families, many do not take advantage of these services. Although the total amount of federal money for child care doubled in recent years, fewer than one-quarter of eligible children received a subsidy. Among low-income parents, only about 30 percent using center-based care and 15.5 percent using an in-home care center (what is often referred to as "family day care") received a government subsidy. Take-up rates are low in part because public child care subsidies are often low and unstable (Williams and Boushey 2010). Child care vouchers for women who have left welfare to enter the job market pay only $2 an hour, and families often receive the subsidies only briefly, for an average of three to seven months.

Another powerful explanatory factor is that many states ration ECEC by implementing policies that depress demand (such as high copayments and long waiting lists) or supply (such as low provider reimbursements). This explains why Head Start does not fill the gap in pre-primary enrollment that exists between low- and high-income children. The Head Start program is intended to serve poor children, but with income eligibility capped at a stringent $17,170 for a family of three for at least 90 percent of enrollees, it excludes many families in the bottom third of the income distribution. Further, states have no legal obligation to serve all income-eligible children. As a result, a recent GAO study found that 90 percent of more than 550 Head Start programs surveyed had wait lists, and eligible families often waited months to be placed in the program (General Accountability Office 2010b). In total, Head Start serves less than half of all income-eligible four-year-olds and far fewer eligible children below that age (U.S. Department of Health and Human Services/ACF/OHS 2010).

Middle-income families also face serious difficulties, because they do not qualify for government assistance. High-quality care, which can cost as much as $12,000 a year, lies out of reach. Yet the care services they do purchase, costing on average about $126 per week, account for about 11 percent of total family income (Williams and Boushey 2010, 46–47). The Child and Dependent Care Tax Credit (CDCTC) provides a federal tax benefit to offset out-of-pocket care expenses. However, families can claim only a percentage of the expenses incurred, subject to a ceiling. As a result, the benefits remain modest (National Association of Child Care Resource and Referral Agencies 2009).

Family Leave

As in the case of ECEC, the adequacy of family leave provisions is also stratified by income, for three reasons. First, the coverage and eligibility rules of the Family and Medical Leave Act (FMLA)—the main national policy in the United States that provides family leave rights—disproportionately exclude lower-income workers. Second, access to employer-provided leave rights and benefits—and particularly to paid leave benefits—is distributed regressively, rising with both workers' earnings and their household income. Third, workers in low-income families are less likely than others to utilize unpaid leave because they cannot afford to go without a regular paycheck.

A number of weaknesses in the FMLA cut across income groups, compromising its protections even for the most advantaged workers and their families. The definition of family members is narrow—many states limit leaves to the care of spouses, children, and parents, excluding domestic partners and other relatives (such as in-laws). In addition, in most states FMLA-covered medical leave is limited to "serious illness," so routine doctor visits are not grounds for leave-taking, and leaves for other (nonmedical) family care needs, such as attending school meetings, are not covered.

The millions of low-income workers who are not covered under the FMLA negotiate a "high-wire balancing act" (Newman 2000, 90). Access to FMLA leave depends on several factors. First, employees must work in a covered establishment—that is, one with at least fifty employees (employed within a seventy-five-mile radius). Thirty-four million American workers—about 30 percent of the workforce—are not covered by the FMLA because their employers are too small (U.S. Small Business Administration 2010). Second, eligibility requires a record of at least twelve months with the current employer, including at least 1,250 hours worked during the previous year; more than one-fifth of those in covered establishments are ineligible on this count (U.S. Department of Labor 2000). Low-earners are less likely than high-earners to work for larger employers and are also less likely to meet the employment history requirements; as a result, they are overrepresented among those not covered or not eligible for FMLA leave.

Disparities in FMLA coverage and eligibility are compounded by low levels of compliance with the law, which recent estimates place at less than 77 percent and possibly as low as 54 percent (Gerstel and Armenia 2009). Workers who know their FMLA rights can sue employers that violate the law, but such suits are risky and expensive; as a recent study shows, low-wage workers in the United States are particularly vulnerable to labor law violations (Bernhardt et al. 2009). In addition, research in California shows that low-income workers are much less likely to be aware of the FMLA and other leave benefits than are middle-income or high-income workers (Milkman and Appelbaum 2004).

Currently, only about 8 percent of private-sector workers are offered paid leave benefits by their employers (Levine 2009). Employer-provided rights and benefits in the private sector may be offered as part of a standard employee benefit package or may be negotiated on a case-by-case basis. Highly paid private-sector workers are more likely than their low-wage counterparts to enjoy some bargaining power with employers because replacing them is often difficult and costly. Accordingly, access to paid leave declines with wages and household income and is also correlated with educational attainment. Employed women with less than a high school degree, for example, are half as likely to have paid maternity leave as women with a high school diploma, and one-fourth as likely as women with a college degree or higher (Smith, Downs, and O'Connell 2001).

Including the public-sector workforce, where access to paid leave benefits is much more prevalent, only 22 percent of poor families have access to four weeks of paid leave some or all of the time, compared to 59 percent of non-poor families (Heymann 2001). The share of working parents with access to any paid leave is less than 46 percent for those with poverty-level income but over 83 percent for those with incomes at or above 200 percent of the poverty threshold (Ross Phillips 2004). And women with earnings in the top decile are seven times as likely as those with earnings in the bottom decile to have employer-provided paid family leave (Levine 2009).

In addition to these limitations on access to paid and unpaid leave benefits, economic constraints reduce the likelihood that parents will use the unpaid leave time to which they are entitled. Among those parents who take FMLA-guaranteed leaves to care for newborns, more than two-thirds take fewer than half of their allowable days. Nearly 80 percent of employees who do not take FMLA leave when needed report that the reason was that they "could not afford to take leave" (U.S. Department of Labor 2000). The data do not indicate what respondents mean by "could not afford"; some might be in low-income families, while others could be higher earners deterred by opportunity costs. Nevertheless, it is clear that the absence of wage replacement seriously disadvantages low-income workers and their families. As of 2000, about 10 percent of FMLA users who did not receive full pay went on public assistance during their leaves (U.S. Department of Labor 2000). Analysis of vital statistics data shows a small but significant reduction in infant mortality rates among college-educated married mothers attributable to unpaid family leave provisions. No such benefits are apparent for children of other mothers, largely as a result of low take-up rates (Rossin 2011).

Foster Care

Foster care, like many other areas of child welfare policy, is "universal," with state child welfare agencies legally required to protect and serve all children regardless of income. Nevertheless, the foster care system predominantly serves children from low-income families—and too often reproduces their economic disadvantages. Although the foster care system serves children from a wide range of family backgrounds, children from low-income families are far more likely to be placed in foster care than their higher-income counterparts. Children in families with incomes below $15,000 are twenty-two times more likely to be the subject of reported abuse and neglect—and forty-five times more likely to be victims of substantiated neglect—than children in families with incomes above $30,000 (Hutson 2001; Lindsey and Klein Martin 2002). These disparities may be due, to some extent, to inequalities in reporting and investigation of abuse and neglect claims, but poor children are understood to be at higher risk for physical and sexual abuse than children from middle-class and afflu-ent families (Stukes Chipungu and Bent-Goodley 2004). Their higher risk may be the result of basic differences in resources or time, family structure, work-force participation, the criminal justice system involvement of parents or other involved adults, or the stress associated with poverty (Paxson and Waldfogel 1999; Waldfogel 2000; Hutson 2001).

In addition, important income disparities emerge among foster parents, espe-cially between kin and nonkin foster parents. Kin care, which currently makes up roughly 20 percent of formal foster care placements, refers to the placement of a child either with a family member or with someone with whom the child has a significant relationship. Because foster children are disproportionately poor, and because poor children often have poor extended families, kin fos-ter parents are, on average, more economically disadvantaged than are nonkin foster parents. One study estimated that 39 percent of kin foster parents have incomes below the federal poverty line (FPL), compared to only 13 percent of nonkin foster parents (Ehrle and Geen 2002). Kin caregivers are also much more likely than nonkin caregivers to have less than a high school degree (24 versus 13 percent), to be single (58 versus 27 percent), and to be over sixty years old (20 versus 11 percent) (Macomber, Geen, and Main 2003; Grimm and Darwall 2005; U.S. Department of Health and Human Services/ACF 2010). Yet kin foster parents often receive lower levels of public support than foster parents who are not biologically related to the children they care for. (See the later discussion of foster care disparities by geography for details.)

A third key issue concerns the outcomes of the estimated 30,000 youth who age out of foster care each year (U.S. Department of Health and Human Services/ ACF/ACYF 2008). Researchers and policymakers have long been concerned about the degree to which tenure in foster care is linked to substantial hardship and poor life outcomes, including a significantly increased likelihood that former fos-ter children will become impoverished adults relative to their peers, even those from similar backgrounds. The system's capacity to provide for the health, educa-tion, and developmental needs of the children in its care and to help them tran-sition into adulthood is of particular concern with respect to those who are in foster care for a substantial part of their childhood. In making the transition from the foster care system to independent living, many of these youth find it difficult to find and keep a job or a place to live, and many become pregnant at an early age. An increased likelihood of mental health or substance abuse problems and of insufficient education or job preparedness compounds their difficulties, and a disproportionate number wind up poor, homeless, or incarcerated (U.S. General Accountability Office 1999; Lenz-Rashid 2004).

Many studies have found that there is a direct relationship between partici-pation in the foster care system and employment and criminal justice outcomes for former foster children. Youth aging out of foster care are less likely than other young adults to work during the two years following their emancipa-tion, and when they do work they have significantly lower earnings (George et al. 2002). Another study found that former foster children age twenty-three and twenty-four are less likely than their age-comparable counterparts to be employed and more likely to be poor, and that those who have jobs earn less. Fewer than half of the former foster youth surveyed had a checking or savings account, and almost one-third had low or very low food security. Three-quarters of the women and one-third of the men received benefits from one or more need-based government programs. They also had much higher levels of criminal justice involvement than their peers: 20 percent of women and 42 percent of men reported having been arrested, and 8 percent of women and 23 percent of men reported having been convicted of a crime (Courtney et al. 2010). Other studies document similarly bleak results (Tweddle 2007).

Services for Children with Disabilities

Services for children with disabilities come closer to meeting their needs and mitigating income disparities than do most other services targeted toward children—or toward adults with disabilities. One of two key services, Medicaid's Early and Periodic Screening, Diagnosis, and Treatment (EPSDT), is a means-tested program (see description in chapter 6). However, many states have either set their income eligibility thresholds and income disregards high enough to cover a substantial number of children under EPSDT or have created state-financed programs to serve children whose household incomes are too high to qualify for EPSDT.

States have the option to set income eligibility levels for EPSDT as high as 300 percent of the federal poverty line, and other federal programs provide them with incentives to do so. Both Medicaid and the Children's Health Insurance Program (CHIP) give states some flexibility when they evaluate income eligibility, allowing them to create deductions and disregards for parents of children with disabilities. Further, the individual educational plans (IEPs) for school-age children and individual family services plans for preschool children required by the Individuals with Disabilities Education Act (IDEA) can include medical and therapeutic services for children with developmental delays. As a consequence, IDEA provides an incentive for states to set higher income eligibility thresholds or income disregards so that Medicaid EPSDT will share in the cost of providing mandated medical and therapeutic services (Rosenbaum 2008). As will be discussed in the following section, Medicaid coverage for adults is more limited because there are no similar incentives to raise income eligibility levels for adults.

Certainly disparities are linked to family income, but these are mitigated by the design and accessibility of services for children with disabilities. A recent study found that lower-income children with disabilities who are enrolled in EPSDT actually fare better than middle-income children with private health insurance. The study found no significant differences between the two groups in use of either supportive services for the family (personal care, respite, and transportation) or therapeutic services for the children (speech therapy, therapies for learning disabilities and behavioral problems, and physical therapy), both in and out of school. However, children who had public EPSDT insurance were two to three times more likely to use these services than either children without insurance or children with private insurance, after controlling for numerous other factors that would affect service use (Benedict 2006).

Another key program for children with disabilities, special education, is an entitlement for all children regardless of income. However, as will be discussed in more detail later, huge differences in spending both across and within states prevent all children from having equal access to its services, and inequalities by income play a significant role alongside differences across geography. Federal allocations for special education are made using a formula that takes into account both the number of children enrolled in special education and the state poverty rate. Within states, spending is based on a range of formulas, some of which result in local allocations that are not proportionate to the level of need among school districts (Parrish 2010).

Policies for Adults with Disabilities and the Frail Elderly

Support for long-term care for adults is more stratified by income than is support for the care and education of disabled children. As with ECEC, many upper-income people in need of care (and their families) can afford to purchase private services, and many are able to purchase high-quality care consistent with their preferences (such as home-based rather than institutional care). Low-income people in need may receive long-term care services through the means-tested Medicaid program, the largest purchaser of long-term care services in the United States, but they are more likely than those paying privately to be placed in a nursing home. As with ECEC, middle-income families are largely left to "make do" and typically cobble together a patchwork of unpaid care and purchased services or spend down their assets and rack up expenses until they qualify for Medicaid. This spend-down and the resulting access to benefits often happens only as a result of placing a family member in a nursing home: while only one-fifth of nursing home residents are Medicaid recipients when they enter, Medicaid is the primary payer for four-fifths of residents who stay longer than three years (Kaye, Harrington, and LaPlante 2010).

Upper-income families clearly have the most options, but they still face constraints and challenges. Many find it difficult to arrange care for a parent, spouse, or child because of the demands of jobs with long work hours and inflexible schedules. And for all but the most affluent families, the costs are a substantial burden. The average cost of a year in a nursing facility in 2009 was $79,935 for a private room and $69,715 for a shared room; one year in an assisted living facility cost $37,572. Home health care purchased through an agency cost $21 per hour on average, and "homemakers/companions" cost about $19 per hour in 2009 (Metlife Mature Market Institute 2009).

Low-income people in need of care face a substantially different landscape because many of them are eligible for Medicaid. Although Medicaid provides coverage for long-term care services, drawing on Medicaid to pay for long-term care can put other members of a family in financial jeopardy because they are forced to choose between their own comfort and that of their loved one. For example, for the last twenty years the Centers for Medicare and Medicaid Services has allowed spouses of Medicaid recipients in nursing homes to retain some of their assets, but in many states there is no spousal asset protection if a Medicaid recipient opts for home- and community-based care (O'Brien and Merlis 2007). This has created a perverse incentive: many people who are low-income but who hold some assets choose nursing home care when they would prefer to stay at home (and staying at home would mean lower costs to the state) in order to avoid impoverishing their spouse.

Many middle-income families (who, for the most part, fail to qualify for Medicaid) face an especially restricted set of options. Some have no health insurance coverage, and even for those who do, many health insurance plans—including Medicare—do not include many long-term care benefits. Unfortunately, most middle-income families encounter the need for long-term care as a sudden and catastrophic event for which they have done little, if any, planning, and they are left to navigate a confusing and fragmented system on their own. Unlike other large expenses in people's lives that are likely to be financed through long-term borrowing (such as houses and cars), paid for with insurance (damage from floods, fires, or automobile accidents), or planned for and financed with savings (retirement), most Americans have little idea how they will pay for long-term care if and when they need it. A 2006 survey by AARP showed that 59 percent of Americans over the age of forty-five believed that Medicare would pay for an extended stay in a nursing home, and 52 percent believed that Medicare covers assisted living costs, neither of which is true. Only 11 percent had long-term care insurance (Barrett 2006). Yet people who earn too much to qualify for Medicaid and do not have long-term care insurance must either pay for care out-of-pocket, rely on unpaid care from family members, or both, forcing many to do without needed care.

In addition, even unpaid care can strain a family's finances, since family caregivers must often give up a paying (or better-paying) job or reduce the hours they work for pay in order to care for a relative. That lost income can threaten the economic security of all but the most affluent families.

DISPARITIES BY GEOGRAPHY

Several factors lead to widespread variation across states in access to, and receipt of, care services and supports. The most powerful factor is the federalist governmental structure in the United States, which leaves a substantial degree of policymaking to the states. As we reported in chapter 6, some care-related policies are purely federal, but the vast majority of care-related policies and programs have large state components. Some policies operate as federal-state matching programs, while others function as federally funded block grants. Some state programs extend the eligibility and benefits granted through national policies, while others operate as autonomous state programs. In some cases, uniform rules about eligibility and benefits are set at the national level, but variation across states in administrative and implementation practices leads to extensive cross-state variation in take-up—which, in turn, results in state-to-state variability in de facto access to and receipt of care.

In practice, nearly all elements of early childhood education and care have large state-based components. Paid family leave policies are devised almost entirely at the state level, and many states have expanded access to unpaid leave beyond the protections provided under the federal FMLA. Although the federal government plays a role in funding and influencing some aspects of foster care policy, many key features, such as the maintenance rates paid to families and the treatment of kin care, are determined at the state level and vary widely from state to state. And even though national Medicaid rules require that all state Medicaid programs provide nursing home care and medically necessary home health care, states vary greatly in the other publicly funded long-term care services and supports that they provide for children and adults with disabilities and for the frail elderly.

Furthermore, state-to-state variation in demographic, labor market, and other economic factors can compound state policy differences. All in all, the adequacy and availability of supports for those in need of care, and for their families, varies enormously depending on their state of residence. In short, where one lives matters—and it matters a lot.

Early Childhood Education and Care

The adequacy of ECEC services for America's young children, especially those in low-income homes, depends in no small part on where a child lives. As described in chapter 6, most governmental support for ECEC comes in one of two forms: means-tested child care subsidies for low-income parents or public prekindergarten programs (including the federal Head Start program and state-level prekindergarten programs). Provisions for both vary markedly across the states.

Expenditures on means-tested assistance for child care, including the Child Care and Development Fund (CCDF) and additional funding allocated from the Temporary Assistance for Needy Families (TANF) program, totaled nearly $11 billion in 2006. With about 2 million low-income children served, spending per child served totaled just under $5,400. However, per child spending varied enormously across the fifty states, from a high of $13,972 in Connecticut to a low of $2,066 in

Mississippi—a nearly sevenfold difference (see table 7.1). Nationwide, about one-fifth of poor children under the age of fourteen receive child care services subsidized through CCDF or TANF. That percentage also varies sharply across the states. As of 2006, in three high-enrollment states (Vermont, Wyoming, and Delaware) 35 percent or more of poor children were served, while in another five states (Colorado, South Carolina, Texas, Nevada, and Arkansas) fewer than one-tenth were served.

The adequacy of public early education programs is also largely determined by the state in which a young child lives (see table 7.1). Public expenditures on early education (Head Start and public prekindergarten programs together) amounted to nearly $10 billion in 2006. About 2 million children were served, for an average expenditure of just over $5,400 per child, but state average expenditures per child ranged from a high of $13,717 in New Jersey to a low of $2,860 in Kansas.

The share of young children served in these early education programs also varies considerably by state. Nationwide, about one-tenth of all children under the age of five are enrolled in either Head Start (which is means-tested) or a state-based prekindergarten program (most of which have some income requirements).[2] Again, enrollment levels vary sharply across the states. On the high end, nearly one-fifth of young children in three states—Kentucky, Oklahoma, and Vermont—were served in publicly funded programs as of 2006, while fewer than 5 percent were served in Nevada, Utah, and Oregon.

The regulation of ECEC quality also varies. Although American families pay substantial amounts for ECEC, recent research suggests that the quality of much of the care that they purchase is not very good. A recent study of ECEC recipients up to age four and a half indicates that only 17 percent experienced high-quality care, while another 24 percent received care that was moderately high-quality. More than one-third (35 percent) experienced low-quality care, and 24 percent encountered moderately low-quality care. In other words, more than half experienced low- or moderately low-quality care, and twice as many experienced low-quality as high-quality care (Vandell et al. 2010). This uneven care quality is due in part to the weakness and variability of state regulation.

Because informal babysitters and small family day care homes are exempt from regulation in most states, most nonparental care for young children is provided in settings with little or no public oversight. Many states exempt certain types of child care centers from regulation, such as religious centers (thirteen states) and half-day nursery schools (twenty-two states) (U.S. General Accountability Office 2004). Licensing rules are even more inconsistent. Only twelve states require that all family day care centers be licensed; others exempt providers who care for only a few children or providers who receive no public funds (U.S. General Accountability Office 2004). State resources for enforcing these requirements are limited, so an unknown number of family day care homes operate illegally, even in states that require licensing.

Family Leave

With no national law granting paid family leave, public provision of paid leaves has been left entirely to the states. Five states (California, Hawaii, New Jersey,

TABLE 7.1 / Child Care and Early Education, 2006

	Child Care Assistance Subsidies (CCDF and TANF)				Head Start and Prekindergarten Programs			
	Total Spending (in millions of Dollars)	Total Children Served	Spending per Child Served	Poor Children (Under Age Fourteen) Served	Total Spending (in Millions of Dollars)	Total Children Served	Spending per Child Served	Young Children (Under Age Five Served)
United States[a]	$13,550	2,518,077	$5,381	21%	$9,698	1,876,295	$5,439	9%
Alabama	114	29,610	3,857	14	112	20,246	5,507	7
Alaska	51	7,365	6,896	38	115	27,578	4,157	6
Arizona	173	39,176	4,416	13	161	21,673	7,419	11
Arkansas	85	7,381	11,620	5	18	3,412	5,398	7
California	2,256	310,323	7,271	20	1,088	218,290	4,987	8
Colorado	98	16,564	5,909	11	105	34,374	3,065	10
Connecticut	164	11,748	13,972	12	122	20,703	5,882	10
Delaware	63	14,510	4,338	57	24	2,733	8,653	5
Florida	820	181,700	4,512	32	489	81,631	5,995	7
Georgia	264	70,531	3,740	16	457	62,826	7,269	9
Hawaii	48	12,366	3,910	38	23	4,535	5,078	5
Idaho	37	10,226	3,609	22	24	5,738	4,194	5
Illinois	897	217,478	4,125	48	506	114,915	4,401	13
Indiana	172	35,990	4,778	14	95	24,379	3,903	6
Iowa	104	20,527	5,080	21	83	15,965	5,173	8
Kansas	107	26,119	4,112	24	64	22,409	2,860	12
Kentucky	198	31,941	6,191	15	192	52,610	3,655	19
Louisiana	118	39,100	3,012	17	235	45,932	5,106	15
Maine	56	7,695	7,319	19	38	6,236	6,115	9
Maryland	172	28,193	6,100	19	200	36,021	5,554	10
Massachusetts	614	70,913	8,654	39	214	37,694	5,670	10
Michigan	553	135,500	4,084	34	317	53,320	5,942	8

Minnesota	201	32,799	6,141	24	90	22,651	3,984	7
Mississippi	82	39,930	**2,066**	21	160	29,342	5,450	14
Missouri	205	47,303	4,340	20	130	38,378	3,383	10
Montana	27	5,100	5,230	15	21	3,723	5,566	6
Nebraska	69	14,453	4,802	28	50	12,013	4,188	9
Nevada	50	6,364	7,784	8	27	5,691	4,753	**3**
New Hampshire	32	8,748	3,673	45	13	4,163	3,238	6
New Jersey	270	42,001	6,432	19	583	42,534	***13,717***	8
New Mexico	80	22,408	3,584	23	58	13,303	4,338	9
New York	1,004	137,679	7,296	18	683	93,467	7,312	8
North Carolina	470	114,822	4,096	30	199	35,564	5,595	6
North Dakota	**15**	**4,698**	3,121	24	17	3,330	5,101	9
Ohio	745	100,099	7,443	20	263	68,795	3,826	9
Oklahoma	153	30,468	5,013	19	323	47,852	6,741	***19***
Oregon	95	22,627	4,133	17	114	9,951	11,468	4
Pennsylvania	650	119,836	5,421	28	265	46,325	5,723	6
Rhode Island	81	11,632	6,950	33	24	4,899	4,812	8
South Carolina	77	20,801	3,711	12	155	34,100	4,533	12
South Dakota	18	5,135	3,412	21	19	4,075	4,569	8
Tennessee	268	54,036	4,962	20	153	28,720	5,329	7
Texas	541	132,783	4,078	10	958	***280,012***	3,420	15
Utah	64	13,985	4,542	14	37	9,332	4,003	4
Vermont	40	8,477	4,669	**62**	23	5,860	3,926	18
Virginia	245	33,017	7,425	15	159	34,070	4,668	7
Washington	396	73,470	5,385	45	140	20,272	6,888	5
West Virginia	73	18,179	4,030	21	148	15,079	9,839	14
Wisconsin	414	66,001	6,270	37	193	47,359	4,069	13
Wyoming	21	6,270	3,323	41	12	**2,215**	5,524	6

Source: Authors' compilation of Meyers et al. (2011); U.S. Census Bureau (2000, 2007).

Note: Within columns, minimum values are marked in **bold**; maximum values are ***bolded and italicized***.

[a]Averages are unweighted fifty-state averages.

New York, and Rhode Island) have TDI programs that grant workers some wage replacement in conjunction with pregnancy and childbirth (see table 7.2). Because TDI programs operate within a disability framework, they only offer benefits related to pregnancy or childbirth; they pay no benefits to fathers caring for infants or to workers caring for ill family members.

Two of these five states—California and New Jersey—have also enacted paid family leave programs. Both programs grant infant-care leaves to mothers and fathers, and both grant family leaves for the care of seriously ill family members. A third state, Washington, recently enacted a paid family leave law as well, although it remains unfunded and will not be implemented until 2012. When Washington's program is up and running, it will grant short periods of paid leave to workers, but only to care for infants (see table 7.2).

Although the federal FMLA grants most workers the right to twelve weeks of unpaid family leave per year to care for infants or for ill family members, states also play an important role in unpaid family leave because several supplement the FMLA with more generous unpaid leave laws of their own (see table 7.2). Seventeen states currently extend FMLA protections to firms with fewer than fifty employees, lengthen the leave period to more than twelve weeks a year, relax the job tenure and hours requirement to less than twelve months and/or fewer than 1,250 hours, and/or broaden the definition of family members beyond child, spouse, or parent.

Some states extend unpaid leaves related to pregnancy or childbirth, some extend leave provisions for caring for seriously ill family members, and some do both. (In table 7.2, the former are reported as "maternity leave" and the latter as "family leave.") For example, Hawaii and Montana impose no firm size minimum for workers taking unpaid maternity leaves; Connecticut, Louisiana, and Tennessee extend the unpaid leave duration from three to four months; and Iowa, Montana, New Hampshire, and Washington have no work tenure requirements for maternity leaves. Maine extends unpaid leaves for care of coresident siblings (who are not covered by the FMLA), and Hawaii grants unpaid leaves to care for several uncovered categories of family members: nondependent adult children, grandparents, parents-in-law, grandparents-in-law, stepparents, and so-called reciprocal beneficiaries (persons who have declared their intent to marry but are not legally eligible to do so).

Foster Care

Nationwide, nearly half a million children are cared for in the public foster care system each year. More precisely, 495,816 children were in foster care on the last day of 2006, constituting 7.3 children per thousand (children under the age of eighteen).[3] However, that rate varies notably by state. Fewer than five children per thousand were in foster care in nine states (Utah, New Hampshire, Mississippi, Virginia, New Mexico, Idaho, South Carolina, Texas, and Louisiana) in 2006. In another nine states (West Virginia, Vermont, Alaska, Wyoming, Oregon, Rhode Island, Iowa, Oklahoma, and Nebraska), the prevalence was twice as high, with ten or more children per thousand in foster care (see table 7.3). Some of this variation can be explained by demographic, economic, social, and behavioral differences

TABLE 7.2 / Family Leave, 2010

	Paid Leave for Private-Sector Employees		Unpaid Leave: Extension of FMLA Rights				
	Paid Maternity Leave Benefits	Paid Family Leave Benefits	FMLA Expansion: Firm Size	FMLA Expansion: Leave Length	FMLA Expansion: Tenure or Hours Required	FMLA Expansion: Definition of Family Members Who Can Be Cared For
United States	No	No	FMLA: 50 or more employees	FMLA: 12 weeks	FMLA: 12 months and 1,250 hours	FMLA: child, spouse, parent
Alabama	No	No	No	No	No	No
Arizona	No	No	No	No	No	No
Arkansas	No	No	No	No	No	No
Arkansas	No	No	No	No		No
California[a]	Yes	Yes	No	No	No	Domestic partner and child of domestic partner; stepparent
Colorado	No	No	No	No	No	No
Connecticut	No	No	No	16 weeks (family and maternity)	1,000 hours (family and maternity)	Civil union partner; parent-in-law; stepparent
Delaware	No	No	No	No	No	No
Florida	No	No	No	No	No	No
Georgia	No	No	No	No	No	No
Hawaii	Yes	No	No firm size requirement (maternity leave)	No	6-month tenure regardless of hours (family leave); no tenure requirement (maternity leave)	Nondependent adult child; grandparent; parent-in-law; grandparent-in-law; stepparent; reciprocal beneficiary (persons who have declared their intent to marry but are ineligible legally)
Idaho	No	No	No	No	No	No
Illinois	No	No	No	No	No	No
Indiana	No	No	No	No	No	No

(Table continues on p. 156.)

TABLE 7.2 / *Continued*

| | Paid Leave for Private-Sector Employees | | Unpaid Leave: Extension of FMLA Rights | | | |
	Paid Maternity Leave Benefits	Paid Family Leave Benefits	FMLA Expansion: Firm Size	FMLA Expansion: Leave Length	FMLA Expansion: Tenure or Hours Required	FMLA Expansion: Definition of Family Members Who Can Be Cared For
Iowa	No	No	4 or more employees (maternity leave)	No	No tenure requirement (maternity leave)	No
Kansas	No	No	No	No	No	No
Kentucky	No	No	No	No	No	No
Louisiana	No	No	26 or more employees (maternity leave)	4 months (maternity leave)	No tenure requirement (maternity leave)	No
Maine	No	No	15 or more employees (family and maternity)	No	12-month tenure regardless of hours worked (family and maternity)	Domestic partner and child of domestic partner; nondependent adult child; sibling who lives with employee
Maryland	No	No	No	No	No	No
Massachusetts	No	No	6 or more employees (maternity leave)	No	Full-time employees with 3-month tenure (maternity)	No
Michigan	No	No	No	No	No	No
Minnesota	No	No	21 or more employees (family leave)	No	12-month tenure half-time (family leave)	No
Mississippi	No	No	No	No	No	No
Missouri	No	No	No	No	No	No

State					
Montana	No	No	No firm size requirement (maternity leave)	No tenure requirement (maternity leave)	No
Nebraska	No	No	No	No	No
Nevada	No	No	No	No	No
New Hampshire	No	No	6 or more employees (maternity leave)	No tenure requirement (maternity leave)	No
New Jersey[b]	Yes	Yes	No	No	Civil union partner and child of civil union partner; parent-in-law; stepparent
New Mexico	No	No	No	No	No
New York	Yes	No	No	No	No
North Carolina	No	No	No	No	No
North Dakota	No	No	No	No	No
Ohio	No	No	No	No	No
Oklahoma	No	No	No	No	No
Oregon	No	No	25 or more employees (family and maternity)	180-day tenure at 25 hours or more per week (family and maternity)	No
Pennsylvania	No	No	No	No	No
Rhode Island	Yes	Yes	13 weeks (family and maternity)	No	Nondependent adult child; parent-in-law
South Carolina	No	No	No	No	No
South Dakota	No	No	No	No	No
Tennessee	No	No	4 months (family and maternity)	No	No
Texas	No	No	No	No	No
Utah	No	No	No	No	No

(Table continues on p. 158.)

TABLE 7.2 / Continued

	Paid Leave for Private-Sector Employees		Unpaid Leave: Extension of FMLA Rights			
	Paid Maternity Leave Benefits	Paid Family Leave Benefits	FMLA Expansion: Firm Size	FMLA Expansion: Leave Length	FMLA Expansion: Tenure or Hours Required	FMLA Expansion: Definition of Family Members Who Can Be Cared For
Vermont	No	No	10 or more employees (family and maternity)	No	No	Civil union partner and child of civil union partner; nondependent adult child; parent-in-law
Virginia	No	No	No	No	No	No
Washington[c]	No	Yes	8 or more employees (maternity)	No	No tenure requirement (maternity leave)	Domestic partner and child of domestic partner
West Virginia	No	No	No	No	No	No
Wisconsin	No	No	No	No	1,000 hours (family and maternity)	Registered or unregistered domestic partner; parent-in-law
Wyoming	No	No	No	No	No	No

Source: Authors' compilation of National Partnership for Women and Families (2012); State of California / EDD (2010a); State of New Jersey / EPBAM (2010); State of New Jersey / DOLWD (2010b).

[a]California enacted paid family leave in 2002; it came into effect in 2004. The FMLA extension provisions reported here refer to the state's unpaid leave law, which predated the paid leave law and which remains in force. The state's paid leave law has no minimum enterprise size; it also has a less stringent tenure requirement than specified in the FMLA.

[b]New Jersey enacted paid family leave in 2008; it came into force in 2009. The FMLA extension provisions reported here refer to the state's unpaid leave law, which predated the paid leave law and which remains in force. The state's *paid* leave law has no minimum enterprise size; it also has a less stringent tenure requirement than specified in the FMLA.

[c]Washington enacted paid family leave (infant care only) in 2007; the program has not been funded.

TABLE 7.3 / Foster Care, 2004 to 2006

	Population in Foster Care on Last Day of Year (2006)	Children in Foster Care per 1,000 Children Under Age Eighteen (2006)	Children in Out-of-Home Care Who Were Placed in Kinship Care (2004)	Monthly Maintenance Payments: Regular Foster Care, Children Age Nine (2004)	Monthly Maintenance Payments: Specialized Foster Care, Children Age Nine (2004)	Children Waiting for Adoption As Percentage of Children in Foster Care (2006)	Adoptions As Percentage of Children in Foster Care Waiting for Adoption (2006)
United States[a]	495,816	7.3	19%	$450	$950	26%	42
Alabama	7,157	6.4	14	434	1,065	23	**23**
Alaska	1,919	10.7	30	580	808	38	29
Arizona	9,767	6.0	32	n/a	n/a	27	53
Arkansas	3,434	5.0	4	435	**2,625**	27	42
California	**76,405**	8.0	33	494	n/a	24	41
Colorado	8,139	7.0	14	n/a	n/a	26	46
Connecticut	6,359	7.8	19	**717**	2,496	21	48
Delaware	**1,074**	5.3	9	391	1,050	28	31
Florida	29,229	7.3	**44**	364	n/a	26	41
Georgia	13,175	5.4	14	405	n/a	17	54
Hawaii	2,357	7.9	39	529	570	32	53
Idaho	1,850	4.7	16	300	n/a	29	32
Illinois	18,815	5.8	34	n/a	n/a	16	57
Indiana	11,401	7.2	13	468	961	29	35
Iowa	9,040	12.7	**1**	n/a	n/a	16	69
Kansas	6,237	9.0	19	568	2,129	33	26
Kentucky	7,606	7.6	9	591	1,110	27	36
Louisiana	5,213	4.8	11	365	**365**	21	43

(Table continues on p. 160.)

TABLE 7.3 / *Continued*

	Population in Foster Care on Last Day of Year (2006)	Children in Foster Care per 1,000 Children Under Age Eighteen (2006)	Children in Out-of-Home Care Who Were Placed in Kinship Care (2004)	Monthly Maintenance Payments: Regular Foster Care, Children Age Nine (2004)	Monthly Maintenance Payments: Specialized Foster Care, Children Age Nine (2004)	Children Waiting for Adoption As Percentage of Children in Foster Care (2006)	Adoptions As Percentage of Children in Foster Care Waiting for Adoption (2006)
Maine	2,076	7.4	15	n/a	n/a	33	48
Maryland	9,051	6.6	33	n/a	n/a	n/a	n/a
Massachusetts	11,499	7.9	17	546	n/a	24	32
Michigan	20,142	8.1	32	n/a	n/a	31	42
Minnesota	6,827	5.4	21	524	524	20	49
Mississippi	3,126	4.1	32	355	700	29	28
Missouri	10,181	7.2	21	**277**	657	27	46
Montana	1,909	8.8	34	450	764	32	45
Nebraska	6,187	*13.9*	16	292	n/a	16	55
Nevada	5,068	8.0	20	n/a	n/a	36	24
New Hampshire	1,146	3.8	13	381	n/a	22	54
New Jersey	10,740	5.1	10	453	n/a	*44*	28
New Mexico	2,357	4.6	24	441	620	36	39
New York	29,973	6.6	17	504	1,007	27	35

North Carolina	11,115	5.2	22	$440	n/a	28	40
North Dakota	1,331	9.3	17	397	632	24	47
Ohio	16,631	6.0	15	n/a	n/a	24	45
Oklahoma	11,736	13.1	25	400	900	31	32
Oregon	10,661	12.4	21	393	568	26	39
Pennsylvania	21,135	7.5	19	n/a	n/a	17	54
Rhode Island	2,998	12.6	25	409	n/a	*13*	65
South Carolina	4,920	4.7	6	n/a	n/a	36	24
South Dakota	1,648	8.5	17	415	693	31	30
Tennessee	8,618	6.0	14	495	545	21	56
Texas	30,848	4.7	18	608	1,369	40	28
Utah	2,427	**3.1**	7	418	510	20	n/a
Vermont	1,379	10.3	9	571	900	18	65
Virginia	7,672	4.2	4	365	n/a	23	31
Washington	10,457	6.8	33	446	174	23	51
West Virginia	4,018	10.3	4	600	1,521	26	39
Wisconsin	7,459	5.7	31	329	n/a	16	**73**
Wyoming	1,304	10.8	15	400	400	16	27

Source: Authors' compilation of data from Child Welfare League of America (2005); U.S. Census Bureau (2007); U.S. Department of Health and Human Services/ACF/ACYF/CB (2009a, 2010).

Note: Within columns, minimum values are marked in **bold**; maximum values are ***bolded and italicized***.

n/a = not available

[a]U.S. value represents the unweighted fifty-state averages.

across states that affect the need for care, but some is clearly explained by variability in the performance of public foster care systems. However, drawing direct connections between the variation in foster care utilization and the specific practices of given states or localities is beyond the scope of this book.

That said, one especially consequential aspect of foster care policy varies markedly across the states and deserves attention, not least because it relates directly to income disparities: that is, the funding available to foster parents to provide for the children in their care. Recent research indicates that these so-called maintenance rates are often inadequate, particularly the regular (nonspecialized care) rates. Inadequate maintenance rates make it difficult to attract and retain high-quality foster care homes (National Association of Public Child Welfare Administrators 2007; DePanfilis et al. 2007). Maintenance payments vary widely from state to state (see table 7.3). In 2004 regular foster care payments for nine-year-old children average from $277 in Missouri to $717 in Connecticut. (These payment rates are cost-of-living-adjusted.) That same year, specialized foster care payments for nine-year-olds with special needs were substantially higher, averaging $980 a month across the states and ranging from less than $500 in Louisiana and Wyoming to more than $2,000 in Kansas, Connecticut, and Arkansas.

One of the most crucial and complex issues in foster care policy concerns the placement of children in kin care. Historically, many child welfare agencies were hesitant to embrace kin care, both because it makes adoption more difficult and because it was believed that children in kin care could remain vulnerable to abuse from their biological parents. However, child welfare analysts have increasingly called for expanding and supporting kin care options, on the grounds that kin care can lessen the trauma of removal, help maintain family connections, and add caregivers and flexibility to a system in which foster homes are often in limited supply, especially on short notice (Center for Law and Social Policy/ABA 2010). Policies promoting and supporting kin care have been adopted by many states, and a preference for it is stated in the 1996 federal welfare reform law (Jantz et al. 2002; Child Welfare League of America 2005; DiNitto and Cummins 2005; Geen 2004).

In 2004 kin care made up about one-fifth (19 percent) of all formal foster care placements nationwide. This percentage varied from 35 percent or more in Hawaii and Florida to less than 5 percent in Iowa, Arkansas, West Virginia, and Virginia (see table 7.3). These official foster care placements do not include the more than 2 million children nationwide living with relatives other than their parents in informal kinship care arrangements (Geen 2004).

States may use waivers and variances to relax foster care rules associated with federal (Title IV-E) payments in order to better incorporate kin care into their foster care programs—and many do. As of 2003, kin were required to meet the same standards as nonkin foster parents in only fifteen states, while twenty-three applied nonkin licensing standards to kin but waived or modified one or more standards for nonkin parents. Twelve of these states allowed waivers concerning minimum household space, eleven waived some or all training requirements, and eight waived minimum age requirements. A few waived requirements related to transportation resources (for example, owning a car), family structure, and educational attainment. Other states offered an entirely separate approval process for kin, which was almost always less stringent than that for nonkin (Geen 2003).

Unfortunately, relaxed licensing requirements for many kin foster parents often go hand in hand with lower maintenance payments—or none at all. Foster parents who do not meet all the Title IV-E licensing standards established in a state's plan are not eligible for federal foster care payments. States often use state or local funds to offer maintenance payments of their own, but these may not be equivalent to their maintenance payments for licensed caregivers (Center for Law and Social Policy/ABA 2010). In twenty-six states, at least some kin are not eligible to receive maintenance payments. Six states provide state-funded foster care payments to kin who meet standards that are different from those for nonkin foster parents (Geen 2003).

Finally, children in foster care face markedly different outcomes across the states with respect to their exit from the foster care system, particularly as regards adoption. In 2006, 26 percent of the children in foster care were designated as waiting to be adopted, ranging from as low as 13 percent in Rhode Island to as high as 44 percent in New Jersey. In that same year, across the states, 44 percent of children in foster care who were waiting for adoption were in fact adopted. Rates of adoption (among those waiting for adoption) also varied widely, from just under one-quarter (23 percent) in Alabama to a remarkably high three-quarters (73 percent) in Wisconsin (see table 7.3).

Very little research has been conducted on the factors that shape these cross-state differences in adoption rates out of foster care, so it is difficult to discern the extent to which policy variation across the states explains these widely varied outcomes. However, a team of social policy researchers recently surveyed state adoption managers about barriers to the adoption of children in the foster care system (Wilson, Katz, and Geen 2005). This survey, to which forty-three states responded, produced some tentative explanations and showed that states vary markedly with respect to several factors thought to be consequential. These include the number of public agency staff assigned to adoption, the structure of the outreach process, and the relative balance struck by state administrators between encouraging prospective parents and screening out those judged to be inappropriate.

Policies for Children with Disabilities

As discussed earlier, children's participation in Medicaid EPSDT and/or CHIP, and in the non-means-tested Early Intervention (IDEA: Part C) and Special Education programs (IDEA: Part B) is high, in part because these programs use a much broader definition of disability than adult programs and in part because enrollment is encouraged through the public school system. Nonetheless, there is still considerable variability in enrollemnt across states.

COMPREHENSIVE HEALTH CARE—MEDICAID EPSDT AND CHIP   Nationally, 36 percent of children age zero to eighteen are enrolled in Medicaid and/or CHIP (see table 7.4). However, statewide participation rates range from highs of 66 percent

TABLE 7.4 / Medicaid Programs for Children: Early and Periodic Screening, Diagnosis, and Treatment (EPSDT) and Children's Health Insurance Program (CHIP), 2007 to 2009

	Medicaid-CHIP Participation (FY 2007) As Percentage of Population Age Eighteen and Younger (2008–2009)	Medicaid-CHIP Participation As Percentage of Eligible Population (FY 2007)	Medicaid-CHIP Payments per Enrollee (FY 2007)	Income Eligibility Levels for Children's Regular Medicaid and Children's CHIP-Funded Medicaid Expansions As Percentage of Federal Poverty Level (2009)[b]		
				Infants Age Zero to One	Children Age One to Five	Children Age Six to Nineteen
United States[a]	36%	82%	$2,298	133%	133%	100%
Alabama	37	85	2,155	**133**	**133**	**100**
Alaska	38	74	**4,261**	150	150	150
Arizona	37	77	4,092	140	150	**100**
Arkansas	50	88	1,846	**133**	**133**	**100**
California	43	82	1,445	200	**133**	**100**
Colorado	25	69	1,723	**133**	**133**	**100**
Connecticut	32	85	2,527	185	185	185
Delaware	36	84	2,225	185	**133**	**100**
District of Columbia	**66**	**95**	2,740	185	**133**	**100**
Florida	34	70	1,665	185	**133**	**100**
Georgia	36	81	2,000	200	**133**	**100**
Hawaii	31	91	2,111	**133**	**133**	**100**
Idaho	30	74	1,728	**133**	**133**	**100**
Illinois	39	88	2,602	**133**	**133**	**100**
Indiana	35	81	1,899	**133**	**133**	**100**
Iowa	30	87	1,675	**133**	**133**	133
Kansas	27	81	2,234	150	**133**	**100**
Kentucky	36	90	2,399	185	**133**	**100**
Louisiana	52	89	**1,192**	**133**	**133**	**100**
Maine	43	92	2,698	**133**	**133**	125
Maryland	27	87	2,590	185	185	185
Massachusetts	29	**95**	4,064	185	**133**	114

State						
Michigan	41	90	1,622	185	150	150
Minnesota	30	81	2,714	275	275	275
Mississippi	45	81	1,659	185	**133**	**100**
Missouri	36	85	2,807	185	**133**	**100**
Montana	26	69	2,406	**133**	**133**	**100**
Nebraska	30	83	2,579	**133**	**133**	**100**
Nevada	19	**55**	1,938	**133**	**133**	**100**
New Hampshire	28	86	2,816	185	185	185
New Jersey	23	81	2,305	200	**133**	**100**
New Mexico	***56***	81	2,664	185	185	185
New York	42	89	2,344	200	**133**	**100**
North Carolina	35	85	2,525	200	200	**100**
North Dakota	23	75	1,908	**133**	**133**	**100**
Ohio	37	83	1,672	150	150	**100**
Oklahoma	44	81	2,251	**133**	**133**	**100**
Oregon	29	75	2,061	**133**	**133**	**100**
Pennsylvania	32	86	2,656	185	**133**	**100**
Rhode Island	37	84	***3,542***	185	**133**	**100**
South Carolina	40	79	2,036	150	**133**	**100**
South Dakota	35	82	2,182	**133**	**133**	**100**
Tennessee	46	87	2,165	185	**133**	**100**
Texas	37	75	2,400	185	**133**	**100**
Utah	**17**	66	2,434	**133**	**133**	**100**
Vermont	49	***94***	2,209	***300***	***300***	***300***
Virginia	23	81	2,015	**133**	**133**	**100**
Washington	38	83	1,927	200	200	200
West Virginia	45	89	2,348	150	150	**100**
Wisconsin	30	87	**1,269**	***300***	185	**100**
Wyoming	36	78	2,038	**133**	**133**	**100**

Source: Authors' compilation of data from Kaiser Family Foundation (2010).
Notes: Children are individuals from birth to age nineteen. Within columns, minimum values are marked in **bold**; maximum values are ***bolded and italicized***.
[a] Unweighted fifty-state averages.
[b] U.S. figure is the federal minimum eligibility level.

in the District of Columbia, 52 percent in Louisiana, and 49 percent in Vermont to lows of 19 percent in Nevada and 17 percent in Utah. The second column in table 7.4 reports the percentage of children eligible for public medical insurance who participate in the programs. That number ranges from a high of 95 percent in the District of Columbia and Massachusetts to the very low rate of 55 percent in Nevada. (Six more states—Hawaii, Kentucky, Maine, Massachusetts, Michigan, and Vermont—report participation rates of 90 percent or higher.)[4]

State-to-state differences in eligibility requirements and in the efforts made to enroll eligible candidates account for state variability in enrollment rates for eligible children.[5] Under Medicaid regulations, state Medicaid agencies must not only pay for preventive and corrective care for children but also ensure that children actually get needed care by providing administrative care management in concert with other public agencies—especially maternal and child health, other public health agencies and schools, and other means-tested programs such as the Supplemental Nutrition Assistance Program (SNAP, or food stamps). This outreach is effective: one study found a participation rate of 93.5 percent among eligible poor children who lived in households that received food stamps, compared to 72.9 percent among those who did not (Kenney et al. 2010). There is also a fairly high positive correlation between the proportion of schoolchildren who are receiving special education and the participation rate of eligible children in Medicaid. As explained in chapter 6, if a child enrolled in special education has special health care needs that are cited in the IEP, and that child is eligible for Medicaid, Medicaid must pay for treatment. Thanks to compulsory education and the universal entitlement to special education, children with special health care needs or disabilities have a very good chance of getting the care they need.

The data reported in table 7.4 on spending per enrollee captures average payments for all children enrolled in the Medicaid and CHIP programs. Medicaid-CHIP spending per enrollee in 2007 ranged from a high of $4,261 in Alaska (with Arizona, Massachusetts, and Rhode Island not far behind) to a low of $1,119 in Louisiana (followed closely by Wisconsin and California). No available public data disaggregate state spending on children enrolled in EPSDT and CHIP into those with disabilities and those without. But it seems likely that variation in per-enrollee spending across states derives from considerable variation in the level of services covered and the proportion of children with special health care needs enrolled in EPSDT (Kenney et al. 2010).[6]

Public insurance is especially critical for children with special health care needs. Even after controlling for age, race-ethnicity, income, gender, family structure, primary language, severity of limitation, and whether parents cut back or stopped working because of the child's condition, children who do not have public insurance are far more likely to report that they are unable to get the services they need (that is, to be underinsured), even if they have private insurance. Similarly, underinsurance rates are higher in states with more stringent Medicaid income eligibility requirements, which makes it more difficult to get public insurance. Children in states where the maximum income eligibility level is

100 percent of the federal poverty line are 24 percent more likely to be under-insured than children living in states where income eligibility is set at 200 percent of the FPL (Kogan et al. 2010).

The final three columns in table 7.4 report Medicaid income eligibility levels for EPSDT in each of three age groups. As discussed in the first section of this chapter on disparities in care by income, states must set EPSDT income eligibility require-ments at no more than 300 percent of the FPL. Income eligibility is higher for CHIP than for EPSDT in most states, because CHIP was meant to expand health insurance coverage to uninsured children, either as an expansion of the Medicaid program or as a separate program. However, children enrolled in CHIP do not receive the range of preventive, corrective, and personal care services included under EPSDT; those services have proven critical to the mainstreaming and education of children with disabilities in the most integrated setting possible (Rosenbaum 2008). EPSDT income eligibility levels are therefore a better indicator of the likelihood that children with special health care needs are adequately covered.

States offer targeted services through a wide variety of Medicaid waivers, for which eligibility may be limited to groups with specific disabilities or other char-acteristics. The utilization of waivers for specific populations varies widely across states. For example, of Colorado's eleven waivers, four are targeted to different groups of children, including two for children with developmental disabilities— one for children with autism spectrum disorders and one for children with physical disabilities. But in Florida, which has twelve waivers, none are targeted specifically to children (Kaiser Family Foundation 2010).

EARLY INTERVENTION AND SPECIAL EDUCATION   As shown in table 7.5, about 2.3 percent of infants and toddlers and 8.7 percent of school-age children were enrolled in early intervention and special education (IDEA) programs nationwide in 2004. Participation in early intervention programs among chil-dren under age three ranged from 7.1 percent (in Hawaii) to a low of 1.3 percent (in Alabama, the District of Columbia, Nevada, and Georgia). Enrollment in special education programs for children age three through twenty-one varied from a high of 12.2 percent (in the District of Columbia, closely trailed by Maine and Rhode Island) to a low of 6.7 and 6.8 percent (in California and Colorado). Nationally, 13.4 percent of public school children were in special education pro-grams, ranging from about one-fifth of students (19.7 percent) in Rhode Island to about one-tenth (10.1 percent) in Texas.

Federal support for special education is estimated by using a formula based on a combination of each state's prior funding level, its share of students receiv-ing special education, and its poverty rate (Parrish 2010).[7] Federal support per student does not vary dramatically across states, but the federal share of total spending on special education varies considerably because there is so much variation in state and local contributions. Total spending per pupil ranged from $8,196 in Mississippi to $34,529 in Hawaii, for a national average of $17,439. Other states with high expenditures per student included Connecticut, New Hampshire, New York, and Vermont. Notably, New York and Vermont were

TABLE 7.5 / Special Education and Early Intervention for Children: Individuals with Disabilities Education Act (IDEA): Parts B and C, 2004 to 2008

	Children (Birth to Age Three) Enrolled in Early Intervention Services (IDEA: Part C) As Percentage of Population (2004)	Students (Age Three to Twenty-Two) Enrolled in Special Education (IDEA: Part B) As Percentage of Population (2004)	Students Enrolled in Special Education As Percentage of Public School Enrollment (2007–2008)	Federal Special Education Appropriations per Student[a] (FY 2008)	Estimated Total Federal, State, and Local Spending per Special Education Student[b] (FY 2007–2008)	Federal Share As Percentage of Estimated Total Spending (2007–2008)[c]
United States	2.3%	8.7%	13.4%	$1,740	$17,439	10%
Alabama	1.3	8.0	11.4	2,175	17,439	12
Alaska	2.0	8.9	13.4	2,153	12,556	17
Arizona	1.5	7.5	12.1	1,435	17,613	8
Arkansas	2.9	9.4	13.8	1,756	14,474	12
California	1.8	6.7	10.6	1,873	15,172	12
Colorado	1.7	6.8	10.4	1,877	18,311	10
Connecticut	3.1	8.2	12.1	1,961	26,158	7
Delaware	3.1	9.1	15.9	1,804	17,962	10
District of Columbia	1.3	12.2	13.9	1,685	n/a	n/a
Florida	1.9	9.5	14.7	1,636	12,207	13
Georgia	1.3	8.1	11.5	1,733	19,008	9
Hawaii	7.1	7.1	11.4	2,008	34,529	6
Idaho	2.7	7.2	10.3	2,004	13,951	14
Illinois	2.9	9.5	15.2	1,605	20,404	8
Indiana	4.2	10.3	17.1	1,454	11,161	13

Iowa	2.1	9.9	14.3	1,789	21,973	8
Kansas	2.6	8.8	14.0	1,669	22,322	7
Kentucky	2.3	10.2	16.4	1,516	16,044	9
Louisiana	2.3	8.2	12.9	**2,179**	20,927	10
Maine	2.9	11.9	17.5	1,645	22,496	7
Maryland	2.8	7.6	12.4	1,954	22,671	9
Massachusetts	5.8	10.4	17.3	1,720	17,265	10
Michigan	2.2	8.9	14.0	1,714	13,079	13
Minnesota	1.5	8.6	14.2	1,632	22,496	7
Mississippi	1.7	8.6	13.3	1,851	**8,196**	**23**
Missouri	1.5	9.6	15.1	1,660	15,172	11
Montana	2.1	8.3	12.7	2,116	14,474	15
Nebraska	1.7	9.8	15.7	1,658	19,532	8
Nevada	**1.3**	7.6	11.3	1,472	17,090	9
New Hampshire	2.7	9.5	16.1	1,511	28,251	**5**
New Jersey	2.2	10.9	18.1	1,461	23,368	6
New Mexico	3.4	9.7	14.1	1,997	17,265	12
New York	4.3	9.3	16.4	1,715	28,600	6
North Carolina	1.7	8.7	12.9	1,714	15,172	11
North Dakota	2.8	9.2	14.3	2,104	20,055	10
Ohio	1.8	8.7	14.8	1,641	14,300	11
Oklahoma	2.0	10.2	14.8	1,567	17,962	9
Oregon	1.6	8.4	13.8	1,675	14,126	12
Pennsylvania	3.1	9.2	16.3	1,477	19,357	8
Rhode Island	3.6	11.9	**19.7**	1,562	21,101	7
South Carolina	1.4	10.2	14.6	1,729	14,126	12
South Dakota	2.8	8.6	14.8	1,904	18,485	10
Tennessee	1.7	8.3	12.5	1,956	13,951	14
Texas	1.8	7.9	**10.1**	2,069	12,033	17

(Table continues on p. 170.)

TABLE 7.5 / Continued

	Children (Birth to Age Three) Enrolled in Early Intervention Services (IDEA: Part C) As Percentage of Population (2004)	Students (Age Three to Twenty-Two) Enrolled in Special Education (IDEA: Part B) As Percentage of Population (2004)	Students Enrolled in Special Education As Percentage of Public School Enrollment (2007–2008)	Federal Special Education Appropriations per Student[a] (FY 2008)	Estimated Total Federal, State, and Local Spending per Special Education Student[b] (FY 2007–2008)	Federal Share as Percentage of Estimated Total Spending (2007–2008)[c]
Utah	1.8	7.8	10.9	1,757	12,556	14
Vermont	3.2	9.2	n/a	n/a	29,123	n/a
Virginia	1.8	9.0	13.7	1,703	20,927	8
Washington	1.7	7.7	12.0	1,834	14,474	13
West Virginia	3.3	12.0	16.9	1,625	15,172	11
Wisconsin	2.8	9.0	14.5	1,693	17,788	10
Wyoming	4.0	10.3	16.5	2,048	15,869	13

Source: Authors' compilation of data from U.S. Department of Education/NCES/IES (2009), tables 35, 52, 178, and 182; U.S. Department of Education/OSERS/OSEP (2009), tables 1 through 10; Parrish et al. (2004); Parrish (2010); and Chambers, Parrish, and Harr (2004).

n/a = not available.

[a] Includes grants to states, preschool grants, and grants for infants and families (Titles B and C).

[b] Estimated as total national spending per enrolled student (U.S. Department of Education/NCES/IES 2009, tables 178 and 35) multiplied by the ratio of the cost to educate special education students to the cost to educate regular students (Parrish et al. 2004), multiplied by the index of relative state spending (Parrish 2010). Per pupil expenditures to educate special education students = average spending per regular student in 1999–2000 multiplied by the inflation factor multiplied by the ratio of spending on special education to regular students. Average spending per regular student in 1999–2000 = $6,556 (Chambers, Parrish, and Harr 2004, exhibit 2 and table B.3); the inflation factor of 1.40 is estimated by total expenditures per pupil in fall enrollment in 2006–2007 divided by total expenditures per pupil in fall enrollment in 1999–2000, in unadjusted dollars (U.S. Department of Education/NCES 2009, table 182). Ratio of spending per special education student to spending per regular student:

1.9 (Chambers et al. 2004, 5). The number of special education students in 2006–2007 is based on column 1.

[c] "Federal Special Education Appropriation per Student" divided by "Estimated Total Federal, State, and Local Spending per Student" (column 4 divided by column 5).

among the states that used Medicaid funds to finance significant amounts of state spending on special education.

Policies for Adults with Disabilities and the Frail Elderly

Assessing the adequacy of long-term care supports is difficult, but three principle metrics help to clarify the picture: the number of people served relative to the population; the amount spent per program participant in each state; and the balance between home- and community-based and institutional care. All three metrics vary widely across the states both for adults with intellectual and developmental disabilities (ID/DD) and for those with non-ID/DD disabilities.

LONG-TERM CARE FOR ADULTS WITH DISABILITIES OTHER THAN ID/DD AND THE FRAIL ELDERLY In 2006, 10.8 elders and people with disabilities for every thousand in the national population were receiving long-term care services (see table 7.6). Some states, such as Utah, Nevada, and Virginia, provided well below average coverage at only 3.3 to 5.4 people per thousand, while others, such as Arkansas (18.9), New York (16.1), Minnesota (14.4), and California (13.8), covered far more than the national average. States also spent hugely different amounts per participant on long-term services and supports in 2006, ranging from a low of $12,912 in Alabama and Arkansas to a high of $63,812 in Alaska. Variation in actual per-participant spending across states depends both on differences in the amount spent per participant in the same type of setting (nursing homes or non-institutional settings) and on variation in the proportion of long-term care provided in each setting. To capture a measure of relative spending that controls for the latter, state spending per participant is measured as the average spending per participant in each setting, weighted by the national average share of participants in each setting (47 percent in home- and community-based services [HCBS] and 53 percent in nursing homes). Nationally, the weighted average spent per Medicaid participant was $20,451.

Most states moved significantly away from their almost total reliance on nursing homes in the 1960s to a more balanced system that includes extensive agency-provided home care services. The last decade has seen a movement to expand consumer-directed care as well. In consumer-directed care programs, care recipients have the option to control their own service budgets and/or to hire, fire, and supervise their care providers. By 2008, fourteen states offered consumer-directed home care as an alternative to agency-supplied services under the state personal care services (PCS) option, and thirty-five offered some consumer direction through HCBS waivers (Harrington, Ng, and Watts 2009). In other states, consumer direction is being introduced through demonstration projects. The Cash and Counseling program, for example, offers a cash budget that Medicaid consumers can use to pay for a combination of home modifications, assistive devices, or personal care and homemaking services.[8]

Though all states have made at least some progress in this area, there is huge variability among them in terms of the balance between institutional and non-institutional care, as reported in table 7.6. In five states (Alaska, California, Idaho,

TABLE 7.6 / Medicaid Long-Term Services and Supports, for Adults Eighteen to Sixty-Four with Disabilities Other Than Intellectual and Developmental Disabilities and Adults Age Sixty-Five and Over, 2006 to 2008

| | Long-Term Care Participants per 1,000 Population (2006) | Spending per Participant, Weighted Average of Nursing Home and HCBS[a] (2006) | Percentage of Home- and Community-Based Services in Total Long-Term Care | | Spending per State Resident (2008) |
			Participants (2006)	Spending (2008)	
United States	10.8	$20,451	47%	27%	$220
Alabama	7.7	$12,912	26	11	$201
Alaska	13.1	63,812	86	63	293
Arizona[b]	n/a	n/a	n/a	n/a	n/a
Arkansas	18.9	12,912	46	21	250
California	13.8	19,261	69	51	210
Colorado	7.0	18,943	48	23	132
Connecticut	15.0	21,853	25	9	392
Delaware	5.8	30,808	27	9	221
District of Columbia	13.0	30,125	44	40	513
Florida	8.7	14,005	27	12	149
Georgia	5.9	21,850	27	19	170
Hawaii	5.6	30,948	31	19	212
Idaho	11.6	18,787	70	39	169
Illinois	9.8	14,063	42	24	151
Indiana	8.3	15,328	8	5	206
Iowa	10.5	15,136	34	16	186
Kansas	11.7	15,647	48	36	200
Kentucky	9.5	17,342	29	8	205
Louisiana	10.3	15,201	28	27	222
Maine	14.1	19,813	53	24	249
Maryland	6.1	27,188	24	12	201
Massachusetts	12.3	25,837	29	21	314
Michigan	11.8	17,684	55	19	183
Minnesota	14.4	21,496	58	51	313

Mississippi	11.9	16,704	34	1	244
Missouri	18.8	13,329	65	30	205
Montana	10.6	20,956	49	28	220
Nebraska	10.2	22,001	37	19	231
Nevada	5.4	21,191	64	35	96
New Hampshire	7.7	29,146	28	15	268
New Jersey	8.7	29,213	38	20	267
New Mexico	10.4	22,995	64	**64**	242
New York	16.1	29,613	34	29	**525**
North Carolina	12.5	19,566	61	41	201
North Dakota	12.5	18,548	28	9	287
Ohio	11.9	21,451	29	18	269
Oklahoma	12.7	14,959	52	29	205
Oregon	11.4	20,720	76	53	184
Pennsylvania	8.8	34,552	23	11	349
Rhode Island	13.0	21,041	22	13	323
South Carolina	6.7	20,051	44	23	145
South Dakota	9.7	15,587	26	8	187
Tennessee	5.8	20,752	**5**	**4**	174
Texas	11.6	13,193	64	33	118
Utah	**3.3**	14,963	30	12	**68**
Vermont	15.5	14,057	41	32	268
Virginia	5.4	21,078	32	30	136
Washington	12.1	19,733	72	59	213
West Virginia	11.8	24,522	47	19	302
Wisconsin	12.4	20,381	50	28	218
Wyoming	8.5	15,806	36	16	155

Sources: Authors' compilation of Burwell, Sredl, and Eiken (2009); Harrington, Carillo, and Blank (2009); and Harrington, Ng, and Watts (2009).
Note: Within columns, minimum values are marked in **bold**; maximum values are ***bolded and italicized.***

n/a = not available.

[a]Per-participant spending is the state average per-participant spending on nursing homes weighted by the national average share of participants in nursing homes (53 percent) plus the state average per-participant spending on HCBS weighted by the national average share of participants in HCBS (47 percent).

[b]Data for Arizona are not available. Medical care for older adults is provided through a managed care program, which includes both acute and long-term care services. Data are not published for these services separately.

Washington, and Oregon), more than two-thirds of people receiving paid long-term care live in their own homes or in community settings. In Tennessee and Indiana, in contrast, fewer than 10 percent of Medicaid long-term care recipients receive home- and community-based services (Howes 2010; Harrington et al. 2009). In Alaska, fully 86 percent of adult long-term care recipients receive HCBS, compared to the national average of 47 percent (Harrington, Ng, and Watts 2009; Harrington et al. 2009).

If tipping the balance toward the use of HCBS has increased the choices and autonomy available to Medicaid consumers, it has also helped slow the growth of per capita costs in states. For example, California and Rhode Island have similar levels of participation in Medicaid-provided long-term care (13.8 per thousand and 13 per thousand, respectively) and of spending per participant ($19,261 and $21,041, respectively), after controlling for differences in the mix between institutional and non-institutional care. Yet because California has a far larger share of people in home care (69 percent of its participants, compared to 22 percent for Rhode Island), it spends far less per state resident on Medicaid long-term care services: $210 compared to Rhode Island's $323.

LONG-TERM CARE FOR ADULTS WITH INTELLECTUAL AND DEVELOPMENTAL DISABILITIES   In 2007, 328.3 people with intellectual and developmental disabilities for every 100,000 in the U.S. population were getting services—again, with a significant variation across states.[9] Four states (Texas, Georgia, Alabama, and Tennessee) provided services to fewer than 150 per 100,000, while eight (Alaska, California, Iowa, Idaho, Massachusetts, Minnesota, New York, and Vermont) provided services to more than 450 per 100,000 (see table 7.7). On the national level, only 6 percent of those with mental disabilities received paid care through these programs, with state averages ranging from 2 percent in Alabama, Kentucky, Mississippi, Tennessee, and Texas to 20 percent in Idaho. Even after controlling for differences in settings, the average amount that states spent on each participant in 2007 varied enormously, from a low of $28,476 in California to a high of $111,310 in Delaware.

As discussed in chapter 6, great progress has been made in recent years in deinstitutionalizing people with intellectual and development disabilities. As of 2007, only 6 percent—61,000—of the 990,000 beneficiaries of publicly funded services were living in residences with sixteen or more residents, including 38,000 in large state hospitals (down from 228,000 in state hospitals in 1967). But a person's likelihood of remaining in a large institution is still high in certain states. In 2007, 38 percent of people in Mississippi with intellectual and development disabilities were housed in five large state hospitals with 100 to 400 residents each, as were 22 percent of those in Texas and 30 percent in Arkansas. By contrast, seven states have eliminated large institutions entirely in favor of small residential settings and family homes (Prouty, Alba, and Lakin 2008).

State policies also vary enormously in unmet need for home- and community-based care for persons with intellectual and developmental disabilities. As of the end of 2007, residential service capacity for persons who wanted to live outside

TABLE 7.7 / Medicaid Long-Term Services and Supports for Adults with Intellectual and Developmental Disabilities, 2007

	Participants per 100,000 Population	Persons with Mental Disabilities Receiving Services	Spending per Participant (Including Residential and Home and Community-Based Services)	Participants in Family Homes	Participants in Small Residential Settings	Participants in Large Residential Settings	Spending per State Resident
United States	328.3	6%	$55,015	52%	41%	6%	$166
Alabama	140.1	2	52,378	49	48	3	67
Alaska	629.2	12	70,252	82	18	0	152
Arizona	403.6	9	30,934	84	15	1	113
Arkansas	192.8	3	48,198	29	41	30	156
California	474.4	10	28,476	69	28	3	140
Colorado	219.7	5	41,029	37	62	1	94
Connecticut	386.4	9	80,395	57	37	6	380
Delaware	341.5	7	111,310	66	30	5	175
District of Columbia	331.5	6	78,660	31	69	0	179
Florida	270.9	5	35,733	72	22	6	91
Georgia	126.1	3	36,150	50	41	9	54
Hawaii	257.5	6	42,256	67	33	0	124
Idaho	1016.2	20	50,197	74	23	3	185
Illinois	246.3	6	51,182	35	45	19	134
Indiana	227.5	4	51,968	26	71	3	175
Iowa	458.1	9	38,094	37	51	12	250
Kansas	264.2	5	40,768	34	60	6	164
Kentucky	151.8	2	88,333	38	52	10	84
Louisiana	352.4	5	51,656	54	34	13	198
Maine	274.5	4	104,105	9	90	1	313

(Table continues on p. 176.)

TABLE 7.7 / *Continued*

	Participants per 100,000 Population	Persons with Mental Disabilities Receiving Services	Spending per Participant (Including Residential and Home and Community-Based Services)	Participants in Family Homes	Participants in Small Residential Settings	Participants in Large Residential Settings	Spending per State Resident
Maryland	173.1	4	52,987	25	72	3	132
Massachusetts	485.5	10	71,689	64	33	3	221
Michigan	334.3	6	44,360	49	50	0	115
Minnesota	540.2	12	62,837	49	48	3	334
Mississippi	175.5	2	65,151	34	27	38	132
Missouri	246.3	4	52,495	56	36	8	122
Montana	432.1	8	35,668	56	42	2	123
Nebraska	212.3	5	53,614	12	73	15	153
Nevada	158.2	4	55,428	64	34	2	54
New Hampshire	171.5	3	44,201	22	77	1	152
New Jersey	424.8	10	88,176	69	20	10	186
New Mexico	167.1	3	69,290	33	67	0	177
New York	641.9	13	97,257	64	34	3	453
North Carolina	294.6	5	66,811	56	35	9	162
North Dakota	418.7	10	33,890	28	66	6	323

Ohio	341.6	6	61,577	47	42	11	236
Oklahoma	256.1	4	56,100	54	33	13	143
Oregon	299.8	5	40,234	49	50	1	152
Pennsylvania	413.5	8	58,796	***100***	**0**	**0**	214
Rhode Island	281.3	5	80,661	29	70	1	285
South Carolina	395.7	7	51,530	73	21	5	126
South Dakota	378.8	9	37,452	26	69	6	166
Tennessee	146.3	**2**	90,876	42	50	8	153
Texas	**116.5**	**2**	56,810	18	60	22	89
Utah	185.9	4	35,916	39	46	15	87
Vermont	457.4	7	51,020	51	49	0	208
Virginia	214.0	5	71,904	59	32	9	112
Washington	321.9	6	42,279	66	28	6	117
West Virginia	247.7	3	61,097	56	43	1	182
Wisconsin	364.0	8	40,876	30	65	5	162
Wyoming	410.0	8	49,859	35	61	4	239

Sources: Authors' compilation of Prouty et al. (2008) and U.S. Census Bureau (2009b).

Notes: Within columns, minimum values are marked in **bold**; maximum values are ***bolded and italicized.*** Participants include some children, all adults, and some older adults; long-term care services for most children with intellectual and development disabilities are covered under Early and Periodic Screening, Diagnosis, and Treatment (EPSDT); some older adults move from ID/DD programs to those aimed at persons over sixty-five when they become eligible. Most children live at home; only 1,600 children were living in large institutions in 2007 (Prouty, Alba, and Lakin 2008); only 6.2 percent of out-of-home placements were children in 2005 (Lakin et al. 2009); children represent only a small percentage of the population in this table.

their family home, either in their own home or in a congregate care setting, would have had to expand by 46 percent nationwide to clear the waiting lists (not shown in table 7.7). In Washington, capacity would have had to expand by only 4 percent, and there were no waiting lists at all in many other states, including New York and Rhode Island. In contrast, Texas, Indiana, and Ohio would all have had to triple capacity to clear their waiting lists (Prouty, Alba, and Lakin 2008). The great volume of complaints against states that have been filed with the U.S. Department of Justice since the Supreme Court's 1999 *Olmstead v. L.C.* decision offers poignant testimony to the inadequacy of home- and community-based services (Ng, Wong, and Harrington 2009).

Just as with long-term care for the elderly and for younger adults with disabilities, per capita costs to the state vary depending on how many people are covered, how adequate the coverage is, and what percentage of the program recipients are living in home- and community-based settings rather than in larger institutions. For example, though Maine and Minnesota each spend just over $300 per state resident on services for people with intellectual and developmental disabilities, Minnesota is able to serve twice as many people because 49 percent of its program participants live in family homes, in contrast to just 9 percent of Maine's.

SUMMARY

Our first conclusion is that money matters. People at all income levels are served by various care policies in the United States, but the adequacy of the supports available to those in need of care and to their families varies dramatically depending on their household income. The affluent turn to private markets and generally have access to higher-quality care services, have more options, and are able to preserve more of their independence and autonomy. The poor linger on waiting lists until rationed care becomes available or rely on means-tested public programs for care that is often meager or low-quality and more likely than privately financed care to be institutional. Middle-income families frequently face the most limited options, since they lack the resources to buy private care yet earn too much to qualify for means-tested public programs. If they cannot afford the long-term supports and services that they need, they must spend themselves and their immediate family members into (income and asset) poverty in order to qualify for Medicaid. And when they do, their choice of services in many states is limited to nursing homes.

One exception to the rule that better services and more autonomy can be purchased in the private market is Medicaid's EPSDT program, which requires states to provide an exceptionally broad range of services to low-income children in order to ensure that they all receive needed health care services and that those who have developmental delays or other disabilities get early intervention and treatment to increase their chances of succeeding in school and in later life. Services are delivered in child care centers and in prekindergarten and elementary and secondary schools, greatly increasing the likelihood that they will reach their targets. Because EPSDT provides for preventive care as well as treatment, and for both acute and long-term care needs, it is perhaps the closest that we have to a model of adequate health care, but it is not available to middle- and higher-income children. The private medical insurance system that these children and their families are left to rely on is not designed to provide the diagnosis and early treatment needed by children with developmental delays or disabilities. Recognizing this fact, a few states have expanded eligibility for EPSDT into the middle class, setting higher income eligibility thresholds or disregarding family income that would be spent on care services.

Our second conclusion is that geography matters. Policies that shape the adequacy of ECEC, family leave, foster care, and services and supports for children, frail elders, and adults with disabilities vary sharply across the fifty states. Most of the care policies under consideration are financed through federal-state partnerships, or at the state level. Although federal support is critical for these programs, states nevertheless spend about one-third of their budgets on care services, including ECEC, early intervention and special education services, comprehensive medical services for children with developmental delays or disabilities, foster care, and long-term care supports and services for adults who need personal assistance. A significant portion of the federal support for various care services comes through nondedicated funding streams such as TANF and the Social Services Block Grant. As a consequence, ECEC, foster care, and some services for the elderly and younger adults with disabilities compete for limited resources at the state level. State supplemental funding for these services competes with funding for schools and infrastructure.

Many states try to limit demand for care services, using a well-worn set of tools. They may set caps on expenditures and enrollment, maintain long waiting lists even for entitlements, or set high copayments to discourage service use. Some states offer a limited array of relatively appealing services, while others set unusually low income and asset thresholds for eligibility. Some observed differences in policy outcomes are certainly attributable to factors other than policy variation, such as demographic and workforce differences across states. However, dramatic cross-state variations in policy rules also play a significant role in producing marked geographic disparities in the receipt of care services in the United States.

Despite the temptation for all states to cut costs by limiting services, some states are relatively generous in providing support for care in one or more policy areas. These states may in some cases provide significantly more generous benefits than the national average, may have substantially higher participation rates, or may make more choices available to families in terms of the types and settings of services supported. For low-income parents of young children in Vermont, for example, the likelihood of receiving child care assistance subsidies or of having one's child enrolled in Head Start or a publicly supported prekindergarten program is twice the national average. Moreover, Vermont has expanded unpaid family leave, allowing workers in small firms to take job-protected leaves and extending the definition of family members to include civil union partners for purposes of caring leaves. Foster care monthly maintenance payments in Vermont are among the highest in the country. In terms of providing health care benefits for children, Vermont is the only state that sets the income threshold for EPSDT eligibility at the maximum allowable 300 percent of the federal poverty line ($54,930 for a family of three in 2010) for all children younger than nineteen. Vermont is also relatively generous in its policies with regard to serving adults with disabilities and older adults; the state is in the top tier in terms of rates of receipt of publicly funded long-term supports and services among these two populations.

As might be expected, this sort of policy generosity with regard to care is most common in northeastern and Pacific coast states, but is not restricted to them. In addition to the "usual suspects," such as New York, Washington, California, and Massachusetts, other states, including Alaska, Minnesota, and Oklahoma, are among the states that are particularly generous in many (although not all) of the care policy areas discussed in this volume. Some states simply exhibit generosity in terms of higher expenditures per recipient or policies that provide expanded access to services, but policy innovation also plays a significant role. Many of these states are particularly innovative in the design and implementation of their programs, and many offer a range of options for families, such as encouraging kinship care in the foster care sphere or providing access to long-term care choices through home- and community-based services.

On the other hand, another set of states—including mostly (but not only) southern and western states such as Alabama, Nevada, Tennessee, and Utah—are generally problematic places to live with respect to the availability of supports for care of children, the disabled, and the frail elderly. For working parents who need help obtaining child care, families of children with special health care needs, those responsible for caring for an ill family member, and those in need of long-term supports and services, these states, among others, provide relatively meager benefits. These less generous states consistently fall into the bottom tier in take-up and spending in most of the care support programs discussed here and, unsurprisingly, also tend to have care policies that are less expansive and less innovative with regard to eligibility, access, and choice.

Although there are clearly some states that are consistently generous in their care policies and some that are consistently less generous, perhaps more notable than the policy variation *between* states is the policy variation *within* states. For example, some states are particularly generous in some of the care policy areas outlined earlier but particularly restrictive in others. These disconnects between policy areas belie the straightforward conclusion that some states are simply more generous with regard to care supports and others simply less so. Some states are particularly generous in one policy area; Georgia, for example, is a leading state in implementing universal prekindergarten but is less generous in other care policy areas. Some states, such as Maryland and Texas, seem to prioritize the needs of children and parents, while providing relatively meager support to the elderly and disabled. Others, such as Maine and Oregon, seem to have the reverse priorities. In some states, there is no consistent policy with regard to children as opposed to the elderly and disabled; for example, Florida is one of the most generous states in terms of care policy for the disabled and foster children, but one of the least generous in terms of care of the frail elderly and support for child care. Moreover, there is often a disconnect within policy areas; for example, spending per beneficiary may be high, but the take-up of benefits among eligible residents may be low. To the extent that benefits and take-up are determined by state policies and administration, these disconnected policy features may indicate a lack of consistency in state policy design and implementation.

The strengths and limitations of our care policies provide clues to what a better care system would entail. Although our country's federalism provides the opportunity to learn from diverse types of policies, the states do not always move quickly to build on the experiences of their more successful neighbors. Residents of many states remain vulnerable to significant shortfalls in care provision, and current policies exert an uneven impact across lines of both income and geography, with unfortunate consequences for caregivers as well as care recipients. Improving access to care and the quality of care will require national policy reform.

NOTES

1. As in chapter 6, we use the term "early childhood education and care" to encompass two types of programs: child care programs, which are primarily intended to provide substitutes for parental care, and early education programs, such as Head Start and prekindergarten programs, which have an explicit educational purpose.
2. In their study of state preschool programs, Barnett et al. (2009) reported that as of 2008–2009, thirty-eight states funded public prekindergarten programs separate from special education services and Head Start. Of these, thirty-two states imposed income requirements. Although the income requirement is set at the federal poverty line in some states, more typically it is set higher, often between 185 and 300 percent of the federal poverty line.
3. This estimate of the number of children in foster care differs modestly from the estimate reported in chapter 6. This may be partly because the two estimates come from different sources, but the more important factor is probably the difference in time periods, as the small decline between 2006 and 2008 is consistent with widespread reports of declining foster care caseloads.
4. There are some regional patterns. Five of the six states in the New England census division were in the top two quintiles. No mountain or west-north-central states were in the top quintile. Seven of the ten states in the lowest quintile were in the west region, and five were in the mountain division of the west region (Kenney et al. 2010).
5. There are also fewer eligible children in states with higher income levels and lower poverty rates.
6. Using pooled data from the 2002 to 2005 Medical Expenditure Panel Survey, Genevieve Kenney, Joel Ruhter, and Thomas Seldon (2009) found that annual expenditures on children in the highest spending decile of EPSDT/CHIP enrollees was more than seven times that of mean spending, and thirty-five times that of median spending on children. Sixty-six percent of children in the top decile had special health care needs, and 68 percent had chronic conditions, roughly three times the rate of the rest of the EPSDT/CHIP enrollees. The top spending decile of children accounted for 72 percent of all EPSDT/CHIP spending.

7. The U.S. Department of Education does not maintain data that can be used to compare total spending on special education across states. However, Parrish (2010) has developed a method for estimating expenditures based on employment costs, which he argues represent about 85 percent of total costs (Parrish, personal communication, November 3, 2010). Using his index of relative expenditures across states, we have estimated spending per capita in each state.

8. The Cash and Counseling program, jointly sponsored by the Robert Wood Johnson Foundation, the Assistant Secretary for Policy and Evaluation and the Administration on Aging, made initial grants to seventeen states over a ten-year period. Many of these states have continued to support the program.

9. Most discussions of disability policy for intellectual and developmental disabilities report coverage as number of participants per 100,000 population, while most discussions of long-term care services for aged adults and adults with disabilities report coverage as number of participants per 1,000 population.

Chapter 8

A Care Policy and Research Agenda

Nancy Folbre, Candace Howes, and Carrie Leana

In preceding chapters, we have developed a unified analysis of unpaid and paid care for three groups with particularly intense needs: children, individuals with disabilities, and the frail elderly. We have shown that the costs of care provision continue to be divided unequally between men and women, and that shortfalls in public support for care provision reduce living standards and intensify social inequality. In this conclusion, we summarize our analysis of care work and explain its implications for public policy. We also outline an agenda for policy-relevant research.

THE IMPORTANCE OF CARE WORK

We have offered three theoretical reasons for an emphasis on care work as an important category of analysis and a significant sector of the economy:

- Care work has distinctive features that make intrinsic motivation and emotional attachment particularly consequential. Indeed, we define care work as work whose quality is likely to be affected by the caregiver's concern for the well-being of the care recipient.

- Care work contributes to the development and maintenance of human capabilities that represent a "public good." Human capabilities have intrinsic value and also yield important positive spillovers for living standards, quality of life, and sustainable economic development.

- The family, community, market, and state are all important sites of care provision, and with good reason: we cannot rely entirely on familial or community altruism, on market forces, or on public support. We need to devise ways to improve and coordinate care provision through all four types of institutions.

We have offered empirical substantiation and illustration of this approach to care work by demonstrating that:

- Survey data (including the nationally representative American Time Use Survey) can be used to categorize and measure inputs of unpaid care.
- Conventional labor force categories of "industry" and "occupation" illustrate both differences and similarities in paid care employment.
- Both labor hours and imputed market values can be used to trace shifts in care provision across time, examine relative quantities of labor inputs, and explore interactions across the unpaid-paid boundary.
- Federal and state care policies can be defined and critically assessed as a package, which implies the possibility of building political coalitions to improve them.

The Increasing Cost of Care

Continuing increases in the costs of care are likely to drive attention to this sector of the economy. Early childhood education is now widely considered a necessity for children; regardless of maternal employment, enrollment rates are high. The incidence of some childhood disabilities, such as autism and asthma, has increased in recent years.[1] The aging of the population has combined with increases in average life expectancy to increase the likelihood that an elderly family member will suffer a debilitating injury or illness. Medicare and Medicaid pay some of the bills, but they do not adequately cover long-term care. Women's increased participation in paid employment has reduced the time they devote to unpaid work, partly by making the costs of such work (such as forgone wages) more visible, and has also led to increases in men's unpaid work, perhaps enhancing their appreciation of both its benefits and its costs.

The advent of new information technologies has belied the predictions of economist William Baumol (1967) that the cost of services would inevitably grow faster than the costs of manufacturing. However, the very definition of care work dictates less substitutability between capital and labor and less potential for cost savings from automation and offshoring than in other forms of work. The price of care services has risen more rapidly than personal consumption expenditures (Folbre 2008c). Technological innovation may have the potential to improve the quality of care services, but it is unlikely to substantially reduce cost escalation, because most vulnerable individuals will continue to require hands-on, face-to-face, personal, and emotional attention.

The Distribution of the Costs of Care

Care provision imposes costs and risks on those who provide it, whether in unpaid or paid form. Rather than taking norms and preferences relevant to the supply of care as a given, researchers should ask how such norms and preferences are socially constructed. Some important aspects of contemporary feminist discourse can be interpreted as an effort to individually and collectively renegotiate the distribution of the costs of care between men and women. For instance, feminists challenge the notion that caring is a "naturally" feminine obligation and raise issues of fairness within the family. Likewise, feminists support policies such as publicly subsidized child care and paid family leaves that shift some of the costs of family care away from women toward taxpayers in general.

Negotiations over the cost of care call attention to other dimensions of collective conflict over the distribution of costs of care, including conflict between rich and poor, high-wage and low-wage workers, citizens and noncitizens, old and young, and those with and without dependents. Social insurance for care provision is efficient because it helps pool risks, but some individuals will always have more to gain from it than others. As the role of the public sector in care provision for children and the elderly grows—along with public subsidies for health care—the scope for distributional conflict intensifies, often leading to political stalemate.

The needs of children are often pitted against the needs of elders and people with disabilities. In an effort to counter this polarization, policy could focus instead on principles of lifetime productivity, risk pooling, and shared commitments to the well-being of dependents. To this end, we need to develop stronger principles of public responsibility and a better picture of intergenerational as well as cross-sectional flows of time and money (Generations United 2010). We also need to improve the economic efficiency, sustainability, and fairness of our larger care system.

In the United States, in particular, several dimensions of collective conflict intersect in ways that help explain why many low-income families face a care crisis. Many single mothers work in jobs that provide little or no flexibility to tend to family needs, resulting in job instability, high turnover, and low earnings. Many families caring for a disabled or aging relative suffer from low income. Many women working in low-wage care occupations lack opportunities to improve their earnings or develop new skills. These problems spill over onto society as a whole, both through their negative effects on children growing up in low-income families and through the low and uneven quality of paid care services, which is caused in part by high turnover rates. Meanwhile, racial-ethnic and class differences make it difficult to build successful political coalitions to improve public support for care provision.

Policy Barriers and Strategies

Institutional barriers are also apparent. The federal structure of U.S. public policy creates programmatic complexities that few social scientists, much less voters, can master. Administrators face perverse incentives to shift costs between federal, state, and local programs. States often promise more than they deliver, and the result is long waiting lists for subsidized assistance for both child care and home- and community-based care for adults. In nursing homes and other predominantly government-funded institutions, the quality of services may even be kept intentionally low to reduce demand.

Government benefits are often means-tested, which exacerbates social divisions and may undermine solidarity and trust among voters (Rothstein 2005). Many state and federal benefits start phasing out somewhere between the poverty line and twice that line (from $22,000 to $44,000 for a family of four in 2009), and losing access to government benefits has the same effect on household budgets as paying more taxes. Taking both income taxes and the loss of benefits into account, marginal tax rates in that range of the income distribution are often higher than the rate of 35 percent applied to the taxable income over $373,650 of married couples filing jointly. An innovative study of households that merged data from tax returns and state administrative data shows that some low-income families faced a combined state and federal marginal tax rate of 44 percent in 2000. Some "fell off a cliff" when they earned just enough income to disqualify them from the state's public health insurance program, the added expense of paying for their own insurance making it difficult for them to meet their other monthly expenses (Holt and Romich 2007).

Many households with children face a hefty marriage penalty in the form of higher marginal tax rates because the pooled income of husband and wife reduces their eligibility for benefits (Carasso and Steuerle 2005). The new health care bill includes subsidy phaseouts that will increase marginal tax rates, with a particularly sharp spike for families with taxable income between $40,000 and $50,000. Pell grants targeted at students from low-income families leave middle-income families in the lurch as tuition and fees at public universities go up. The marginal tax rate built into that program ranges from 22 to 47 percent. It is difficult to estimate the size of the resulting disincentives to work longer hours or to get married. But even if these are small, they may contribute to widespread resentment of government programs targeted narrowly at the poor.

For these reasons, we favor relatively universal care policies, where taxpayers can clearly see what they are getting for their money. Indeed, we think it is important to highlight the private costs of care in order to explain the benefits of increased public provision. Precisely because care provision relies on cultural norms of obligation and gendered preferences, it is easy to take it for granted. Many people seem to believe that care problems could easily be solved if women had better priorities or if low-income families had better values. Indeed, a common criticism of public care provision is that it will undermine private provision of care or create other perverse incentives. In our view, however, "crowding-out" poses a less significant threat than shortfalls in care provision that not only hurt our most vulnerable citizens but also penalize those who take responsibility for the care of others. Individuals unencumbered by any obligations to dependents typically enjoy more disposable income and leisure time than those who make and keep care commitments. Many current economic and demographic trends, including greater family instability and increased geographic mobility, create obstacles to care.

Since altruism often involves sacrifice, we should not be surprised to find evidence of distributional conflict over who should bear the costs of care. One way to reduce such conflict is to clearly demonstrate the collective benefits of improved care provision. Investments in human capabilities—or, to use the more conventional terms, human and social capital—represent a key contribution to economic development. A "care movement" is already under way in the United States, characterized by a variety of grassroots efforts and political initiatives (Engster 2010). A set of clear, comprehensive, and universal care policies could help build the types of political coalition needed to achieve critical mass.

A CARE POLICY AGENDA

Ten years ago, Deborah Stone published a short article entitled "Why We Need a Care Movement" in which she made a case for joining "three corners of the care triangle: people who need care, families who care for and about their members, and people who give care for a living" (Stone 2000b, 14). We hope to strengthen this case here. As our review of existing policies in chapters 6 and 7 indicated, we see substantial shortcomings in all three aspects of U.S. policy.

The moral urgency of meeting care needs is deeply rooted in the logic of reciprocity. Whether provided by the family, the community, or the state, care represents a fundamental aspect of social reproduction and cohesion. As the political scientist Daniel Engster (2007, 15) writes, "Because we all claim care from others at one time or another during our lives, we owe care to others when we can provide it to them." From an evolutionary standpoint, altruism that is likely to help kin or be reciprocated offers clear benefits to a species characterized by physical dependency at the beginning and end of the life cycle. From an economic standpoint, care represents a form of social insurance that is particularly important for dependents.

Economic change requires institutional adjustment. Women now represent almost half of employees on non-agricultural payrolls. As a recent report from the Sloan Foundation emphasizes, "The vast majority of American workers have family caregiving responsibilities outside of work and no full-time caregiver at home." In about 70 percent of American families with children, all adults engage in paid employment. About 25 percent of workers currently report elder-care responsibilities; about 40 percent are likely to report such responsibilities by 2020 (Sloan Foundation 2009). American families increasingly rely on both government and the market to help them meet their care needs.

Care recipients and care workers are not natural allies in every respect, but they share a common interest in quality of care. Women are disproportionately represented both among those who need care services and among those who provide them. As more women have entered paid employment, both the costs and the benefits of unpaid care time have become more apparent. Yet the pace of institutional efforts to help both women and men balance the demands of paid employment with those of family and community life has remained remarkably slow. Women married to high-earners or with highly paying managerial or professional jobs of their own can purchase substitutes for unpaid care that increase their flexibility. Women without husbands, especially those in low-wage jobs, often find it extremely difficult to meet family needs.

Some jobs in the care sector—those that are highly credentialed—pay quite well. But workers providing hands-on care for both children and adults earn low wages with little reward for their education or experience and scant opportunity for advancement. They seldom enjoy a very supportive work environment and tend to cycle in and out of full-time employment. Adult care workers are also vulnerable to high rates of physical injury. Poor regulation of "gray market" employment, in which caregivers are hired and supervised directly by the people they care for or their families, puts these workers in a vulnerable position, particularly if they are undocumented and hence afraid to report financial or other abuse. All of these factors contribute to high rates of turnover among both child and adult care workers, which lowers the quality of services provided.

As previous chapters have emphasized, both intrinsic and extrinsic motivation play an important role in both unpaid and paid care provision. Given the unique character of care work, it is difficult to conceive of a sustainable system of paid care that does not consider both types of rewards. Thus, while many of the policy initiatives discussed here are aimed primarily at enhancing extrinsic *or* intrinsic motivation, we also emphasize the relationship between them. Just as higher wages in themselves cannot guarantee worker satisfaction and fulfillment, even the highest levels of intrinsic motivation will erode over time without adequate compensation and support.

Emerging Care Technologies

New information technology can improve the productivity of many functional aspects of care provision through innovations such as standardized medical records and online education. Improved communication technology is already delivering important benefits. But technological change does not offer a panacea for problems of the care sector and promises little regarding empathetic aspects of care. A high priority should be placed on policy efforts to train unpaid and paid caregivers to better use state-of-the-art technologies and improve their capacity for collaboration with medical professionals.

A recent meta-analysis of assessments of an innovative Veterans Administration program providing telemedicine (the exchange of medical information across geographic sites via electronic communication) substantiates significant improvements in the success of decentralized health care, especially in the treatment of chronic health and mental health conditions such as diabetes and cancer. However, the success of this program was largely determined by its effective integration into a community care provision infrastructure that ensured high levels of personal interaction (Hill et al. 2010).

Research on "carebots" designed to automate some aspects of elder care is well under way (Pineau et al. 2003). Long-distance monitoring of blood pressure and blood sugar and video surveillance for physical accidents or medical crises offer obvious benefits. But such technologies do not provide a substitute for human contact and emotional support. The psychologist Sherry Turkle (2011) explicitly challenges the notion that carebots can become effective "buddies." In her visits to nursing homes where residents had been given robot dolls such as Paro, a seal-shaped stuffed animal programmed to purr and move when held or talked to, she found that residents were pathetically starved for human contact. Robots can make good helpers, but "programming for love" is not the same as delivering the real thing (Young 2011).

Meeting People's Needs

It costs money to meet needs. Not surprisingly, definitions of need are almost always contested. Yet it should be easier to agree on basic needs for individuals unable to care for themselves than for others. Indeed, current social policies in the United States provide fallback care for children, the disabled, and the elderly. Our cultural tradition and political history reveal a pattern of increased public support for care needs over time, from the expansion of public education to the more recent growth of state-funded early education for four-year-olds, from the advent of Medicare and Medicaid to the 1999 Olmstead Act nudging public agencies to provide services to the disabled in home- and community-based settings.

The U.S. electorate expresses consistently strong approval of policies aimed at both unpaid and paid care provision. For instance, a 2007 poll by Lake Research Partners found that paid family and medical leave enjoyed support across party lines, with only 11 percent of Democrats, 17 percent of Independents, and 23 percent of Republicans opposed.[2] An increasing percentage of parents—57 percent in 2010 versus 49 percent in 2006—describe child care as an economic necessity.[3] Almost 70 percent of voters polled in 2008 wanted state and local governments to provide voluntary prekindergarten education for all children.[4]

Political support weakens when explicitly linked to tax increases, but public provision can help reduce private expenditures and reduce family burdens. About 66 percent of Americans believe that they will provide care for an adult family member or friend in the future, and about half of these say that they feel unprepared to help with the more intimate activities of daily living, such as bathing, dressing, and toileting. About one-third worry that caregiving will interfere with their paid work responsibilities.[5] Many worry about their ability to help their parents in the future.[6] According to a recent poll, "76 percent of respondents believe publicly funded programs targeted to a specific age group such as K-12 education or Social Security are not burdensome responsibilities to certain age groups, but investments that benefit all generations" (Generations United 2010, 4).

Yet public funding for care provision is buckling. The recession of 2008–2009 increased fiscal pressures on states that were only temporarily reduced by the American Recovery and Reinvestment Act (ARRA). Major cuts to state programs for older individuals and adults with physical disabilities are currently under way. A recent report by the AARP Public Policy Institute finds that thirty-one states cut non-Medicaid aging and disability services programs in 2010, and twenty-eight states were expecting to cut these programs in 2011. Yet more than half of states reported increased demands for information and referrals, home-delivered meals, respite, case management, personal care assistance, family care-giver support, transportation, and homemaker services (Walls et al. 2011). No clear procedures are in place for monitoring the effects of such budget cuts on the vulnerable. Research shows that states rarely specify uniform standards for pro-viding backup for personal care service breakdowns or quality assurance (Seavey and Salter 2006).

Children and adults who cannot care for themselves need developmentally appropriate assistance from their families, their communities, and/or the state, and the burdens of providing such assistance should be equitably distributed. Forms of support should be flexible and customizable while meeting minimum standards of accessibility, reliability, and quality. When private or public agencies set out to provide care services, one of the first tools they deploy is a care needs assessment based on consideration of specific circumstances. Children have differ-ing needs based on age and ability, and families have differing capacities to care for them based on resources of money and time. As pointed out in earlier chap-ters and the appendix, adult needs are often assessed based on ability to perform ADLs or IADLs. In the United Kingdom, all adults who believe they need care are entitled to a community needs assessment, as are their caregivers.[7]

What would a care needs assessment for the United States as a whole look like? From the point of view of children, adults with disabilities, and the frail elderly, a general list of high priorities includes:

- Public policies to facilitate and support family care
- Expanded and reliable provision of affordable, high-quality child care and early education
- High-quality foster care for children and for those adults with disabilities or frail elderly who would benefit from it
- Expanded and reliable public provision of adult care services in home- and community-based settings and (where necessary) in nursing homes
- Improved wages, benefits, training, and working conditions for child care and adult care workers

POLICIES FOR UNPAID CARE PROVIDERS

Policies to provide support and recognition for unpaid care providers can take several different forms, including income supports and tax credits for depen-dent care. Some reduce the opportunity cost of care provision by making it easier to combine unpaid with paid work, by providing public services, and by encouraging a more equitable gender division of labor in family care. In exploring some of these avenues, we highlight features that could help reduce the impact of income inequality and gender stereotypes.

Family Leave

The federal Family and Medical Leave Act (FMLA) guarantees some American workers the right to twelve weeks of job-protected unpaid leave from paid employment in order to cope with their own illness, that of a spouse or parent, or the birth or adoption of a child. However, the FMLA, as discussed in chapter 6, leaves many workers ineligible for unpaid leave, either because their employers are not covered by the law or because the person requiring care does not fit the criteria stipulated (such as a gay or lesbian partner, an in-law, or another extended family member). Even when they are eligible, workers are often unable to take advantage of unpaid leave for financial reasons. And although some workers enjoy paid maternity or paternity leave, such coverage is concentrated at the high end of the job market.

The United States stands out among affluent countries for its failure to provide federally guaranteed paid leave (Gornick and Meyers 2003). We could build on the experience of other countries and of California and New Jersey, which have limited paid family leave policies, to develop a national paid family leave program. Janet Gornick and Marcia Meyers have offered a detailed proposal for a six-month parental leave (Gornick, Meyers, and Wright 2009). Each employed parent would have his or her entirely nontransferable leave entitlement, increasing incentives for paternal participation. Payment would be determined by a percentage of earnings, with a cap on the level of earnings that could be replaced (which would reduce the impact of earnings inequality). Parents would be allowed to take up their benefits either full-time or in combination with part-time employment, allowing them to draw their entitlements incrementally. A more concerted effort to promote gender equality in parenting would make the amount of leave available to mothers contingent on the length of leave taken by fathers (Brighouse and Wright 2009).

Paid parental leave could have the effect of encouraging mothers to take so much time out of paid employment that they reduce their wage-earning capabilities (Bergmann 2009). However, there is little evidence that paid leave of modest duration would have negative effects. Indeed, it can improve earnings by increasing job stability and job tenure. One analysis from the 1996 and 2001 Survey of Income and Program Participation (SIPP) shows that access to leave for the birth of a child had either positive or no effects on wages (Boushey 2005a).

Sick Leave and Flexibility

Parental leave alone, however, leaves much unpaid care provision uncovered. Although permanent or near-permanent disability is covered by the federal Social Security program, over 40 percent of all employees in the United States—and a much higher percentage in low-wage jobs—lack access to paid time to care for themselves or an ailing family member (IWPR 2010). Models for paid sick leave programs include a federal initiative introduced in June 2007 that would provide up to eight weeks of paid leave for a worker's serious health or family care needs. Such a program would tend to reduce transmission of infectious disease (a serious problem with food-service workers in particular), dampen worker turnover, and reduce public spending on paid care services and public assistance (Hartmann and Lovell 2009).

Regulation of work time is also an important issue. When individual workers compete with one another for approval and promotion, they can create "rat-race" pressures to increase the length of total work hours (Folbre 2004). Many full-time workers in the United States put in far more than forty hours per week. Increases in the quality and availability of reduced-hour and part-time work would help families successfully combine unpaid and paid work. Jane Waldfogel (2010) describes such measures taken in Great Britain over a decade that resulted in positive changes in the welfare of children. Individuals who enjoy flexible work arrangements typically report more work-life balance, greater mental health, and increased life satisfaction (Jones 2006).

Many part-time jobs pay extremely low wages with limited or no benefits, but more workers might opt for part-time employment if wages and benefits were strictly prorated according to hours worked. Other measures to improve regulation of work time include the right to formally request a shift to reduced-hour or flexibly scheduled work, which employers would be required to provide unless they could show adverse economic impact (Gornick, Meyers, and Wright 2009, 24).

Family Responsibility Discrimination

Intensified efforts to educate workers and employers about family responsibility discrimination (FRD) could improve workplace outcomes. No federal statute expressly prohibits this form of discrimination, but it is often linked to discrimination on the basis of gender, and several states and local jurisdictions have passed laws that address it (Williams and Bornstein 2008). Lawsuits filed by individuals who believed they were treated unfairly by supervisors because they stated a need to provide care for a family member increased almost 400 percent between 1996 and 2005, and they are getting increasing publicity (Still 2006). Verdicts in these cases have reached $11.6 million for an individual (*Schultz v. Advocate Health and Hosp. Corp*) and $250 million in a recent class-action suit (*Velez v. Novartis*) (Calvert 2010).[8]

Family Caregiver Support

The National Family Caregiver Support Program, enacted in 2000, provides resources for giving support and advice to caregivers of people with disabilities and elders. It emphasizes the need to assess caregivers' own needs in order to tailor services and expanded opportunities for consumer direction (Feinberg, Wolkwitz, and Goldstein 2006). Greater coordination with health care providers can help reduce fragmentation and discontinuity of care as people transition from hospitals to extended-care facilities or to home. A number of transitional care programs, including the United Hospital Fund's Next Step in Care campaign, provide sets of practical tools, including guides and checklists. A variety of new procedures are being monitored for their effects on quality enhancement (Levine et al. 2010).

With foster care in particular, a case can be made for "investing in prevention." Efforts to help families better meet their children's needs are often cost-effective and lead to better child outcomes than forced separation. Similarly, birth families seeking reunification often need assistance to successfully make the transition back to in-home care (Bass, Shields, and Behrman 2004).

Community-Based Care Provision

Many communities have developed collaborative strategies for sharing and bartering care. Local cooperatives in the San Francisco Bay Area, Washington, D.C., and New York City provide a template that could be promoted in other areas. Elder care communities such as Senior Citizen Match have developed systems for exchanging services denominated in terms of labor hours. Religious congregations often mobilize to help provide care services for their members (Harris 1995). The "social economy" of Quebec provides a model for public promotion of democratically organized care provision (Mendell and Neamtan 2008).

Financial Support for Family Caregiving

U.S. policies currently offer substantial financial support for child-rearing through income tax deductions, the Child Tax Credit, the Child and Dependent Care Tax Credit (CDCTC), and the Earned Income Tax Credit (EITC). These benefits add up to a subsidy comparable to that provided by many European countries in the form of family allowances. These benefits are unevenly distributed across income levels, however, and represent a relatively small share of the total costs of raising children—no more than about 10 percent if the market value of parental time is taken into account (Folbre 2009).

The Child and Dependent Care Tax Credit, which is currently limited to 35 percent of expenses, can be used to help defray costs of paid care for an adult family member, but only if that care recipient lives with an employed caregiver for more than half the year. One legislative proposal introduced in Congress in 2009 would expand this definition to include parents or grandparents not residing with the caregiver (Mulvey and Scott 2010). Elders and people with disabilities are eligible for a tax credit, but their unpaid caregivers are not. There is no counterpart to the Child Tax Credit for the care of an adult, nor is there any increment to the Earned Income Tax Credit based on financial responsibility for a dependent adult. Some family caregiver advocates advocate an extension of the Child Tax Credit to cover care for adults in need of assistance, whether family members or friends.[9] A federal bill introduced to Congress by Rep. Christopher Carney of Pennsylvania would provide a refundable tax credit of $2,500 for caregivers of family members or dependents with long-term care needs.[10]

During the 2000 presidential campaign, candidate Al Gore proposed modifications to calculations of Social Security benefit credits to help offset the loss of retirement benefits when mothers take time out of paid employment to care for children.[11] This proposal has been extended to include caregivers for adults in need of assistance. Congress has considered legislation along these lines but has not yet passed such a law.[12] Another proposal would allow parents and other caregivers to draw down Social Security benefits, either as an addition to or a postponement of retirement benefits, if they withdraw from paid employment to provide care (Rankin 2002; Ferree 2009).

Foster Care

Both kin and nonkin foster care can rightly be considered unpaid care work, since basic maintenance payments (the payments that are available for the care of most foster children) are targeted to meet the costs of the foster child's material needs, not to compensate foster parents for their care work. These low rates make it extremely challenging to attract and retain quality foster parents. Although it may be difficult to frame parenting—even foster parenting—as care that should be compensated by public resources, the expectation that the foster care system, which serves hundreds of thousands of children with intensive and complex needs each year, can provide an adequate supply of consistently high-quality care without any real compensation for caregivers may simply be unrealistic. Research indicates that increasing payment rates would substantially improve the likelihood of children being placed in foster homes rather than institutional care and decrease the number of placements they experience (Duncan and Argys 2007).

Concerns about the inadequate supply of nonkin foster homes have led to increased mobilization of family members to take on parental roles. Legal rulings dictate parity in foster care payments to kin, but in practice many kin foster parents receive no public support. Reliance on "informal" placements and alternative licensing policies provide flexibility and can reduce the administrative hurdles to placing children with willing kin caregivers who do not meet (or have not yet met) the technical requirements for licensure. When kin caregivers can provide care that would otherwise be provided by nonkin, society theoretically obtains more quality care (if we believe that there is added value to kin caregiving) at lower or no cost.

However, from the caregiver's perspective, the costs are significant. Kin caregivers, many of them poor, elderly, single women, are asked to become unpaid caregivers and are not provided with even the minimal subsistence-level payments that basic monthly foster care maintenance rates represent. Moreover, even among kin caregivers who are eligible for foster care payments, many are unaware that they are eligible for public support. Equalizing maintenance payments for kin foster parents operating under alternative licensing standards or even informal care arrangements would represent an important step to providing adequate support to family caregivers (Bass, Shields, and Behrman 2004).

POLICIES FOR PAID CARE PROVIDERS

A foundational assumption in this book is that the effective delivery of care requires a significant level of intrinsic motivation on the part of caregivers, both paid and unpaid. However, our current system of care, facing new economic and demographic stresses, may depend too heavily on intrinsic motivation to be sustainable. Extrinsic supports can range from paid family leave for unpaid caregivers in the home to better pay and working conditions for paid caregivers. The goal of policy to enact or enhance such supports is not to displace but to fortify the intrinsic motivation upon which good caregiving depends.

In their classic discussion of the contemporary American workplace, Stephen Herzenberg, John Alic, and Howard Wial (1998, 149) point to our "collective failure to imagine ways of improving the economic performance of much of the service sector." This collective failure is particularly apparent in low-wage care jobs, where managers implement short-term cost minimization strategies that reinforce a low-quality equilibrium. Only a concerted effort to strengthen labor market institutions can alter the incentives currently facing employers and help move us toward a high-performance/high-pay regime that could benefit care recipients as well as workers. Such an effort dovetails with the policies described earlier to improve unpaid care provision, which would increase the flexibility and bargaining power of workers who assume considerable responsibilities for family care.

Low-wage care workers represent an important component of the overall low-wage labor force, and as the preceding chapters have shown, their absolute and relative numbers are projected to increase significantly over time. As traditional jobs in manufacturing, mining, and utilities decline, the quality of service-sector jobs, including those involving direct care provision, will have important implications for the overall distribution of earnings and social welfare in the United States (Holzer et al. 2011). The global trend toward increased health care provision for aging populations creates enormous pressure for cost minimization, which can be risky when service quality is difficult to measure. For instance, increased reliance on certified nursing assistants rather than nurses can be problematic unless CNAs are treated as members of a larger care team rather than merely cheap and disposable inputs into service provision. Cross-national research clearly shows that national policies profoundly affect job quality and compensation standards (Appelbaum 2010).

Low-wage care work represents an important venue for efforts to improve job quality. High-performance work practices (management practices that develop and leverage employees' knowledge and ability to create value) can foster the development of human capital, including the motivation and commitment of workers, and they can also enhance social capital, facilitating knowledge sharing and work coordination (Kochan et al. 2009). Such practices include training and mentoring of workers, knowledge-sharing among workers and management, and mechanisms to promote shared decision-making between management and workers (Appelbaum, Grittell, and Leana 2008). As Herzenberg and his colleagues (1998) emphasize, job performance in service jobs depends heavily on the "soft" technologies of interpretation, teamwork, and communication.

Job Training

Low-wage care workers seem to be largely stuck on treadmills, without much opportunity to climb a ladder toward better working conditions or job opportunities. Concern about poor labor market outcomes has fueled interest in training both outside and inside the workplace. High-quality career and technical education that offers access to good jobs after high school without shutting off post-secondary options has a potentially important role to play. Career academies, which provide occupational training and work experience in specific economic sectors within high schools, could target care occupations (Holzer et al. 2011). Community colleges have developed promising initiatives targeting particular occupations, though their efforts seem fragmented and inadequate (Benner et al. 2001). Recent initiatives to improve and expand community college programs, however, could speak to this problem. For-profit colleges are also playing a role in this area, though their success rates remain controversial.[13]

In general, programs that enhance skill development through education enjoy more support than broader workforce development policies like raising wages and unionization. Public investments in employment and training have declined significantly over time, however, largely because they have not been deemed cost-effective. But many evaluations show modest gains from carefully designed and well-managed efforts, especially for adult women workers (Holzer 2009). A sectoral approach to skill development could increase the productivity of both unpaid and paid care. Indeed, measuring gains in productivity due to increased education and training in unpaid work—which are currently ignored in most cost-benefit analyses—could tip the balance in favor of greater public investment (Haveman and Wolfe 1984).

Changing Work Culture

Several intervention programs have taken aim at the corrosive work culture in many facilities and proposed models of culture change aimed at promoting the inclusion of direct care workers in care planning. The Better Jobs Better Care program has involved several large- and small-scale studies of culture change in nursing homes

(Institute of Medicine 2008; Stone and Dawson 2008). As part of this program, the Robert Wood Johnson Foundation is collaborating with the Hitachi Foundation and the U.S. Department of Labor in funding seventeen job-training and upgrading demonstration projects in Jobs to Careers: Promoting Work-Based Learning for Quality Care, a program of broad-based local partnerships of employers, educational institutions, and other community organizations. Although details vary from site to site, all include some effort to promote work-based learning, improve work and career outcomes, change organizational culture, and improve quality outcomes. Evaluation of these efforts has not included any randomized trial-based comparisons, but significant and measurable gains, including improved worker morale and reduced turnover, have been demonstrated (Morgan et al. 2010).

These studies cumulatively show that interventions aimed at improving supervision and better integrating interactive care workers into decision-making can significantly improve the quality of care. At the same time, several studies report mixed feelings on the part of care workers regarding the programs. On the one hand, participants typically reported enhanced feelings of satisfaction and discretion and a broader understanding of the work. On the other hand, many found that the new responsibilities made it more difficult to complete their other job duties, suggesting the need to redesign the whole job rather than just a part of it.

Unionization

Unionization offers another strategy for improving job quality, although its political viability seems to be declining in conjunction with steadily declining unionization rates.[14] Although highly adversarial labor-management relations can be problematic, union membership is often associated with high-performance work practices because, among other things, it increases the extent to which workers' voices are heard. Low-wage workers are particularly likely to benefit. One study based on analysis of national data from 2003 to 2007 found that unionization was associated with a 20.6 percent wage premium for workers in the lowest tenth percentile of earnings, compared to 13.7 percent in the fiftieth percentile (Schmitt 2008). In service-sector jobs, the union wage premium—calculated after controlling for observable differences among workers in education and experience—amounts to 10.1 percent, or about $2 per hour. The differentials are even more striking for benefits: unionized service-sector workers are about nineteen percentage points more likely to have health insurance and about twenty-five percentage points more likely to have a pension than their non-union counterparts (Schmitt 2009).

Low-wage care workers fit this pattern. Between 2003 and 2006, unionized child care workers were paid an average of $11 per hour, compared to $8.27 for non-unionized workers, and 56.6 percent had heath care benefits, compared to 13.7 percent of non-unionized workers. Differences for home care aides and nursing and home health aides were smaller in terms of wages, but still significant ($9.87 per hour compared to $9.00 an hour, and $11.52 compared to $10 per hour, respectively). Almost 50 percent of unionized home care aides had health care benefits, compared to less than 22 percent of non-unionized aides, and almost 80 percent of nursing and home health aides enjoyed such benefits, compared to 37 percent of their non-unionized counterparts (Schmitt et al. 2007, 6). However, as indicated in chapter 4, union membership in low-wage care occupations is significantly lower than in relatively high-wage care occupations such as teaching and nursing.

State policies hold significant implications for both the likelihood and the form of unionization, particularly where home care and family day care providers are involved. The public authority model that establishes states as employers of record has proved remarkably successful. In California, for example, quasi-public intermediary organizations have been established for home care workers that act as the employers with which workers can collectively bargain (Howes 2005). The California model is promising not only because it improved worker pay and benefits and reduced turnover, but also because it increased consumer choice and improved the viability of home- and community-based care services (Howes 2004). Evidence suggests that higher wages and benefits made it easier for consumers to hire the care providers they preferred, including their own family members (Howes 2004, 2005).

A variant of the public authority model has been applied to family day care providers, based on state-level executive orders that allow these providers to meet and negotiate with the state on specific issues such as reimbursement rates. Illinois has taken the lead in this area. Family child care workers are also organized in Washington, while organizing efforts are ongoing in Oregon, Iowa, New Jersey, New York, and Michigan (Dresser 2008, 130).

Minimum Wage Policies

Although most low-wage care workers earn more than the minimum wage, the floor provided by the legislative minimum has a significant impact on overall wage contours. The relatively low level of the U.S. federal minimum wage ($7.25 per hour in 2011), measured by historical standards, helps explain the trend toward increasing wage inequality. State and local efforts to increase minimum wages through "living wage" campaigns have enjoyed success in many areas, although statewide minimum wage requirements that exceed the federal floor are rare, with only nine states (California, Connecticut, District of Columbia, Illinois, Massachusetts, Nevada, Oregon, Vermont, and Washington) requiring wages to be higher than the $7.50 federal minimum.

Other countries have often adopted minimum wage standards for specific occupations. For example, in Germany minimum wages are collectively bargained based on occupational groupings. This approach deserves consideration in the United States, where "prevailing wage" laws have been primarily applied in construction jobs. Several states have mandated prevailing wages and benefits for service workers employed by businesses that supply services to state agencies (Sonn and Luce 2008, 276). Because the public sector provides considerable support for both child care and adult care, public policies setting higher standards for pay and benefits could have a substantial impact. For instance, government could require that child care and adult care workers financed through Temporary Assistance to Needy Families (TANF) or Medicaid abide by a living wage standard.

Labor Law and Immigration Reform

Low-wage care workers have never enjoyed strong labor law protections. The federal Fair Labor Standards Act does not currently cover home care workers, on the grounds that they provide mere "companionship" services. Hopefully, the rule change proposed by the Obama administration in December 2011 to extend coverage will be approved by the U.S. Department of Labor. However, such a rule change could be reversed by future administrations.

As emphasized in chapter 4, evidence suggests that economic self-interest and tax-filing complexities combine to foster employer preference for "gray market" arrangements in household employment. Workers who lack better opportunities in the labor market often accept under-the-table employment, which can leave them stranded without basic labor market protections, unemployment insurance, workers' compensation, or access to Social Security and Medicare as they grow older. Most domestic workers are equally vulnerable to being left without these protections. New York's Domestic Workers Rights bill, passed in July 2010, will make it easier for that state's household employees to assert their rights.[15] Other states should consider developing and adopting similar bills.

Immigration reform also holds particular significance for care workers. Some health care advocacy groups, including the American Health Care Association and the National Center for Assisted Living, have called for expanded visa programs for nurses and long-term care workers.[16] Such policies could alleviate short-term labor shortages, but they could also discourage investment in the education and training of U.S. workers. The danger of creating a "brain drain" from developing countries such as Ghana and the Philippines is also worrisome.

Workers Based in Institutions Versus Clients' Homes

Care provided in institutional settings such as nursing homes and child care centers differs from that provided in people's own homes along almost every significant dimension, including wages, training, and unionization rates. Aging adults and people with disabilities generally prefer home-based care. Many paid care workers also prefer home-based work, because of the additional autonomy and the one-on-one care it makes possible. At the same time, however, they recognize the risks of social isolation. There is no "water cooler" where workers can gather to solve problems or build relationships (Dresser and Pagnac 2010).

Because of the intense interdependence between caregiver and care recipient and the intimacy of the home setting, home-based workers may be even more prone than those in institutional settings to form deep emotional attachments to their clients. This can mean a stronger commitment to the job and higher-quality care, but it can also make workers more vulnerable. Client needs may change on a weekly or even a daily basis, leading to unpredictable work hours, and adequate health and retirement benefits are seldom forthcoming. Thus, although home-based adult care may be particularly rewarding in terms of intrinsic motivation, it tends to be particularly deficient with regard to extrinsic rewards.

A CARE WORK RESEARCH AGENDA

The collaborative process of writing this book has generated an extensive research agenda enriched by synergies between analysis of unpaid and paid care work and connections among theoretical, empirical, and policy-related concerns. We began this book with a consideration of the distinctive nature of care work: concern for the well-being of the care recipient is likely to affect the quality of services provided. This definition highlights the importance of a particular subset of social preferences and a particular process of emotional attachment. It also calls attention to the formation and reproduction of cultural norms of responsibility or obligation.

These issues fall clearly within the purview of several behavioral science disciplines aimed at understanding work motivation, individual preferences, and the expanding literature on altruism and prosocial behavior. Within economics, there is scope for developing more formal theoretical models of the individual decisions that lead to making a commitment to care work, models that would embed individual decision-making within a larger social context and pay particular attention to gender roles. Such research can be aimed at examining how decisions to make care commitments can alter existing preferences and norms, both through unintended spillover effects and through individual and collective bargaining over the distribution of the costs of care. One result of weakening norms of family responsibility may be increased reliance on individual resources, which puts some people at a disadvantage. High-earning women seem to be able to negotiate relatively stable partnerships, for instance, while low-earning women suffer considerable relationship instability. Further, inequality itself may exert a destabilizing effect on low-income families. The links between relative income and family resilience deserve detailed exploration.

A variety of longitudinal and experimental research designs could help reveal the distribution of propensities to provide care. For instance, working group member Douglas Wolf has proposed and designed a survey that would use biomarkers to determine if variability in response to stress helps explain why some family members are more willing than others to take on responsibilities for the care of an elderly parent. Working group members Catherine Eckel and Angela de Oliveira have designed experiments to explore the possibility that paid care workers reveal higher levels of altruism than others in specific contexts. Working group member Paula England plans to collaborate with Maria Charles of Stanford University on a longitudinal analysis of occupational mobility, asking whether parental employment in a caring occupation increases the likelihood that a child will enter a caring occupation. Since relatively little attention has been devoted to occupational "inheritance" among women, the link between mothers' and daughters' choices will be of particular interest.

Scholars who study work organization and management also have many insights on paid care work to offer. The signs of failure to effectively manage the care workforce are evident. Employers face labor shortages and high turnover. As described in previous chapters, workers face low wages and few opportunities for skill development and enhancement. Working group member Carrie Leana is doing research that addresses these concerns. For example, her current work focuses on how different sources of work motivation may result in different outcomes regarding the quality of care and worker attachment to care jobs. In earlier work, she and her colleagues followed groups of nursing assistants over a two-year period and found different types of motivation between those who stayed on the job ("stayers"), those who switched to new jobs in care work ("switchers"), and those who left the field ("leavers"). Stayers reported the same level of dissatisfaction with their pay as switchers and leavers, but they also reported greater attachment to the elderly people in their care, as well as a sense of "calling" for their work more generally. These results provide tangible evidence of the role of altruism and prosocial motivation in care work occupations.

Increases in the burden of family care over time may be intensifying the economic anxiety caused by persistently high unemployment and declining family income. Yet we do not systematically measure either the level of cash expenditures or the value of time devoted to dependents, treating these as just another form of personal consumption. Standard equivalence scales used to adjust for household size and composition ignore changes in the costs of children and elderly relatives to working-age adults, as well as transfers to family members who are not living in the same household. Further, they typically weight children less than adults simply because the cost of feeding children is lower. This assumption is conspicuously out of date.

Food is now a relatively small portion of family budgets compared to the costs of services such as child care and education. Trends in real wages are typically adjusted for changes in the cost of living, as measured by the Consumer Price Index (CPI), but trends in family income are never adjusted for changes in the cost of caring for dependents. The U.S. Department of Agriculture regularly estimates family expenditures on children but ignores both the costs of college and the value of parental time (Folbre 2008a). More systematic efforts to measure trends in the cost of caring for dependents could improve assessments of inequity in real living standards.

We know that time reallocated from paid employment to family care lowers lifetime earnings, but we do not yet have a clear picture of how this care penalty varies among different socioeconomic groups, or how it is changing over time. One recent study suggests that low-earning women suffer the most adverse effects (Budig and Hodges 2010). Another suggests that high-skilled women (as assessed by scores on the Armed Forces Qualification Test) pay the highest penalty (Wilde, Batchelder, and Ellwood 2010). Further research is also required on the pay penalty associated with entering a caring occupation, net of its other characteristics. In both cases, the ideal methodology entails examination of longitudinal data using fixed effects to control for unobservable characteristics.

The valuation of nonmarket work has significant implications for estimates of the level and distribution of extended income. Further research in these areas—even if based on approximations or simulations—could call attention to the profound differences between market income and consumption of goods and services. It could also help clarify the impact of increases in married women's labor force participation on inequality in living standards. There is a pressing need to improve upon existing replacement and opportunity-cost approaches to valuation and include consideration of factors of production other than labor. Advances in this area will require development of new surveys that combine estimates of time use with consumer expenditure and consumption of publicly provided services, moving beyond the existing segregation of these topics in the American Time Use Survey, the Consumer Expenditure Survey, and the Survey of Income and Program Participation.

Many descriptive questions concerning the low-wage care labor force remain unanswered. Why do child care workers earn lower wages, on average, than adult care workers, but have higher family incomes? What do the job trajectories of child care and adult care workers look like over time? How do home- and community-based workers spend their workdays? In particular, how much time do they devote to unpaid travel, to domestic tasks, to medical care tasks, and to the "companionship" activities that have become a bone of contention in exemptions from the Fair Labor Standards Act?

Part-timers make up a sizable and growing percentage of the paid care workforce. For example, while 20 percent of all workers work part-time, 39 percent of all child care workers and 32 percent of adult care workers are employed part-time. There have been some empirical comparisons of differences between full-time and part-time workers on factors ranging from demographics to job attitudes to working conditions (Holtom, Lee, and Tidd 2002; Kalleberg 2000; Lee and Johnson 1991), but we know little about the variability within the part-time workforce. How many prefer part-time work, and how many are involuntarily underemployed? Do motivations differ between these two groups? Are part-time jobs in care necessarily "Bad Jobs in America" (Kalleberg, Reskin, and Hudson 2000)? If not, how could they be improved?

Many employment policy questions are also pressing: Are differences across states in minimum wage rates and employment rights reflected in differences in job quality or turnover rates? Which education, job training, and job enhancement efforts have proved most successful? Which efforts to raise wages and improve benefits have gained significant traction, and how are these likely to be affected by a period of prolonged long-term unemployment? Why has there been an upswing in the use of part-time versus full-time paid workers as a percentage of the total? Part-timers may be cheaper in terms of benefits, but their higher turnover rates often entail added expenses. Institutions like hospitals or nursing homes appear more amenable to full-time work than agency-based and consumer-directed home care. Why?

Extreme differences across states in the provision of early childhood education and also home- and community-based care for elderly and disabled individuals remain a puzzle. Why has Oregon developed the best coverage and balance in long-term care, while Georgia has become the cutting edge of innovation in early childhood care and education? The AARP Public Policy Institute is developing a set of data indicators designed to evaluate each state's performance in delivering long-term care services and to measure progress over time.[17] Assessment and ranking should be accompanied by efforts to develop and test hypotheses explaining these differences. In particular, it is important to ask how differences in racial, ethnic, and class inequality may drive state policies. Looking beyond the United States to Europe, what can we learn from distinctive features of care work in other countries, and what implications can we draw regarding their impacts on the quality of care?

As we conclude this book, the future of the Affordable Healthcare for Americans Act (the health care reform act signed into law by President Barack Obama in 2009) remains in doubt, and the Community Living Assistance Services and Supports Act (CLASS Act), a subset of the health care act that would have helped families meet the costs of long-term care, has effectively been dropped. The political and economic aftershocks of the 2008–2009 recession seem to have undermined confidence in public policy initiatives. High levels of public debt in Europe have also put pressure on public commitments there, signaling at least some retrenchment.

We need to develop a better explanation of both long-run trends and short-run cycles in the evolving relationship between the family, the market, and the state. At the same time, we should ask how best to mobilize all three institutions toward a better social organization of care.

NOTES

1. See, for instance, Benedict Carey, "Study Finds Increased Prevalence of Autism," *New York Times,* December 18, 2009, available at: http://www.nytimes.com/2009/12/19/health/19autism.html (accessed January 23, 2011), and Tara Parker-Pope, "New Risks Linked to Asthma Rise," *New York Times,* February 12, 2009, available at: http://well.blogs.nytimes.com/2009/02/12/new-risk-factors-linked-to-asthma-rise (accessed January 23, 2011).

2. National Partnership for Women and Families, "Key Findings from Nationwide Polling on Paid Family and Medical Leave," conducted by Lake Research Partners (September 25), available at: http://www.nationalpartnership.org/site/DocServer/WF_PaidLeave_PollResults_071002.pdf?docID=2521&autologin=true (accessed January 2, 2010).

3. See National Association of Child Care Resources and Referral Agencies, available at: http://www.naccrra.org/publications/naccrra-publications/publications/9890928_Parent%20Poll%20Report-06.pdf (accessed January 1, 2010).

4. See Pew Center on the States, "Pre-K Education," available at: http://www.preknow.org/advocate/opinion/nationalpoll.cfm (accessed January 1, 2010).

5.   See Strength for Caring, "Attitudes and Beliefs About Caregiving in the U.S. Findings of a National Opinion Survey," available at: http://www.strengthforcaring.com/util/press/research (accessed January 2, 1010).

6.   See Mindy Fetterman, "Many Worry About Being Able to Care for Relatives in the Future," *USA Today*, June 27, 2007, available at: http://www.usatoday.com/money/perfi/eldercare/2007-06-24-elder-care-poll_N.htm (accessed January 3, 2010).

7.   See, for instance, the website maintained by the organization Shelter, a "housing and homelessness charity," http://england.shelter.org.uk/get_advice/finding_a_place_to_live/housing_with_support/getting_needs_assessed (accessed March 3, 2011).

8.   For a summary of the Novartis sex discrimination case, see Patricia Hurtado and David Glovin, "Novartis Must Pay Punitive Damages in Sex-Bias Case, Jury Rules," *Business Week*, May 18, 2010.

9.   See Caregiver Credit Campaign, http://www.caregivercredit.org (accessed January 3, 2011).

10. For more details, see Family Caregiver Alliance, "Caregiver Tax Relief Act (2008)," available at: http://www.caregiver.org/caregiver/jsp/content_node.jsp?nodeid=2324&chcategory=43&subcategory=45&chitem=417 (accessed January 3, 2011).

11. James Dao, "Gore Proposes New Benefits for Parents and Widows," *New York Times*, April 5, 2000, p. A19.

12. See Social Security Caregiver Credit Act of 2007 (HR 1161), available at: http://www.govtrack.us/congress/billtext.xpd?bill=h110-1161 (accessed January 3, 2011).

13. Kelly Field, "For-Profit Colleges Could Do More on Shortage of Health-Care Workers," *New York Times*, January 20, 2011.

14. Stephen Greenhouse, "Union Membership in U.S. Fell to a 70-Year Low Last Year," *New York Times*, January 22, 2011.

15. Nicholas Confessore and Anemona Hartocollis, "Albany Approves No-Fault Divorce and Domestic Workers' Rights," *New York Times*, July 1, 2010.

16. See the issue brief of the American Health Care Association and the National Center for Assisted Living, "Immigration Reform Could Ease Workforce Shortages," July 1, 2010, available at: http://www.ahcancal.org/advocacy/issue_briefs/Issue%20Briefs/IBImmigrationReformWillHelpLTC.pdf (accessed April 30, 2012).

17. See Susan C. Reinhard, "Long-Term Services and Supports State Scorecard." Washington, D.C.: AARP Public Policy Institute (September). Available at: http://www.aarp.org/health/health-care-reform/info-11-2010/ltss-scorecard.html (accessed April 30, 2012).

Appendix:
Measuring Care Work

Nancy Folbre and Douglas Wolf

If something is difficult to define, it is likely to be even more difficult to measure. How many people regularly provide unpaid care? How much time do they devote to care tasks? How many people are employed in care occupations? How do the tasks they perform differ from those of other workers? Accurate answers to these questions depend on definitions of care based on observable features of individuals and the work they perform. Although researchers share a general consensus regarding the meaning of care, specific definitions often vary. As a result, different types of care are often studied using different metrics. Even highly specialized studies of child care or adult care apply different criteria from one survey to the next, making it difficult to combine or compare empirical results.

In this appendix, we grapple with the difficulties of translating definitions of care work into quantifiable measures that are applicable to both unpaid and paid domains, analyzing the strengths and weaknesses of the different methodologies applied in empirical research. We begin with a discussion of general measurement problems in the definition of care provision, care needs, and the concept of disability. We then focus on description and evaluation of different types of measurement tools and discuss one overarching problem: the issue of joint production and economies of scale in care provision.

Our critical assessment of the empirical literature informs a list of suggestions for research design that could help calibrate measurements across different types of surveys, improving comparability. It also provides guidance for the practical use of existing data.

FROM DEFINITION TO MEASUREMENT

The need for accurate measures of care work grows out of practical concerns as well as research priorities. At the societal level, policymakers may ask whether the need for care services outstrips the amount they provide, or whether care occupations will be growing rapidly in years to come. Consistent measures of care work can also make it easier to assess the implications of shifts in the allocation of women's time from unpaid to paid work, which may or may not involve a shift out of care work.

At the individual or family level, administrators often need to assess the suitability of home-based versus institutional care or to determine whether a patient can be safely discharged from a hospital into self-care or the care of family and friends. Accurate measures of unpaid and paid care work and the relationship between them would also help assess the extent to which these forms of care work substitute for one another or complement one another. A precise definition of care activities is also needed to determine just how big a "care penalty" people pay for specializing in care work, whether in the home or in the labor market.

Scope of the Measurement Problem

Chapters 1 and 2 identified several attributes and dimensions of care work that are difficult to measure, including face-to-face interaction, types of motivation, and emotional attachment. In this appendix, we focus on more practical concerns: measuring the number of care providers, the number of care recipients, and the time devoted to caring activities. Where possible, we use the categories of interactive care, support care, and supervisory care defined in chapter 1.

For the purposes of counting both people and effort, a second distinction—between the *potential* and the *actual* quantity—is also important. In particular, the aggregate need for care may exceed the aggregate provision of care at any point. In other words, the number of potential care recipients could exceed the number of actual care recipients in both unpaid and paid care.

Addressing Ambiguities

The classification of human activities and interactions is typically based on negotiated compromises rather than some natural consensus (Bowker and Star 1999). Ambiguity is rooted in the very nature of care work and the complexity of human interaction. As emphasized in chapter 1, concepts such as "care" and "dependency" are often culturally contested. Good classification requires ongoing communication and collaboration among stakeholders. For instance, the Nursing Interventions Classification (NIC) system that is now widely used in medical management grew out of years of consultation between researchers and practitioners (Bowker and Star 1999, chapters 7 and 8).

Although wording choices are obviously important when attempting to define concepts such as "care" or "caregiver," they are especially important when designing survey questions or other tools to produce empirical measures of these concepts. The survey researcher's hope is to develop language that will be similarly—ideally, identically—interpreted by any and all potential respondents. That is, of course, a tall order, and problems of meaning and interpretation are particularly acute in the realm of caring and care work. Whether in unpaid or paid care work, differences in perceptions of care can drive a wedge between reports of care provided and care received.

Focus groups provide one vehicle for resolving these issues. One study of family caregiving for disabled and frail elderly, for instance, found that family caregivers were often uncomfortable with survey terminology designating them in those terms (Lake Snell Perry and Associates 2001); many associated the term "caregiver" with paid employees and felt that they were simply fulfilling their responsibilities as a parent or a spouse rather than enacting a separate role. Some went so far as to suggest that an official "title" was self-serving because they were simply fulfilling a family obligation. Such results suggest that family caregiving can easily go underreported.

Another example of possible confusion about what may or may not be considered care is the overlap between care delivery—a response to a need that the care recipient cannot fully address on his or her own—and the normal exchanges of family life (Walker, Pratt, and Eddy 1995). Women typically perform many household tasks that are included in standardized measures of instrumental activities of daily living (IADLs), such as housework and meal preparation. Wives and mothers may not consider such tasks to be "caregiving," but they may be perceived as such by a husband or child, whether or not the beneficiaries could perform those same tasks for themselves.

A final example of ambiguity concerns the differing perspectives of providers and recipients. For example, a family day care provider who looks after three children during an eight-hour day may expend much the same effort as another who looks after four children in the same period. However, from the perspective of the care recipients (or a third-party observer), the "output" is considerably higher. Similarly, the total amount of care received by older family members can be much greater than the average amount provided by any given family member for the simple reason that older care recipients may be receiving help from more than one child simultaneously (Freedman et al. 1991).

The Definition and Relevance of "Disability"

We focus on two particularly vulnerable groups of care recipients, children and adults needing personal assistance as a result of disability or age. Children's care needs vary greatly, of course, whether or not they include special needs associated with physiological problems or mental health or other developmental issues. Further, children's care needs typically change substantially as they grow older. Nonetheless, this part of our target population of care recipients can at least be readily—if crudely—defined with respect to one objective criterion: chronological age. It is far more difficult to define the criteria with which to isolate the population of people with disabilities. Considerable effort has been expended on developing a universally applicable conceptualization of disability. A recent National Academy of Sciences report (Field and Jette 2007) adopts the World Health Organization's International Classification of Functioning, Disability, and Health (ICF), which was released in 2001, but recommends further development and enhancements. The ICF defines "disability" as an umbrella term that encompasses "impairments," "activity limitations," and "participation restrictions." Impairments are problems in body function or structure, which may or may not be a consequence of a health condition (in this scheme, "aging" is a health condition) and are therefore both specific to an individual and independent of the social or environmental context in which the person is located. In contrast, both activity limitations and participation restrictions depend in part on the interaction between the person and his or her environment. Thus, for example, a musculoskeletal condition that interferes with someone's capacity to climb stairs—an impairment—need not imply activity limitations if the person's residence, workplace, and social environment are free of stairs.

Language similar to that used in the ICF is also found in the 1990 Americans with Disabilities Act (ADA). However, in the ADA a disability is defined as a physical or mental impairment with specific *consequences*—substantially limiting a major life activity. The ADA's definition also encompasses having a history of such an impairment and being perceived by others as having such an impairment (Gregory 2004).

The ICF's characterization of impairments, activity limitations, and participation restrictions uses terms like "problems" and "difficulties." Accordingly, there would seem to be a straightforward connection between "disability" and "care": care, using this framework, could be defined as assistance provided by another person in order to help someone cope with or overcome an impairment, diminish or eliminate a difficulty, or overcome a problem. However, for a number of reasons, the presence of disability does not translate neatly into care—neither care needs nor actual care receipt.

First, many impairments or limitations can be addressed by modifying the physical environment with devices such as ramps, handrails, and grab bars or by using special equipment such as canes, walkers, large-format telephones, or motorized wheelchairs. Some people disinclined to make use of assistive devices or technology may instead receive, or wish to receive, assistance from others, while others will adapt their expectations or goals so as to minimize the limiting consequences of their impairments. Thus, a given level of impairment is likely to translate into a broad range of possible care needs.

Second, the definition of disability includes subjective elements. How are we to decide that an activity is a "major" activity, or whether any particular impairment has "substantially" limited that activity? How are we to adjudicate between a person's claims concerning his or her own situation and other people's perceptions of the person's situation? Personal preferences seem to be built into the ADA's definition: there are many potential "major life activities," and one's preferences surely play a large role in judging the consequences for well-being of having an impairment that reduces one's ability to pursue that activity.

The ICF, which attempts to define and classify disability and related theoretical constructs such as the "disablement process" (Verbrugge and Jette 1994), exerts considerable influence on research and policy analysis. However, the design and implementation of public programs intended to address disability demands more specificity than these conceptual schemes provide.

Programmatic definitions and eligibility criteria show a great deal of variety. One survey of U.S. federal programs reveals that there are forty-three different definitions of "disability" in these programs (Adler and Hendershot 2000). One such definition is shown in box A.1, which summarizes the language used to define people with disabilities for the purposes of the Social Security program. This example illustrates many of the problems that must be solved when moving from the general to the specific. Note, for example, the requirements that conditions be "continuous" and last at least twelve months, as well as the very specific earnings test by which "substantial gainful employment" is determined. The difficulty of applying these programmatic definitions comparably across a wide spectrum of geographic locations and bureaucratic actors is suggested by the widespread prevalence of denials of applications—and often-successful appeals of those denials—for Social Security Disability Insurance benefits (Benítez-Silva et al. 1999).

BOX A.1 / U.S. Social Security Program Definitions of Disability

- Disability in adults is defined as a physical or mental condition expected to last continuously for at least twelve months, which prevents the individual from engaging in substantial gainful employment (defined as earning at least $1,000 per month in 2010).
- An intellectual disability or "mental retardation," as it was commonly called, is measured by an IQ of about 70 or lower, combined with substantial limitations on functioning related to independent living and which is manifested prior to age twenty-two (Larson et al. 2005).
- A developmental disability, when applied to adults, is defined as a severe, chronic disability that originated at birth or prior to age twenty-two, is expected to continue indefinitely, and substantially restricts the individual's functioning. Developmental disabilities may be due to mental or physical impairments or a combination of physical and mental impairments. Examples of developmental disabilities include autism, behavior disorders, brain injury, cerebral palsy, Down syndrome, fetal alcohol syndrome, mental retardation, and spina bifida (U.S. Department of Health and Human Services/ASPE/DALTCP 2006).
- People over the age of five are classified as having developmental disabilities and are eligible for services if they have substantial functional limitations in three or more of the areas of major life activity (self-care, expressive or receptive language, learning, mobility, self-direction, capacity for independent living, and economic self-sufficiency). These limitations are expected to last for at least twelve months, with at least one limitation manifested before the age of twenty-two (Larson et al. 2005).
- Developmental disability in infants and young children (individuals age zero to six) is a substantial developmental delay or specific congenital or acquired condition with a high probability of resulting in developmental disabilities if services are not provided.

TOOLS FOR MEASURING CARE

A close consideration of efforts to provide operational measures of care need and care provision enriches our understanding of the theoretical issues at stake and helps inform policy-relevant research. In the remainder of this appendix, we provide a critical review of five empirical tools that are used in care research and that informed the construction of our own estimates in earlier chapters. As we have defined it, care work can vary along several dimensions: care of children versus care of adults who need assistance, unpaid care versus paid care, and care provided versus care received. We do not explore every permutation of these dimensions, but we do address them in a consistent and comprehensive way.

Demographic Measures

Several purely demographic measures can be used to describe the possible size of the populations of potential care providers and potential care recipients. Various dependency ratios are most often used to make comparisons across countries or within countries over time (see the discussion of dependency ratios in chapter 1). However, the ratio is intended to capture economic or financial dependency and is therefore of less value as a guide to care needs. The definition also implies that children and the elderly are equally "dependent," but in fact many of those classified as in the working-age population are unable to work, while the dependent population—especially those age sixty-five and older—includes many employed people. Efforts have been made to address these issues. One approach is weighting the groups most likely to make temporal demands—those under age seven or over age seventy-five—twice as heavily as other children and elderly (Budlender 2008). Another approach applies estimates of probable morbidity (sickness or disability) to the elderly, a particularly useful exercise for estimating the impact of changes in retirement age (Muszynska, Yi, and Rau 2010).

More precise estimates of age-specific demands for care could allow us to further refine dependency ratios. Since people who live together typically share care responsibilities—at least to some extent—households have their own dependency ratios. Coresidence of other adult family members, for instance, can reduce the burden of child care for parents. Older children may help care for younger children, and spouses are typically the most important source of care for elderly adults. The health heterogeneity of the elderly represents a distinct challenge, however. When elderly adults such as grandparents coreside with working-age adults, it is difficult to determine whether they represent a care demand or a potential supply of care for young children.

Since women typically provide more unpaid and paid care than men, measures of the female working-age population are often considered particularly important. One widely circulated measure of the "care gap" compares the population of women age twenty-five to sixty-four to the population of all individuals over age sixty-five (Turnham and Dawson 2003). More precise measures of the likelihood that either women or men with specific characteristics are likely to provide specific types of care would provide more plausible estimates of the potential supply of unpaid care.

Kinship also has a profound impact: individuals who have married and raised children typically receive more assistance from family members than those who have not. As a result, changes in family structure have significant implications for the future supply of family caregivers. Demographers have developed several models for "kin counts" in an attempt to describe the availability of potential caregivers—or the claims on potential caregivers—at the family or kin-group level (Tomassini and Wolf 2000). These models have been used to show how changes in fertility, mortality, divorce, and remarriage tend to increase the within-family "elder care dependency ratio." Although the older population of the future will have fewer biological children and grandchildren, they will have more stepchildren and grandchildren (Wachter 1997). Similarly, the adult children of the future will have fewer siblings, but more step- and half-siblings with whom to share the burdens of caring for older parents.

Need-Based Measures of the Demand for Care

Publicly funded programs providing or regulating care must rely on some formalized and standardized assessment of applicant needs, and they must have some way of determining eligibility for services based on those assessments. An example is the Long-Term Care Placement Form (Form DMS-1) used to determine eligibility for New York State's Long-Term Home Health Care Program (LTHHCP). The DMS-1 form must be filled out by a registered nurse, and only applicants with a score of 60 or higher are eligible for LTHHCP services. The DMS-1 score depends on numerous factors, including functioning problems, mental status, sensory impairments, and the patient's ability to administer medications and other therapies. Although the total score produced by the DMS-1 form establishes eligibility for services, it does not determine the level (that is, hours per week by category of provider) of the services to be provided. For that, a separate form must be jointly completed by a nurse representing the service provider and a staff representative of the local government agency that administers the program. It seems likely that a given severity score could translate into a broad range of hours per week of care time, depending on the applicant's circumstances and the perceptions and predispositions of the professionals who make the determinations.

However one might judge the objectivity and reasonableness of the components of a numeric scoring system like that of the DMS-1, it is evident that disability measures are much more easily standardized in a bureaucratic, professionally administered, highly structured system than in a population survey. Yet it is only through large-scale surveys—in which information is provided by respondents on either their own behalf or as a proxy for someone else—that the prevalence of disability and of the care needs implied by disability can be measured.

In the United States, there is no one population-level disability monitoring survey, but a large number of surveys devote varying degrees of attention to producing disability measures. These surveys include some that cover people of all ages (for example, the Medical Expenditure Panel Survey [MEPS] and the American Community Survey [ACS]), some that cover all adults (for example, the Current Population Survey [CPS] and the Behavioral Risk Factor Surveillance System [BRFSS]), and some that cover only the older population (the Health and Retirement Survey [HRS], the National Long-Term Care Survey [NLTCS] between 1982 and 2004, and, beginning in 2011, the National Health and Aging Trends Study [NHATS]).[1]

Most disability surveys include questions about respondents' difficulties with, or limited capacity to perform, specific *activities*. Health researchers have developed standard inventories of such activities, which are usually classified as activities of daily living and as instrumental activities of daily living. The most commonly included tasks of each type are listed in box A.2.[2] Some surveys ask about ADLs or IADLs individually, while others group them into just one or two global questions. For example, the HRS asks separately about "dressing," "walking across a room," "bathing or showering," "eating," "getting in or out of bed," and "using the toilet, including getting up and down." In contrast, the American Community Survey (ACS) has two questions that cover a subset of the tasks normally considered to be ADLs: "Does this person have serious difficulty walking or climbing stairs?" and "Does this person have difficulty dressing or bathing?" The ACS includes a

---

BOX A.2 / Activities Typically Included in Disability Scales

Activities of Daily Living (ADLs)
- Feeding
- Continence
- Transfer (into or out of bed or chair)
- Using the toilet
- Dressing
- Bathing
- Indoor mobility

Instrumental Activities of Daily Living (IADLs)
- Managing personal finances
- Meal preparation
- Shopping
- Traveling–outdoor mobility
- Housework
- Using the telephone
- Medication management

Sources: Fillenbaum (1995); Gallo (2006).

---

third question that captures some, but not all, of the tasks normally associated with IADLs: "Because of a physical, mental, or emotional condition, does this person have difficulty doing errands alone such as visiting a doctor's office or shopping?" These two approaches have unknown consequences for estimates of the prevalence of disability. The item-by-item approach taken by the HRS gives respondents more chances to report the presence of a problem and might therefore produce more reports than the narrower approach taken in the ACS. On the other hand, the somewhat generic reference to "errands" in the ACS's IADL question—even with the specific illustrations of doctor's visits and shopping—may allow respondents to interpret this question broadly, producing more reports of difficulty than in a closed-ended, item-by-item inventory.

Several studies have attempted to "cross-walk" the estimates of disability prevalence produced by different survey designs, including question wording (Wiener et al. 1990; Freedman et al. 2004). Efforts to harmonize measures suggest that there is reasonably good agreement across survey designs; nevertheless, researchers and their audiences need to be equally careful to recognize the appropriate use of, as well as the limitations attached to, any given measurement approach.

Survey questions directed at measuring disability differ in other important ways as well. For example, the HRS questions mentioned earlier start by asking, "Because of a health or memory problem do you have *any difficulty* with ____ ," whereas the National Health Interview Survey (NHIS) includes a question that asks whether, "because of a physical, mental, or emotional problem, *you need the help of other persons* with ____" (emphasis added). The difference between having difficulty doing something and needing help doing that same thing provides a good illustration of the challenges of mapping theoretical abstractions into empirical measures, whether or not those measures are to be used in determining programmatic eligibility or allocating services. For example, more people are likely to report having "any difficulty" than are likely to report "needing help," because low levels of difficulty may not be viewed as serious enough to warrant external assistance (Freedman et al. 2004).

However, the borderline between having "no difficulty" and having "any difficulty" with a personal care task is a very subjective matter, with unknown threshold differences across individuals. Also, either type of question could produce a negative answer from someone who has a genuine physical or cognitive impairment but has successfully (from the respondent's viewpoint) addressed that impairment through the use of special equipment (such as a cane) or some environmental modification (such as the installation of grab bars in a bathroom or shower). A third approach to question wording is found in the NLTCS, which asks respondents whether they "get help" from others doing ADL tasks. Particularly for ADLs, which tend to be hands-on personal care tasks, it seems reasonable to assume that anyone actually getting help would, if asked, report that they "have difficulty" with, or "need help" with, that task. However, the correspondence between need, difficulty, and receipt of help is surely not perfect.

Another question wording difference across disability surveys concerns the "chronicity" of any reported problems. For example, the NLTCS includes questions aimed at establishing whether any reported difficulties have lasted, or are expected to last, for a total of three months, and the HRS asks respondents to "exclude any difficulties that you expect to last less than three months." However, the American Community Survey's measures are based on questions about "physical, mental, or emotional condition[s] lasting 6 months or more," and the Medicare Current Beneficiary Survey (MCBS) and the NHIS ask about "current," or point-in-time, difficulties. The more stringent the duration requirement built into the disability question, the lower the reported prevalence of disability is likely to be.

Apart from differences in question wording, other aspects of survey methodology have been shown to influence the reported prevalence or severity of disability. There is some evidence that lower rates of disability are found in telephone-based surveys than in in-person surveys (Herzog and Rogers 1988; Wolf, Mendes de Leon, and Glass 2007). Several reasons have been suggested for these differences, including the higher prevalence of hearing problems, higher rates of missing data or nonresponse in telephone interviews, and a greater reliance on interviewer assistance in a telephone interview setting, suggesting more confusion or misunderstanding (Herzog and Rogers 1988). Respondents may also be reluctant to admit or provide details about their everyday difficulties, and they may be better able to conceal those difficulties from a telephone interviewer than from an in-person interviewer. Some population surveys are confined to the non-institutional population, an obvious shortcoming when the goal is to measure disability, since people in nursing homes clearly have higher-than-average levels of need for care and are receiving substantial quantities of care.

Another important methodological issue is that of self- versus proxy-reported responses to disability questions. Past research has shown that proxy-based reports of the prevalence of disability exceed self-reported disability (Andresen et al. 2000; Santos-Eggimann, Zobel, and Bérod 1999; Todorov and Kirchner 2000). Problems with cognition present particularly vexing measurement problems, with the most severely cognitively impaired individuals—for example, those with advanced cases of Alzheimer's disease—the least able to provide their own answers to cognitive tests, necessitating the use of proxy or other secondhand reports.

The accuracy of proxy reports of disability is especially important when considering data on disabilities among children, for whom surveys are usually completed by a proxy reporter—typically the parent. For example, the NHIS asks parents of children less than five years old whether those young children are "limited in the kind or amount of play activities [they] can do because of a physical, mental, or emotional problem." The NHIS also asks, about all household members under age eighteen, whether they "receive Special Educational or Early Intervention Services." The question about personal care needs, quoted earlier, is asked about each household member over age two. At its most abstract level, the conceptualization of disability (such as that laid out in the ICF) is independent of age; what is special about children is the particular activities, and the types of participation, considered appropriate for them.

Measures of Care Based on Time Diary Data

Time diaries can be administered to adults providing care (as in the American Time Use Survey [ATUS]) or to recipients of care (as in the Child Development Supplement of the Panel Study of Income Dynamics [PSID]). Self-reported activities are typically coded into a variety of predetermined categories, only some of which explicitly use the word "care." Researchers exercise considerable discretion in designating which specific activities represent care activities. An activity is typically labeled as care only if it involves helping another person—typically someone who needs help as a result of age or disability.

Time diaries generally yield estimates that are more accurate than those yielded by stylized questions. On the other hand, the focus on a single day in the life of a respondent leads to underrepresentation of activities that are not undertaken on a regular daily basis. Furthermore, virtually all time use surveys are organized around the designation of specific activities, without consideration of who the beneficiary of such activities might be. The American Time Use Survey collects data on "who else was present" while an activity was performed. But it does not ask "for whom" an activity was performed. As a result, some activities conducted for the purpose of caring for others—such as telephoning or shopping—may not be visible because they are not specifically designated as care activities.

It is important to note that the distinction we made between interactive care and support care in chapter 1 is not observed in many surveys of individuals who are asked simply if they "take care of" others—many respondents who say yes may be reporting support care activities that are counted as if they were interactive care. As also pointed out in chapter 1, most national time use surveys collect data only on specific *activities*. The "primary activity" is designated in response to the question "What were you doing?" The "secondary activity" is designated (by some surveys) as a response to the question "What else were you doing at the same time?" But care for dependents is not merely an activity; it is also a responsibility that constrains allocation of time even when no direct care activity is being performed (Budig and Folbre 2004).

Both U.S. and Canadian time use surveys include questions that measure what can be interpreted as supervisory care for children, though the results seem sensitive to small differences in wording (Folbre and Yoon 2007b; Allard et al. 2007). These surveys do not address the issue of supervisory care for adults, although such care is commonly provided by families with a member who suffers from an extreme physical or mental disability such as paraplegia or Alzheimer's disease.

TIME DIARY DATA ON UNPAID CHILD CARE   Time diary surveys typically include questions on care activities that involve direct interaction, such as feeding or bathing children. In general, children are both present and awake during these activities, but some inconsistencies are apparent. Most studies include care-related travel—for example, taking a child to school or to after-school activities—as part of care, even though children are often not present (for example, the child is not in the car on the driver's return trips). Also, tasks such as talking to a child's teacher or doctor are included, even when the child is not present. These are examples of implicit coding of "for whom" the activity was performed. By contrast, cooking a meal for or cleaning up after a child is not coded as an explicit child care activity.

Another measurement issue concerns secondary activities, those conducted simultaneously with primary activities. For instance, a mother might report that her primary activity is cooking dinner, but her secondary activity is talking with her children while she does so. As was observed in one of the first published cross-national comparisons, much child care takes the form of secondary activities, measurement of which is highly susceptible to differences in survey wording and administration (Stone 1972). One study of Australian data suggests that primary activity measures may capture no more than about 25 percent of the time devoted to children (Ironmonger 2004).

But the measurement of child care as a secondary activity seems to be successful only if, as in the Australian case, supervisory care, or "looking after children," is included on the activity list and respondents are primed to report this as an "activity." National surveys are inconsistent on this issue, and numerous problems have been reported with interpretation of data from developing countries (Budlender 2008: Charmes 2006, 58).

This limitation of conventional time use surveys raises a problem of construct validity—"the extent to which an observed measure reflects the underlying theoretical construct that the investigator has intended to measure" (Andrews 1989, 393). A survey question that focuses only on time devoted to specific "activities" without examining how these activities are timed, or what constraints they impose on other activities, sometimes misses the point. Michael Bittman offers a poignant example from a focus-group discussion with Australian respondents who provided care for a sick or disabled family member: a mother who described using a vacuum aspirator to suction mucus out of her daughter's throat on a regular basis. The care activity itself required only about five minutes out of every hour, but the responsibility to provide this care made it virtually impossible for the mother to perform any activities outside the home, even shopping (Bittman, personal communication, 2005).

One could argue that responsibility for young children is a twenty-four-hour-a-day task and that there is therefore little to be gained by measuring it more precisely (Bianchi, Robinson, and Milkie 2006). But such responsibility is typically shared among parents or adults, with important implications for both participation in wage employment and the costs of child care (Presser 2003).

TIME DIARY DATA ON CARE OF ADULTS WITH DISABILITIES AND THE FRAIL ELDERLY   As mentioned earlier, time use surveys tend to limit their definition of child care to direct, interactive care. But elder care takes different forms from child care and tends to be defined in different ways as well. In particular, the distinction between interactive care and support care is less salient when providing assistance to an adult. For instance, going shopping or doing housework on behalf of an adult often entails discussion, negotiation, and interaction even if that adult is not physically present.

Awareness of these complexities has shaped the categories used in ATUS, which includes two different types of categories relevant to the care of adults: *caring* for household adults (or nonhousehold adults) and *helping* household adults (or non-household adults). Yet the list of sample activities for helping household adults implies that such adults are dependent, while the list of activities for nonhousehold adults includes a much longer list of activities such as housework and related activities. In other words, "support care" like housework is not separately tallied for household adults, but it is separately tallied for nonhousehold adults.

These apparently minor differences in definition can have significant implications. For instance, men are more likely than women to provide support care for a nonhousehold adult, such as running errands or doing yard work. Women are probably more likely to provide support care for household adults, but this activity is not distinguished from the larger category of household support work. This definitional inconsistency distorts the picture, making it appear that men provide a greater percentage of elder care relative to women.

Self-Reported Measures of Caregiver or Care Recipient Status

Several large-scale surveys targeting the older population have included questions that elicit information from respondents about unpaid care. Because these surveys in effect ask respondents to label themselves as caregivers or care recipients, they provide measures of actual rather than potential care work. Surveys may ask respondents to identify themselves are "caregivers" or as providers of "care," or they may use less direct language, such as "helping" or "assisting" a family member with specific activities owing to health or disability problems. Some surveys limit their questions about care to what is provided to household members, while others ask about care provided to family members or friends living elsewhere.

Surveys differ greatly with respect to the specificity of the tasks or activities that respondents should count as caregiving, as well as in the language used in the questions. In general, surveys of this type, whether broad or narrow in focus, use a reference period that is much longer than the typical time diary study covers: they may ask about care or assistance provided during the last week or month, and some use a two-year reference period. As a consequence, the estimated prevalence of caregiving activity produced by time diary data may be quite different from what is found in sociodemographic household survey data.

Surveys that are not explicitly focused on measuring caring activity may nonetheless provide useful information about it. For example, labor force surveys targeted at working-age individuals may reveal situations in which respondents were not in the labor force, or recently missed some time from work, because they were meeting family needs—for example, "providing help to a family member because of illness or disability." The Current Population Survey asks respondents who were not working for pay what their main reason was. Among the coded responses are "ill or disabled" and "taking care of home or family." Surveys whose goal is to describe patterns of volunteer work may ask respondents about activities such as making deliveries for the Meals on Wheels program; respondents who engage in this type of volunteer work may not consider themselves to be "caregivers," but from the perspective of those receiving their deliveries, they are doing care work.

The following paragraphs highlight differences in the wording of questions, or the targeting of questions to respondents, that have consequences for the estimates of prevalence and intensity of caregiving provided in chapter 3.

NATIONAL SURVEY OF FAMILIES AND HOUSEHOLDS   The NSFH was originally conducted in 1987, with follow-up interviews from 1992 to 1994 and again from 2001 to 2002.[3] It included extensive questions about family composition, family and household activities, children's well-being, marriage and cohabitation, and "taking care" of seriously ill or disabled relatives. The NSFH data have been used in several studies describing the prevalence of caring and characteristics over the life cycle (Marks 1996), the trade-off between paid work and caregiving (Wolf and Soldo 1994; Ettner 1996), and the role of employment as a factor in the gender gap in parent care (Sarkisian and Gerstel 2004a). These studies all comment on various shortcomings of the NSFH care questions. For example, the "care" questions refer exclusively to nonresident care recipients. Moreover, the twelve-month reference period for caregiving is poorly aligned with questions about hours of work, which refer to the week prior to the interview.

SURVEY OF INCOME AND PROGRAM PARTICIPATION   The SIPP is a family of panel surveys that have been conducted since 1984. New panels have been periodically enrolled and subsequently followed, with interviews every four months over a follow-up period ranging from thirty to forty-eight months (U.S. Census Bureau 2006). For only some of these panels, and in only a selected few of the follow-up interviews, have questions about informal care been included.

For example, the 2001 SIPP panel asked:

> There are situations in which people provide regular unpaid care or assistance to a family member or friend who has a long-term illness or a disability. During the past month, did you provide any such care or assistance to a family member or friend living here or living elsewhere?

This was followed by a series of questions about the provision of specific kinds of assistance: help with dressing, eating, bathing, or using the bathroom; help with medical needs; help with money management; help with shopping or going to the doctor; and an open-ended "other" category. The series also included a question about the usual number of hours of help provided per week in the last month. Additional questions addressed the number of care recipients, the relationship of the care recipient to the respondent, whether the care recipient received help from others besides the respondent, and the duration (in years) of the respondent's period of care provision.

It is evident that the SIPP questions are considerably more detailed than the NSFH questions discussed earlier. Descriptive statistics on caregivers based on the 1996 SIPP can be found in McNeil (1999) and in Alecxih, Zeruld, and Olearczyk (2001); Susan Ettner (1995) used the 1986 to 1988 SIPP panel to analyze how informal caregiving affects the female labor supply.

HEALTH AND RETIREMENT SURVEY AND ASSETS AND HEALTH DYNAMICS AMONG THE OLDEST OLD   These surveys have been conducted since 1992. The HRS is a panel survey of people originally aged fifty-one to sixty-one in 1992, who have been interviewed semiannually since that year. In 1993 an additional panel of people age seventy and older was added. They were reinterviewed in 1995 and 1998. The two cohorts were merged in 1998, and additional cohorts were added, making it a random sample of the fifty-one-and-older population that year.[4] The HRS (as the merged studies are now collectively called) provides considerable detail about health, family situation, economic resources, and intergenerational support, including questions about the provision of care—mainly to parents—and the receipt of care. We focus on the care-provision questions:

- Did you . . . spend a total of 100 or more hours in the last two years helping your parents/father/mother with basic personal activities like dressing, eating, and bathing?
- Roughly how many hours did you yourself spend in the last two years giving such assistance to your [mother/father/mother's husband/father's wife]?

The hours-of-care questions direct respondents to include help given to now-deceased parents if they died during the two-year reference period.

The Health and Retirement Survey (HRS) and Assets and Health Dynamics Among the Oldest Old (AHEAD) data have been used in studies of the division of parent care efforts among siblings (Wolf, Freedman, and Sol 1997); studies of exchanges of financial support for caregiving support in families (Henretta et al. 1997); studies of changes in hours of care received in response to changes in the severity of disability (Freedman et al. 2004); studies of substitution between informal care and nursing home care (Lo Sasso and Johnson 2002; Charles and Sevak 2005); and studies of the mental health consequences of being a caregiver (Amirkhanyan and Wolf 2003, 2006).

NATIONAL ALLIANCE FOR CAREGIVING/AARP CAREGIVING IN THE U.S. 2009 SURVEY   Widely cited, the NAC/AARP survey is the third in a series (earlier surveys were conducted in 1997 and 2004). Of the caregiver surveys featured here, it has the most inclusive criteria for measuring caregivers. It counts as caregivers all those eighteen years or older who answer affirmatively the following question:

In the last 12 months, has _____ provided unpaid care to a relative or friend 18 years or older to help them take care of themselves? Unpaid care may include help with personal needs or household chores. It might be managing a person's finances, arranging for outside services, or visiting regularly to see how they are doing. This person need not live with you.

NATIONAL LONG-TERM CARE SURVEY   In contrast to the four preceding examples, the NLTCS, which was conducted from 1982 through 2004, is a survey of the older population, with special emphasis on those with chronic disabilities. Chronic disabilities are defined as problems with everyday tasks that have lasted three months or are expected to last at least three more months. Respondents with disabilities who do not live in nursing homes are asked about the help they receive with each of a series of six ADL and eleven IADL tasks. One or more "helpers" may be identified for each task. These helpers may be coresident or not; they may be family members, friends, or neighbors; or they may be paid professionals. Of all the surveys reviewed here, the NLTCS provides the most detailed and thorough characterization of care networks, including the presence of unpaid family care providers in those networks; the perspective, however, is that of the care recipient, and the care activity captured is limited to that directed at the chronically disabled sixty-five-and-older population. The NLTCS has been used in several studies of the care needs of the disabled older population and their use of both paid and unpaid care services (Spillman and Pezzin 2000; Spillman 2004; Manton, Gu, and Lamb 2006; Wolff and Kasper 2006).

SUMMARY OF SURVEY EXAMPLES   The preceding examples of surveys have been chosen in part because of the contrasts they present with respect to the problem of measuring unpaid adult care. First, the perspective is in most cases that of the caregiver or potential caregiver, but it is sometimes that of the care recipient. The coverage of the potential caregiver population varies considerably: the NSFH refers to "relatives" who are "seriously ill or disabled," but is limited to nonresident care recipients. The broadest coverage is provided by the SIPP and NAC/ AARP surveys, which ask about care provided to relatives (family members) or friends; at the other end of this spectrum are the HRS questions that ask specifically about help provided to parents or parents-in-law.

The reference periods over which care activities are defined also vary greatly. The SIPP uses a one-month reference period, while the HRS uses twenty-four months. The NLTCS does not refer to a specific time period when it asks respondents to list helpers for each task, but NLTCS questions about hours of help received refer to just the one-week period prior to the interview.

Finally, there is tremendous diversity in the task specificity of the surveys' questions. The NSFH asks people whether they "take care" of relatives, leaving them to determine what is to be counted. The NAC/AARP question is also very broad in scope, listing not only a number of typical daily tasks but also "visiting regularly." Referring to "basic personal activities," the HRS provides some specific examples (dressing, eating, and bathing) but leaves the respondent some latitude on what additional such activities might be counted. The SIPP takes a similar approach, while providing a longer list of illustrative tasks. The NLTCS is the most specific, asking about a particular, and closed-end, list of six specific ADLs and eleven specific IADLs.

These differences in scope, coverage, and specificity lead to large differences in survey estimates of the size and characteristics of the caregiver population, as well as of the aggregate volume of the care work they provide. Beyond this, the various caregiver surveys, to varying degrees, have shortcomings that limit the types of analyses that they can support. For example, long reference periods of twelve or twenty-four months lead to ambiguity about the exact timing of care work; it cannot, for example, be assumed that someone who has done care work at some point over a two-year interval has done such work in each month of that interval. Moreover, it is hard to model trade-offs in the allocation of time to caring and paid employment when the reference periods for these two uses of time are extremely different—for example, twelve or twenty-four months for care work and one week or one month for paid employment.

Also, measures that make no distinctions between help with ADL tasks and help with IADL tasks are less useful than those that do. As we discuss later in this appendix, there is more potential for joint production in IADL than in ADL tasks, with further implications for the valuation of care efforts or for the study of the relative efficiency of family and formal care. Coresidence of the care provider and the care recipient also has implications for the efficiency of care resources and for joint production of household tasks. The NSFH, which asks only about care provided to nonresident relatives, therefore cannot be used to make comparisons of this sort.

Industry and Occupation Classifications of Paid Workers

Standard labor force surveys deploy occupation and industry codes that can be used to create consistent categories of paid care work and to produce measures of the care workforce that include those caring for children or adults. Previous research has defined caring occupations as those in which "workers are supposed to provide a face-to-face service that develops the human capabilities of the recipient" (England et al. 2002, 455). The term "human capabilities" refers to health, skills, or proclivities that are useful to oneself or others. These researchers also define a larger category of occupations that involve interactive service work that may require emotional labor but less genuine emotional connection (England, Budig, and Folbre 2002, table A.1).

Data on industry of employment can be used to designate participation in a care industry even by those not in a care occupation. For instance, Randy Albelda, Mignon Duffy, and Nancy Folbre (2009) apply the distinction between interactive care and support care in unpaid work to paid work, designating employment in a care occupation as interactive care and employment in a care industry, but not a care occupation, as support care. Their list of care industries includes health care, K-12 education, care of children and youth, social services, and private households. A significant number of employees in these industries are not engaged in interactive care occupations. For example, hospitals employ a large number of secretaries, managers, janitors, cooks, and laundry workers.

Our own categorization of care occupations and industries, presented in boxes A.3 and A.4, is similar. Most care jobs are concentrated in five major occupational groups (health care practitioners, health care support occupations, community and social services occupations, personal care and services occupations, and education, training, and library occupations) and in five industry groups (education, health care, social assistance, personal care and services, and private households).[5] There are also large numbers of care workers in employment services, which is part of the larger administrative services sector, and government services, and a significant number of the self-employed are care workers.

BOX A.3 / Care Industries

Educational Services
Elementary and secondary schools
Colleges and universities, including junior colleges
Business, technical, and trade schools and training
Other schools, instruction, and educational services

Health Care and Social Assistance
　Hospitals
　Health services, except hospitals
　　Offices of physicians
　　Offices of dentists
　　Offices of chiropractors
　　Offices of optometrists
　　Offices of other health practitioners
　　Outpatient care centers
　　Home health care services
　　Other health care services
　　Nursing care facilities
　　Residential care facilities, without nursing
　Social assistance
　　Individual and family services
　　Community food and housing, and emergency services
　　Vocational rehabilitation services
　　Child day care services

Other Services
　Religious organizations

Private Households

Public Administration
　Administration of human resource programs

BOX A.4 / Care Occupations

Professional and Related Occupations
Life, physical, and social science occupations
    Psychologists
Community and social services occupations
    Counselors
    Social workers
    Miscellaneous community and social service specialists
    Clergy
    Directors, religious activities, and education
    Religious workers, all other
Education, training, and library occupations
    Postsecondary teachers
    Preschool and kindergarten teachers
    Elementary and middle school teachers
    Secondary school teachers
    Special education teachers
    Other teachers and instructors
    Teacher's assistants
Health care practitioner and technical occupations
    Chiropractors
    Dentists
    Dietitians and nutritionists
    Optometrists
    Pharmacists
    Physicians and surgeons
    Physicians' assistants
    Podiatrists
    Registered nurses
    Audiologists
    Occupational therapists
    Physical therapists
    Radiation therapists
    Recreational therapists
    Respiratory therapists
    Speech language pathologists
    Therapists, all other
    Health diagnosis and treating practitioners, all other
    Dental hygienists
    Emergency medical technicians and paramedics
    Licensed practical and licensed vocational nurses
    Opticians, dispensing

(*Box continues on p. 224.*)

BOX A.4 / *Continued*

Service occupations
  Health care support occupations
    Nursing, psychiatric, and home health aides
    Occupational therapists' assistants and aides
    Physical therapists' assistants and aides
    Massage therapists
    Dental assistants
    Medical assistants and other health care support occupations
  Personal care and service occupations
    Child care workers
    Personal and home care aides
    Recreation and fitness workers
    Residential advisers

Using labor force surveys to identify care workers offers only an approximation of those actually engaged in care work. For instance, not all nurses interact with patients; some may be managers handling scheduling and paperwork. Analysis of the actual content of work performed requires more fine-grained tools, based on time use diaries or ethnographic observation.

The classification of work processes can have momentous policy implications. For example, until an administrative rule change in December 2011, workers paid to care for adults who need assistance in their own homes were not covered by the Fair Labor Standards Act (FLSA), which guarantees minimum wage and overtime pay, on the grounds that they were primarily providing "companionship." In some ways, the issue of "companionship" resembles the issue of supervisory care, discussed earlier, and could be susceptible to analysis using time diary surveys.

OCCUPATION AND INDUSTRY DATA SOURCES   The problem of measuring the number of paid care workers is complicated by the fact that no single data set captures the range of occupational and demographic detail needed to accurately describe the paid care workforce. Establishment surveys—surveys of employers or places of employment—do not capture people working in private households or those who are self-employed, nor do they report demographic information, but they generally use occupational and industry classification schemes with the high level of disaggregation needed to study care work. Household and individual surveys capture the demographic texture of occupations but generally provide insufficient industry or occupational detail. As discussed, several national data sets can and have been used by England, Budig, and Folbre (2002) and Albelda, Duffy, and Folbre (2009) to measure care employment and demographic detail by occupation and industry in all or part of the care sector. In principle, more detailed studies could be carried out at a secure-data "enclave," if researchers were able to link individual- and firm-level data, possibly in conjunction with other restricted-access data sources such as Social Security earnings histories. In general, studies of this sort are quite costly and raise complex access and data security issues.

ESTABLISHMENT SURVEYS   The Occupational and Earnings Statistics (OES) is an annual survey of 400,000 establishments; data are combined over a three-year period to produce a 1.2 million record sample. It covers wage and salary workers in nonfarm establishments but excludes self-employed people, owners and partners in unincorporated firms, household workers, and unpaid family workers. Detailed occupational and industry categories are identified, but there are no demographic or work conditions data. The Current Employment Statistics (CES) survey is a monthly survey covering 140,000 businesses and state agencies and 400,000 work sites. Its strength is its level of geographic disaggregation.

HOUSEHOLD AND INDIVIDUAL-LEVEL SURVEYS   The Current Population Survey is a monthly survey of 50,000 households, with an annual supplement that captures an additional 2,500. Data are available at fine levels of geographic disaggregation, down to metropolitan areas, but the sample size is small and the occupation and industry definitions are not as detailed as in the OES. The CPS includes some demographic and work condition data. The annual March CPS, now known as the American Social and Economic Supplement (ASES), provides important additional demographic and work conditions data on each individual.

NATIONAL LONGITUDINAL SURVEY OF YOUTH   The NLSY is a panel data set constructed from an annual household survey of eligible people that asks about education, employment, and earnings. Using these responses, the census codes individuals into occupations and industries. The data can also be used to determine whether people are self-employed or not. Paula England and her colleagues (2002) used the NLSY for 1983 to 1992 to measure the wage penalty associated with working in a care job.

AMERICAN COMMUNITY SURVEY   The ACS is the largest household survey in the United States, with an annual sample size of 3 million people. The ACS uses the census industry and occupation codes, limiting its usefulness for closer analysis of adult care workers. It permits analysis at a high level of geographic disaggregation, but occupational and industry disaggregation is limited because it uses the census codes. Albelda and his colleagues (2009) used the ACS to measure the size of the care sector in Massachusetts.

ESTABLISHMENT AND HOUSEHOLD SURVEYS COMBINED   The National Employment Matrix is a secondary data set that combines data from the OES, the CPS, and the CES to provide ten-year employment projections by occupation. In combining the three data sets, the National Employment Matrix can be used to get a more complete and detailed measure of employment in the care sector because it breaks industries and occupations down into the greater detail that is possible with establishment surveys, while also including measures of self-employed people and household workers that are only available in household surveys.

CARE INTENSITY, JOINT PRODUCTION, AND ECONOMIES OF SCALE

Time use surveys are typically administered to adults who are supplying care rather than to children or other individuals who are receiving care. Since more than one person often cares for one individual, it is difficult to use time use surveys to ascertain how much care time an individual care recipient has received, without careful analysis of accurate data regarding who else was present (Folbre et al. 2005). Even with excellent data, problems of interpretation remain. From the caregiver's point of view, is it twice as much work to care for two dependents at the same time as to care for one? Obviously not, but the burden is probably somewhat greater. From the care recipient's point of view, does care provided by two adults at once represent twice as much care as by a single adult? Obviously not, but the net effect is unclear.

With respect to adult and elder care, the greatest potential for joint production seems to lie in the areas of IADLs such as housework, meal preparation, and shopping, which is especially relevant in the case of coresidence. For activities such as these, a unit of an informal care provider's time may produce meals or a clean house for the care recipient—someone who presumably cannot conduct housework or meal preparation on his or her own—and for the care provider as well. Wolf (2004) discusses how joint production creates problems for the social valuation of informal care. But joint production also creates problems in the measurement of inputs. For example, it may be important to determine how much of a caregiver's time it takes to jointly produce output, such as the housework or meal preparation outputs just mentioned. And it may turn out that, in some cases at least, it takes no more time to prepare a meal for two than for one. If the alternatives to be compared are for either a family member or a publicly funded paid helper to provide this service, then the small (and possibly zero) incremental time costs of family production seem to favor the family as a more efficient provider of care services. However, if the problem is one of assessing the amount of paid help to allocate to the needy elder, if for some reason the family care provider is incapacitated or no longer available, then the incremental time input previously provided by the family member is clearly inappropriate.

SUMMARY

Inconsistent definitions and varying approaches to measurement of both unpaid and paid care work make it difficult to create a unified picture of care provision. Efforts to forge a stronger consensus on these issues could strengthen this field of research. Our assessment of this literature yields three important recommendations:

- Researchers should define care more consistently across surveys, making distinctions between interactive care, support care, and supervisory care. They should also harmonize other features of measurement such as category thresholds (for example, how much care must someone provide to be characterized as a caregiver).

- Researchers should look for ways of improving the quality of care measurement, including examination of the receipt as well as the provision of care ("double-entry bookkeeping") and mixed-method approaches that use both quantitative and qualitative survey instruments.

- Rather than focusing simply on unpaid or paid care, researchers should examine combinations, trade-offs, and synergies among different types of care provision and develop improved methods—for example, contingent value questions—for estimating the market value of unpaid care.

In the meantime, researchers can move forward with efforts to make the best possible use of existing data, mindful of its many limitations.

NOTES

1. For a more complete list of national surveys that include disability items, see Field and Jette (2007), table 2.1.
2. Assessment of ADLs and IADLs is sometimes supplemented by more specific measures of dependency for profoundly disabled individuals, such as those suffering mental handicaps or dementia (Lohrmann, Dijkstra, and Dassen 2003).
3. For more information about the NSFH, see http://www.ssc.wisc.edu/nsfh/design.htm (accessed April 30, 2012).
4. For more information on the Health and Retirement Survey, see http://hrsonline.isr. umich.edu/index.php?p=dbook (accessed April 30, 2012).
5. These major occupational and industry groups are defined in the Standard Occupational Classification (SOC) and the North American Industrial Classification System (NAICS), both of which are discussed later.

References

Abel, Emily K., and Margaret K. Nelson. 1990. "Circles of Care: An Introductory Essay." In *Circles of Care: Work and Identity in Women's Lives,* edited by Emily K. Abel and Margaret K. Nelson. New York: State University of New York Press.

Abraham, Katherine, and Christopher Mackie, eds. 2005. *Beyond the Market: Designing Nonmarket Accounts for the United States.* Washington, D.C.: National Academies Press.

Abraham, Katharine G., Aaron Maitland, and Suzanne M. Bianchi. 2006. "Nonresponse in the American Time Use Survey: Who Is Missing from the Data and How Much Does It Matter?" *Public Opinion Quarterly* 70(5): 676–703.

Adler, Michele C., and Gerry E. Hendershot. 2000. "Federal Disability Surveys in the United States: Lessons and Challenges." Paper presented to the American Statistical Association. Portland, Oreg. (May 17–21). Available at Proceedings of the Survey Research Methods, http://www.amstat.org/sections/srms/Proceedings/y2000.html (accessed May 19, 2011).

Adler, Paul S., Seok-Woo Kwon, and Charles Heckshur. 2008. "Professional Work: The Emergence of Collaborative Community." *Organization Science* 19(2): 359–76.

Akerlof, George. 1982. "Labor Contracts as Partial Gift Exchange." *Quarterly Journal of Economics* 97(4): 543–70.

Albelda, Randy, Mignon Duffy, and Nancy Folbre. 2009. "Counting on Care Work: Human Infrastructure in Massachusetts." University of Massachusetts research report (September). Available at: http://countingcare.org/documents/counting_on_care_web_0909.pdf (accessed May 19, 2011).

Alecxih, Lisa Maria B., Sharon Zeruld, and BrieAnne Olearczyk. 2001. "Characteristics of Caregivers Based on the Survey of Income and Program Participation." Selected issue briefs. Washington: U.S. Administration on Aging, National Family Caregiver Support Program. Available at: http://www.lewin.com/content/publications/1557.pdf (accessed May 19, 2011).

Allard, Mary Dorinda, Suzanne Bianchi, Jay Stewart, and Vanessa R. Wight. 2007. "Comparing Childcare Measures in the ATUS and Earlier Time-Diary Studies." *Monthly Labor Review* 130(May): 27–36.

Amirkhanyan, Anna, and Douglas A. Wolf. 2003. "Caregiver Stress and Non-Caregiver Stress: Exploring the Pathways of Psychiatric Morbidity." *The Gerontologist* 43(6): 817–27.

———. 2006. "Parent Care and the Stress Process: Findings from Panel Data." *Journal of Gerontology: Social Sciences* 61B(5): S248–55.

Amrein, Audrey L., and David C. Berliner. 2002. "High-Stakes Testing, Uncertainty, and Student Learning." *Education Policy Analysis Archives* 10(18). Available at: http://epaa.asu.edu/epaa/v10n18 (accessed August 16, 2010).

Andreoni, James. 1990. "Impure Altruism and Donations to Public Goods: A Theory of Warm-Glow Giving." *Economic Journal* 100(401): 464–77.

References

Andresen, Elena M., Carol A. Fitch, Patricia M. McLendon, and Allan R. Meyers. 2000. "Reliability and Validity of Disability Questions for U.S. Census 2000." *American Journal of Public Health* 90(8): 1297–99.

Andrews, Frank. 1989. "Construct Validity and Error Components of Surveys." In *Survey Research Methods: A Reader,* edited by Eleanor Singer and Stanley Presser. Chicago: University of Chicago Press.

Angel, Ronald, and Marta Tienda. 1982. "Determinants of Extended Household Structure: Cultural Patterns or Economic Need?" *American Journal of Sociology* 87(6): 1360–83.

Appelbaum, Eileen. 2010. "Institutions, Firms, and the Quality of Jobs in Low-Wage Labor Markets." In *Low-Wage Work in the Wealthy World,* edited by Jerome Gautié and John Schmitt. New York: Russell Sage Foundation.

Appelbaum, Eileen, Thomas Bailey, Peter Berg, and Arne Kalleberg. 2000. *Manufacturing Advantage: Why High Performance Work Systems Pay Off.* Ithaca, N.Y.: ILR Press.

Appelbaum, Eileen, Annette D. Bernhardt, and Richard J. Murnane, eds. 2003. *Low-Wage America: How Employers Are Reshaping Opportunity in the Workplace.* New York: Russell Sage Foundation.

Appelbaum, Eileen, Jody Hoffer Gittell, and Carrie Leana. 2008. "High-Performance Work Practices and Economic Recovery and Performance." *Journal of Applied Behavioral Science* 44(1): 25–47.

Arno, Peter, Carol Levine, and Margaret M. Memmnott. 1999. "The Economic Value of Informal Caregiving." *Health Affairs* 18(2): 182–88.

Autor, David. 2010. *The Polarization of Job Opportunities in the U.S. Labor Market: Implications for Employment and Earnings.* Washington, D.C.: Center for American Progress.

Babcock, Linda, and Sara Laschever. 2003. *Women Don't Ask: Negotiation and the Gender Divide.* Princeton, N.J.: Princeton University Press.

Baca Zinn, Maxine, and Barbara Wells. 2000. "Diversity Within Latino Families: New Lessons for Family Social Science." In *Handbook of Family Diversity,* edited by David H. Demo, Katherine R. Allen, and Mark A. Fine. New York: Oxford University Press.

Badgett, M. V. Lee, and Nancy Folbre. 2003. "Job Gendering: Occupational Choice and the Labor Market." *Industrial Relations* 42(2): 270–98.

Barnett, Steven W., Dale J. Epstein, Allison H. Friedman, Rachel A. Sansanelli, and Jason T. Husdtedt. 2009. *The State of Preschool 2009.* New Brunswick, N.J.: Rutgers University, National Institute for Early Education Research. Available at: http://nieer.org/yearbook/pdf/yearbook.pdf (accessed November 4, 2010).

Barrett, Linda. 2006. "The Costs of Long-Term Care: Public Perceptions Versus Reality in 2006: AARP Fact Sheet." Washington, D.C.: American Association of Retired Persons (December).

Bass, Sandra, Margie K. Shields, and Richard E. Behrman. 2004. "Children, Families, and Foster Care: Analysis and Recommendations." *The Future of Children* 14(1): 4–29.

Batson, Daniel C. 1990. "How Social an Animal? The Human Capacity for Caring." *American Psychologist* 45(3): 336–46.

Baumol, William J. 1967. "Macroeconomics of Unbalanced Growth: The Anatomy of Urban Crisis." *American Economic Review* 57(3): 415–26.

Becker, Gary S. 1993. *A Treatise on the Family,* rev. ed. Cambridge, Mass.: Harvard University Press.

———. 1996. *Accounting for Tastes.* Cambridge, Mass.: Harvard University Press.

Becker, Gary S., and George J. Stigler. 1977. "De Gustibus Non Est Disputandem." *American Economic Review* 67(2): 76–90.

Beere, Carole A. 1990. *Gender Roles: A Handbook of Text and Measures.* New York: Greenwood Press.

Behrman, Jere R., Robert A. Pollak, and Paul Taubman. 1995. *From Parent to Child: Intrahousehold Allocations and Intergenerational Relations in the United States.* Chicago: University of Chicago Press.

Bellah, Robert, Richard Madsen, William Sullivan, Ann Swidler, and Steven M. Tipton. 1985. *Habits of the Heart: Individualism and Commitment in American Life.* New York: Harper & Row.

Bem, Sandra L. 1974. "The Measurement of Psychological Androgyny." *Journal of Consulting and Clinical Psychology* 42(2): 155–62.

Benedict, Ruth E. 2006. "Disparities in Use of and Unmet Need for Therapeutic and Supportive Services Among School-Age Children with Functional Limitations: A Comparison Across Settings." *Health Services Research* 41(1): 103–24. Available at: http://www.ncbi.nlm.nih.gov/pmc/articles/PMC1681537/pdf/hesr041-0103.pdf (accessed May 20, 2011).

Benhabib, Seyla. 1987. "The Generalized and the Concrete Other: The Kohlberg-Gilligan Controversy and Feminist Theory." In *Feminism as Critique: On the Politics of Gender,* edited by Seyla Benhabib and Drucilla Cornell. Minneapolis: University of Minnesota Press.

Benitez-Silva, Hugo, Moshe Buchinsky, Hiu Man Chan, John Rust, and Sofia Sheidvassen. 1999. "An Empirical Analysis of the Social Security Disability Application, Appeal, and Award Process." *Labour Economics* 6(2): 147–78.

Benner, Chris, Bob Brownstein, Laura Dresser, and Laura Leete. 2001. "Staircases and Treadmills: The Role of Labor Market Intermediaries in Placing Workers and Fostering Upward Mobility." Paper presented to the annual meeting of the Industrial Relations Research Association. New Orleans, La. (January 4–8).

Bergmann, Barbara R. 1981. "The Economic Risks of Being a Housewife." *American Economic Review* 71(2): 81–86.

———. 1986. *The Economic Emergence of Women.* New York: Basic Books.

———. 2009. "Long Leaves, Child Well-being, and Gender Equality." In *Gender Equality: Transforming Family Divisions of Labor,* edited by Janet C. Gornick, Marcia K. Meyers, and Erik Olin Wright. London: Verso.

Bernhardt, Annette, Ruth Milkman, Nik Theodore, Douglas Heckathorn, Mirabai Auer, James DeFilippis, Ana Luz Gonzalez, Victor Narro, Jason Perelshteyn, Diana Polson, and Michael Spiller. 2009. "Broken Laws, Unprotected Workers: Violations of Employment and Labor Laws in America's Cities." Available at: http://www.nelp.org/page/-/brokenlaws/BrokenLawsReport2009.pdf?nocdn=1 (accessed May 20, 2011).

Bianchi, Suzanne M. 2006. "Mothers and Daughters 'Do,' Fathers 'Don't Do' Family: Gender and Generational Bonds." *Journal of Marriage and Family* 68(4): 812–16.

———. 2011. "Family Change and Time Allocation in American Families." *Annals of the American Academy of Political and Social Science* 638(1): 21–44.

Bianchi, Suzanne M., V. Joseph Hotz, Kathleen McGarry, and Judith A. Seltzer. 2008. "Intergenerational Ties: Theories, Trends, and Challenges." In *Intergenerational Caregiving,* edited by Alan Booth, Ann C. Crouter, Suzanne M. Bianchi, and Judith A. Seltzer. Washington, D.C.: Urban Institute.

References

Bianchi, Suzanne M., and Sara Raley. 2005. "Time Allocation in Working Families." In *Work, Family, Health, and Well-being,* edited by Suzanne M. Bianchi, Lynne M. Casper, and Rosalind Berkowitz King. Mahwah, N.J.: Lawrence Erlbaum Associates.

Bianchi, Suzanne M., John P. Robinson, and Melissa A. Milkie. 2006. *Changing Rhythms of American Family Life.* New York: Russell Sage Foundation.

Bishop, Christine E., Dana Beth Weinberg, Walter Leutz, Almas Dossa, Susan G. Pfefferle, and Rebekah M. Zincavage. 2008. "Nursing Assistants' Job Commitment: Effect of Nursing Home Organizational Factors and Impact on Resident Well-being." *The Gerontologist* 48(special issue I): 36–45.

Bittman, Michael, Lyn Craig, and Nancy Folbre. 2004. "Packaging Care: What Happens When Children Receive Nonparental Care?" In *Family Time: The Social Organization of Care,* edited by Nancy Folbre and Michael Bittman. New York: Routledge.

Blau, David. 2001. *The Child Care Problem: An Economic Analysis.* New York: Russell Sage Foundation.

Blau, Francine D., Mary C. Brinton, and David B. Grusky, eds. 2006. *The Declining Significance of Gender?* New York: Russell Sage Foundation.

Blau, Joel, and Mimi Abramovitz. 2010. *The Dynamics of Social Welfare Policy,* 3d ed. New York: Oxford University Press.

Blinder, Alan S. 2006. "Offshoring: The Next Industrial Revolution?" *Foreign Affairs* 85(2): 113–28.

Blustein, Jan, Sewin Chan, and Frederico C. Guanais. 2004. "Elevated Depressive Symptoms Among Caregiving Grandparents." *Health Services Research* 39(6p1): 1671–90.

Boaz, Rachel F. 1996. "Full-Time Employment and Informal Caregiving in the 1980s." *Medical Care* 34(6): 524–36.

Boris, Eileen, and Jennifer Klein. 2008. "Labor on the Home Front: Unionizing Home-Based Care Workers." *New Labor Forum* 17(2): 32–41.

Boushey, Heather. 2005a. "Family-Friendly Policies: Boosting Mothers' Wages." Washington, D.C.: Center for Economic and Policy Research (April 6). Available at: http://www.cepr.net/documents/publications/labor_markets_2005_04_06.pdf (accessed January 3, 2011).

———. 2005b. "Are Women Opting Out? Debunking the Myth." Briefing paper. Washington, D.C.: Center for Economic Policy Research.

Bowker, Geoffrey C., and Susan Leigh Star. 1999. *Sorting Things Out: Classification and Its Consequences.* Cambridge, Mass.: MIT Press.

Bowles, Samuel. 1998. "Endogenous Preferences: The Cultural Consequences of Markets and Other Economic Institutions." *Journal of Economic Literature* 36(1): 75–111.

Bowles, Samuel, Herbert Gintis, and Melissa Osborne. 2001. "Incentive-Enhancing Preferences: Personal Behavior and Earnings." *American Economic Review* 91(2): 155–58.

Bowman, Barbara T., M. Suzanne Donovan, and M. Susan Burns, eds. 2000. *Eager to Learn: Educating Our Preschoolers.* Washington, D.C.: National Academies Press.

Brannon, Diane, Teta Barry, Peter Kemper, Andrea Schreiner, and Joe Vasey. 2007. "Job Perceptions and Intent to Leave Among Direct Care Workers: Evidence From the Better Jobs Better Care Demonstrations." *The Gerontologist* 47(6): 820–29.

Braverman, Harry. 1975. *Labor and Monopoly Capital: The Degradation of Work in the Twentieth Century.* New York: Monthly Review Press.

Brighouse, Harry, and Erik Olin Wright. 2009. "Strong Gender Egalitarianism." In *Gender Equality: Transforming Family Divisions of Labor,* edited by Janet C. Gornick, Marcia K. Meyers, and Erik Olin Wright. London: Verso.

Browne, Kingsley. 1999. *Divided Labors: An Evolutionary View of Women at Work.* New Haven, Conn.: Yale University Press.

Brown-Lyons, Melanie, Anne Robertson, and Jean Layzer. 2001. *Kith and Kin: Informal Child Care: Highlights from Recent Research.* New York: Columbia University, National Center for Children in Poverty.

Bubeck, Diemut. 1995. *Care, Gender, Justice.* Oxford: Clarendon Press.

Budig, Michelle J., and Paula England. 2001. "The Wage Penalty for Motherhood." *American Sociological Review* 66(2): 204–25.

Budig, Michelle J., and Nancy Folbre. 2004. "Activity, Proximity, or Responsibility: Measuring Parental Childcare Time." In *Family Time: The Social Organization of Care,* edited by Nancy Folbre and Michael Bittman. New York: Routledge.

Budig, Michelle J., and Melissa J. Hodges. 2010. "Differences in Disadvantage: Variation in the Motherhood Penalty Across White Women's Earnings Distribution." *American Sociological Review* 75(5): 1–24.

Budig, Michelle J., and Joya Misra. 2009. "How Carework Employment Shapes Earnings in a Cross-National Perspective." Department of Sociology, University of Massachusetts at Amherst.

Budlender, Debbie. 2008. "The Statistical Evidence on Care and Non-Care Work Across Six Countries." Paper 4. United Nations Research Institute for Social Development, Gender and Development Program (December). Available at: http://www.unrisd.org/unrisd/website/document.nsf/ab82a6805797760f80256b4f005da1ab/f9fec4ea774573e7c1257560003a96b2/$FILE/BudlenderREV.pdf (accessed May 20, 2011).

Burgio, Louis D., and Michelle Bourgeois. 1992. "Treating Severe Behavioral Disorders in Geriatric Residential Settings." *Behavioral Residential Therapy* 7(2): 145–68.

Burgio, Louis D., Bernard T. Engel, Andre Hawkins, Kathleen McCormick, and Ann Scheve. 1990. "A Descriptive Analysis of Nursing Staff Behaviors in a Teaching Nursing Home: Differences Among NAs, LPNs, and RNs." *The Gerontologist* 30(1): 107–12.

Burke, Sheila P., Judith Feder, and Paul N. van de Water, eds. 2005. *Developing a Better Long-Term Care Policy: A Vision and Strategy for America's Future.* Washington, D.C.: National Academy of Social Insurance. Available at: http://www.nasi.org/sites/default/files/research/Developing_a_Better_Long-Term_Care_Policy.pdf (accessed May 20, 2011).

Burr, Jeffrey A., and Jan E. Mutchler. 1999. "Race and Ethnic Variation in Norms of Filial Responsibility Among Older Persons." *Journal of Marriage and the Family* 61(3): 674–87.

Burton, Alice, Marcy Whitebook, Marci Young, Dan Bellm, Claudia Wayne, Richard N. Brandon, and Erin Maher. 2002. "Estimating the Size and Components of the U.S. Child Care Workforce and Caregiving Population." Human Services Policy Center Reports. Washington, D.C.: Center for Child Care Work Force.

Burton, Lynda C., Jason T. Newsom, Richard Schulz, Calvin H. Hirsch, and Pearl S. German. 1997. "Preventive Health Behaviors Among Spousal Caregivers." *Preventive Medicine* 26(2): 162–69.

References

Burwell, Brian, Kate Sredl, and Steve Eiken. 2009. "Medicaid Long-Term Care Expenditures FY 2008." Cambridge, Mass.: Thomson Reuters (December 1). Available at: http://www.hcbs.org/moreInfo.php/doc/2723 (accessed January 8, 2010).

Buss, David M. 1996. "Sexual Conflict: Evolutionary Insights into Feminism and the "Battle of the Sexes." In *Sex, Power, Conflict. Evolutionary and Feminist Perspectives,* edited by David M. Buss and Neil M. Malamuth. New York: Oxford University Press.

Calvert, Cynthia T. 2010. *Family Responsibilities Discrimination: Litigation Update 2010.* San Francisco: Center for Work Life Law. Available at: http://www.worklifelaw.org/pubs/FRDupdate.pdf (accessed January 2, 2011).

Camilli, Gregory, Sadako Vargas, Sharon Ryan, and W. Steven Barnett. 2010. "Meta-Analysis of the Effects of Early Education Interventions on Cognitive and Social Development." *Teachers' College Record.* Available at: http://www.tcrecord.org/Content.asp?ContentID=15440 (accessed October 12, 2010).

Cancian, Francesca M. 2000. "Paid Emotional Care." In *Care Work: Gender, Class, and the Welfare State,* edited by Madonna Harrington Meyer. New York: Routledge.

Cancian, Francesca M., and Stacey J. Oliker. 2000. *Caring and Gender.* Walnut Creek, Calif.: Alta Mira Press.

Cancian, Maria, Sheldon Danziger, and Peter Gottschalk. 1993. "Working Wives and Family Income Inequality Among Married Couples." In *Uneven Tides: Rising Inequality in America,* edited by Peter Gottschalk and Sheldon Danziger. New York: Russell Sage Foundation.

Cancian, Maria, and Robert Schoeni. 1992. "Female Earnings and the Level and Distribution of Household Income in Developed Countries." Luxembourg Income Study (LIS) Working Paper 84 (September).

Carasso, Adam, and Eugene Steuerle. 2005. "The Hefty Penalty on Marriage Facing Many Households with Children." *The Future of Children* 15(2): 157–75.

Carlson, Marcia J., and Sara S. McLanahan. 2010. "Fathers in Fragile Families." In *The Role of the Father in Child Development,* 5th ed., edited by Michael E. Lamb. Hoboken, N.J.: Wiley & Sons.

Casper, Lynne M., and Suzanne M. Bianchi. 2002. *Continuity and Change in the American Family.* Thousand Oaks, Calif.: Sage Publications.

Center for the Childcare Workforce. n.d. "Worthy Wages: The Worthy Wage Campaign." Available at: http://www.ccw.org/index.php?option=com_content&task=view&id=24&Itemid=53 (accessed February 20, 2012).

Center for Law and Social Policy (CLASP). American Bar Association (ABA). 2010. "Relative Foster Care Licensing Waivers in the States: Policies and Possibilities." September 29. Available at: http://www.clasp.org/admin/site/publications/files/Relative-foster-care-licensing-waivers-in-the-states101810.pdf (accessed February 27, 2012).

Chadiha, Letha Ann, Sheila Feld, and Jane Rafferty. 2010. "Likelihood of African American Primary Caregivers and Care Recipients Receiving Assistance from Secondary Caregivers: A Rural-Urban Comparison." *Journal of Applied Gerontology,* published online May 25, 2010, doi:10.1177/0733464810371099.

Chambers, Jay G., Thomas B. Parrish, and Jenifer J. Harr. 2004. "What Are We Spending on Special Education in the United States, 1999–2000?" Report 1, submitted to the U.S. Department of Education, Office of Special Education Programs. Palo Alto, Calif.: Special Education Expenditure Project, Center for Special Education Finance (June).

Chambers, Jay G., Thomas B. Parrish, Joanne C. Lieberman, and Jean M. Wolman. 1998. "What Are We Spending on Special Education in the United States?" Brief 8. Palo Alto, Calif.: Center for Special Education Finance, American Institutes of Research (February). Available at: http://www.specialed.us/Parents/ASMT%20Advocacy/CSEF/BRIEF8.PDF (accessed May 20, 2011).

Charles, Kerwin Kofi, and Purvi Sevak. 2005. "Can Family Care Substitute for Nursing Home Care?" *Journal of Health Economics* 24(6): 1174–90.

Charles, Maria, and Karen Bradley. 2009. "Indulging Our Gendered Selves: Sex Segregation by Field of Study in 44 Countries." *American Journal of Sociology* 114(4): 924–76.

Charles, Maria, and David B. Grusky. 2004. *Occupational Ghettos: The Worldwide Segregation of Women and Men.* Stanford, Calif.: Stanford University Press.

Charmes, Jacques. 2006. "A Review of Empirical Evidence on Time Use in Africa from UN-Sponsored Surveys." Working paper 73 in *Gender, Time Use, and Poverty in Sub-Saharan Africa,* edited by C. Mark Blackden and Quentin Wodon. Washington, D.C.: World Bank.

Cherlin, Andrew J. 2009. *The Marriage-Go-Round: The State of Marriage and the Family in America Today.* New York: Vintage Books.

Child Trends. 2010. "State Child Welfare Policy Database." Available at: http://www.childwelfarepolicy.org/maps/state (accessed May 20, 2011,).

Child Welfare League of America. 2005. *CWLA State Child Welfare Agency Survey.* Unpublished data formerly available online as part of the Child Welfare League of America National Data Analysis System at: http://ndas.cwla.org/data_stats.

Choi, Jung-Kyoo, and Samuel Bowles. 2007. "The Coevolution of Parochial Altruism and War." *Science* 318(5850): 636–40.

Christakis, Nicholas A., and Paul D. Allison. 2009. "Inter-Spousal Mortality Effects: Caregiver Burden Across the Spectrum of Disabling Disease." In *Health at Older Ages: The Causes and Consequences of Declining Disability Among the Elderly,* edited by David M. Cutler and David A. Wise. Chicago: University of Chicago Press.

Cohen, Philip N. 2004. "The Gender Division of Labor: Keeping House and Occupational Segregation in the U.S." *Gender and Society* 18(2): 239–52.

Cohen, Philip N., and Lynne M. Casper. 2002. "In Whose Home? Multigenerational Families in the United States, 1998–2000." *Sociological Perspectives* 45(1): 1–20.

Cohen, Philip N., and Miruna Petrescu-Prahova. 2006. "Gendered Living Arrangements Among Children with Disabilities." *Journal of Marriage and Family* 68(3): 630–38.

Coleman, Marilyn, and Lawrence Ganong. 2008. "Normative Beliefs About Sharing Housing with an Older Family Member." *International Journal of Aging and Human Development* 66(1): 49–72.

Coltrane, Scott, and Justin Galt. 2000. "The History of Men's Caring." In *Care Work: Gender, Class, and the Welfare State,* edited by Madonna Harrington Meyer. New York: Routledge.

Commission for Children at Risk. 2010. "Adoption Tax Credit Information." Available at: http://www.comission.org/resources/?id=1390 (accessed May 20, 2011).

Commission on the Measurement of Economic Performance and Social Progress. 2009. "Report of the Commission on the Measurement of Economic Performance and Social Progress." Available at: http://www.stiglitz-sen-fitoussi.fr/en/index.htm (accessed March 5, 2012).

Compton, Janice, and Robert A. Pollak. 2009. "Proximity and Coresidence of Adult Children: Description and Correlates." Working paper 2009-215. Ann Arbor: University of Michigan, Institute for Social Research (October). Available at: http://www.mrrc.isr.umich.edu/publications/papers/pdf/wp215.pdf (accessed May 20, 2011).

Congressional Budget Office (CBO). 2004. *Financing Long-Term Care for the Elderly.* Washington, D.C.: Center for the Development of Human Services, Research Foundation of SUNY at Buffalo State College (April). Available at: http://www.cbo.gov/doc.cfm?index=5400&type=0&sequence=0 (accessed May 20, 2011).

Conway, Michael, M. Teresa Pizzamiglio, and Lauren Mount. 1996. "Status, Communality, and Agency: Implications for Stereotypes of Gender and Other Groups." *Journal of Personality and Social Psychology* 71(1): 25–38.

Cooney, Teresa M., and Peter Uhlenberg. 1990. "The Role of Divorce in Men's Relations with Their Adult Children After Mid-Life." *Journal of Marriage and the Family* 52(3): 677–88.

Correll, Shelley J. 2004. "Constraints into Preferences: Gender, Status, and Emerging Career Aspirations." *American Sociological Review* 69(1): 93–113.

Correll, Shelley J., Stephen Benard, and In Paik. 2007. "Getting a Job: Is There a Motherhood Penalty?" *American Journal of Sociology* 112(5): 1297–1338.

Cotter, David A., Joan A. Hermsen, and Reeve Vanneman. 2004. "Gender Inequality at Work." In *The American People Census 2000 Series.* New York: Russell Sage Foundation and Population Reference Bureau.

———. 2011. "The End of the Gender Revolution? Gender Role Attitudes from 1977 to 2008." *American Journal of Sociology* 117(1): 259–89.

Couch, Kenneth A., Mary C. Daly, and Douglas A. Wolf. 1999. "Time? Money? Both? The Allocation of Resources to Older Parents." *Demography* 36(2): 219–32.

Courtney, Mark E., Amy Dworsky, Joann S. Lee, and Melissa Raap. 2010. "Midwest Evaluation of the Adult Functioning of Foster Youth." Chicago: Chapin Hall at the University of Chicago. Available at: http://www.chapinhall.org/sites/default/files/Midwest_Study_Age_23_24.pdf (accessed May 20, 2011).

Cox, Donald, and Oded Stark. 2005. "On the Demand for Grandchildren: Tied Transfers and the Demonstration Effect." *Journal of Public Economics* 89(9–10): 1665–97.

Crocker, Jillian. 2010. "Buying Time: The Importance of Gender in Union Contracts." Unpublished paper, University of Massachusetts at Amherst, Department of Sociology.

Dalenberg, Douglas, John Fitzgerald, and John Wicks. 2004. "Direct Valuation of Personal Care by Households." *Population Research and Policy Review* 23(1): 73–89.

Daly, Martin, and Margo Wilson. 1983. *Sex, Evolution, and Behavior,* 2d ed. Belmont, Calif.: Wadsworth.

Deci, Edward L. 1971. "Effects of Externally Mediated Rewards on Intrinsic Motivation." *Journal of Personality and Social Psychology* 18(1): 105–15.

Deci, Edward L., and Richard R. M. Ryan. 1985. *Intrinsic Motivation and Self-Determination in Human Behavior.* New York: Plenum Press.

———. 2000. "The 'What' and 'Why' of Goal Pursuits: Human Needs and the Self-Determination of Behavior." *Psychological Inquiry* 11(4): 227–68.

Decker, Frederic H., Peter Gruhn, Lisa Matthews-Martin, K. Jeannine Dollard, and Anthony M. Tucker. 2003. "Results of the 2002 AHCA Survey of Nursing Staff Vacancy and Turnover in Nursing Homes." Health Services Research and Evaluation, American Health Care Association, February 12. Available at: http://www.ahcancal.org/research_data/staffing/Documents/Vacancy_Turnover_Survey2002.pdf (accessed June 1, 2011).

Delp, Linda, and Katie Quan. 2002. "Homecare Worker Organizing in California: An Analysis of a Successful Strategy." *Labor Studies Journal* 27(1): 1–23.

DePanfilis, Diane, Clara Dailing, Kevin D. Frick, Julie Farber, and Lisa Levinthal. 2007. "Hitting the MARC Establishing Foster Care Minimum Adequate Rates for Children." New York, Minneapolis, and Baltimore: Children's Rights, National Foster Parents Association, and University of Maryland School of Social Work (October). Available at: http://www.childrensrights.org/policy-projects/foster-care/hitting-the-marc-foster-care-reimbursement-rates/2 (accessed December 14, 2011).

Diamond, Tim. 1992. *Making Gray Gold: Narratives of Nursing Home Care.* Chicago: University of Chicago Press.

DiMaggio, Paul, and Hugh Louch. 1998. "Socially Embedded Consumer Transactions: For What Kinds of Purchases Do People Most Often Use Networks?" *American Sociological Review* 63(5): 619–37.

DiNitto, Diana M., and Linda K. Cummins. 2005. *Social Welfare: Politics and Public Policy,* 6th ed. Boston: Allyn & Bacon.

Dovidio, John F., Judith L. Allen, and David A. Schroeder. 1990. "The Specificity of Empathy-Induced Helping: Evidence for Altruistic Motivation." *Journal of Personality and Social Psychology* 59(2): 249–60.

Doyle, Joseph J., Jr., and H. Elizabeth Peters. 2007. "The Market for Foster Care: An Empirical Study of the Impact of Foster Care Subsidies." *Review of the Economics of the Household* 5(4): 329–51.

Dresser, Laura. 2008. "Cleaning and Caring in the Home: Shared Problems? Shared Possibilities." In *The Gloves-Off Economy: Workplace Standards at the Bottom of America's Labor Market,* edited by Annette Bernhardt, Heather Boushey, Laura Dresser, and Chris Tilly. Urbana-Champaign, Ill.: Labor and Employment Relations Association.

Dresser, Laura, and Adrienne Pagnac. 2010. "Better Jobs for In-Home Direct Care Workers." Policy brief 5. New York: Direct Care Alliance (October). Available at: http://www.directcarealliance.org/_data/global/images/PolicyBrief5_InHome.pdf (accessed April 29, 2012).

Duffy, Mignon. 2005. "Reproducing Labor Inequalities: Challenges for Feminists Conceptualizing Care at the Intersections of Gender, Race, and Class." *Gender and Society* 19(1): 66–82.

———. 2011. *Making Care Count: A Century of Gender, Race, and Paid Care Work.* New Brunswick, N.J.: Rutgers University Press.

Duncan, Brian, and Laura Argys. 2007. "Economic Incentives and Foster Care Placement." *Southern Economic Journal* 74(1): 354–62.

Duncan, Greg, and Jeanne Brooks Gunn, eds. 1999. *Consequences of Growing Up Poor.* New York: Russell Sage Foundation.

Duncan, Greg J., and Rachel Dunifon. 1998. "Long-Run Effects of Motivation on Labor Market Success." *Social Psychology Quarterly* 61(1): 33–48.

Duncan, Greg J., and Saul D. Hoffman. 1988. "What Are the Economic Consequences of Divorce?" *Demography* 25(4): 641–45.

Duncan, Greg J., Aletha C. Huston, and Thomas S. Weisner. 2007. *Higher Ground: New Hope for the Working Poor and Their Children.* New York: Russell Sage Foundation.

Dweck, Carol S. 2008. "Can Personality Be Changed? The Role of Beliefs in Personality and Change." *Current Directions in Psychological Science* 17(6): 391–94.

Early, Diane, Kelly L. Maxwell, Margaret Burchinal, Soumya Alva, Randall H. Bender, Donna Bryant, Karen Cai, Richard M. Clifford, Caroline Ebanks, James A. Griffin, Gary T. Henry, Carollee Howes, Jeniffer Iriondo-Perez, Hyun-Joo Jeon, Andrew J. Mashburn, Ellen Peisner-Feinberg, Robert C. Pianta, Nathan Vandergrift, and Nicholas Zill. 2007. "Teachers' Education, Classroom Quality, and Young Children's Academic Skills: Results from Seven Studies of Preschool Programs." *Child Development* 78(2): 558–80.

Eckel, Catherine C. 1998. "Are Women Less Selfish Than Men? Evidence from Dictator Experiments." *Economic Journal* 108(448): 726–36.

Eckel, Catherine C., and Philip Grossman. 2001. "Chivalry and Solidarity in Ultimatum Games." *Economic Inquiry* 39(2): 171–89.

Economic Opportunity Institute. 2007. "Washington Family Leave Insurance Fact Sheet." December. Available at: http://www.eoionline.org/work_and_family/fact_sheets/FLI FactSheet-Dec07.pdf (accessed May 20, 2011).

Economic Policy Institute (EPI), State of Working America. 2010. "Wages and Compensation Stagnating: Hourly Wage and Compensation for Production/Non-Supervisory Workers, 1959–2009." EPI analysis of Bureau of Economics and Bureau of Labor Statistics Data. December 14. Available at: http://stateofworkingamerica.org/charts/hourly-wage-and-compensation-growth-for-productionnon-supervisory-workers-1959-2009/ (accessed February 20, 2012).

Ehrle, Jennifer R., and Rob Geen. 2002. "Kin and Non-Kin Foster Care: Findings from a National Survey." *Children and Youth Services Review* 24(1–2): 55–78.

Eika, Kari H. 2009. "The Challenge of Obtaining Quality Care: Limited Consumer Sovereignty in Human Services." *Feminist Economics* 15(1): 113–37.

England, Paula. 1982. "The Failure of Human Capital Theory to Explain Occupational Sex Segregation." Journal of Human Resources 17(3): 358–70.

———. 1992. *Comparable Worth: Theories and Evidence.* New York: Aldine.

———. 2004. "More Mercenary Mate Selection? Comment on Sweeney and Cancian (2004) and Press (2004)." *Journal of Marriage and Family* 66(4): 1034–37.

———. 2005. "Emerging Theories of Care Work." *Annual Review of Sociology* 31: 381–99.

———. 2010. "The Gender Revolution: Uneven and Stalled." *Gender and Society* 24(2): 149–66.

England, Paula, Michelle Budig, and Nancy Folbre. 2002. "Wages of Virtue: The Relative Pay of Care Work." *Social Problems* 49(4): 455–73.

England, Paula, and Su Li. 2006. "Desegregation Stalled: The Changing Gender Composition of College Majors, 1971–2002." *Gender and Society* 20(5): 657–77.

English, Ashley, Heidi Hartmann, and Jeff Hayes. 2010. "Are Women Now Half the Labor Force? The Truth About Women in the Labor Force." Briefing paper C374. Washington, D.C.: Institute for Women's Policy Research (March). Available at: http://www.iwpr.org/publications/pubs/are-women-now-half-the-labor-force-the-truth-about-women-and-equal-participation-in-the-labor-force (accessed May 20, 2011).

Engster, Daniel. 2007. *The Heart of Justice: Care Ethics and Political Theory.* New York: Oxford University Press.

———. 2010. "Strategies for Building and Sustaining a New Care Movement." *Journal of Women, Politics, and Policy* 31(4): 289–312.

Epstein, Dale, and Steve Barnett. 2010. "Brief Report: Funding Cuts to State-Funded Prekindergarten Programs in FY10 and 11." New Brunswick, N.J.: Rutgers University,

National Institute for Early Education Research (August). Available at: http://nieer.org/publications/latest-research/Funding-Cuts-to-State-Funded-Prekindergarten-Programs-fy10-11 (accessed April 29, 2012).

Erickson, William, Camille G. Lee, and Sarah von Schrader. 2010. "2008 Disability Status Report: the United States." Ithaca, N.Y.: Cornell University Rehabilitation Research and Training Center on Disability Demographics and Statistics. Available at: http://digital commons.ilr.cornell.edu/edicollect/1285/ (accessed February 18, 2012).

Esping-Anderson, Gøsta. 1999. *The Social Foundations of Postindustrial Economies.* Oxford: Oxford University Press.

———. 2009a. "Economic Inequality and the Welfare State." In *The Oxford Handbook of Economic Inequality,* edited by Wiemer Salverda, Brian Nolan, and Timothy M. Smeeding. Oxford: Oxford University Press.

———. 2009b. *The Incomplete Revolution: Adapting to Women's New Roles.* Cambridge: Polity Press.

Ettner, Susan L. 1995. "The Impact of 'Parent Care' on Female Labor Supply Decisions." *Demography* 32(1): 63–80.

———. 1996. "The Opportunity Costs of Elder Care." *Journal of Human Resources* 31(1): 189–205.

Fass, Sarah. 2009. "Paid Leave in the States: A Critical Support for Low-Wage Workers and Their Families." New York: Columbia University, National Center for Children in Poverty (March).

Fehr, Ernst, and Armin Falk. 2002. "Psychological Foundations of Incentives." *European Economic Review* 46(4–5): 687–724.

Feinberg, Lynn, Susan C. Reinhard, Ari Houser, and Rita Choula. 2011. "Valuing the Invaluable: 2011 Update." Washington, D.C.: AARP Public Policy Institute. Available at: http://assets.aarp.org/rgcenter/ppi/ltc/i51-caregiving.pdf (accessed December 16, 2011).

Feinberg, Lynn, Kari Wolkwitz, and Care Goldstein. 2006. *Ahead of the Curve: Emerging Trends and Practices in Family Caregiver Support.* AARP policy brief 2006-09. Washington, D.C.: AARP Public Policy Institute. Available at: http://assets.aarp.org/rgcenter/il/2006_09_caregiver.pdf (accessed January 3, 2011).

Ferree, Myra Marx. 2009. "An American Road Map? Framing Feminist Goals in a Liberal Landscape." In *Gender Equality: Transforming Family Divisions of Labor,* edited by Janet C. Gornick, Marcia K. Meyers, and Erik Olin Wright. London: Verso.

Field, Marilyn J., and Alan M. Jette, eds. 2007. *The Future of Disability in America.* Washington, D.C.: National Academies Press.

Filer, Randall K. 1981. "The Influence of Affective Human Capital on the Wage Equation." In *Research in Labor Economics,* vol. 4, edited by Ronald G. Ehrenberg. Greenwich, Conn.: JAI Press.

———. 1983. "Sexual Differences in Earnings: The Role of Individual Personalities and Tastes." *Journal of Human Resources* 18(1): 82–99.

Fillenbaum, Gerda G. 1995. "Activities of Daily Living." In *The Encyclopedia of Aging,* edited by George L. Maddox, 2d ed. New York: Springer.

Fiske, Susan, Amy Cuddy, Peter Glick, and Jun Xu. 2002. "A Model of (Often Mixed) Stereotype Content: Competence and Warm Respectively Follow from Perceived Status and Competence." *Journal of Personality and Social Psychology* 82(6): 878–902.

Fisman, Raymond, Sheena S. Iyengar, Emir Kamenica, and Itamar Simonson. 2006. "Gender Differences in Mate Selection: Evidence from a Speed Dating Experiment." *Quarterly Journal of Economics* 121(2): 673–97.

Fitzgerald, John, and John Wicks. 1990. "Measuring the Value of Household Output: A Comparison of Direct and Indirect Approaches." *Review of Income and Wealth* 36(2): 129–41.

Floro, Maria. 1995. "Women's Well-being, Poverty, and Work Intensity." *Feminist Economics* 1(3): 1–25.

Folbre, Nancy. 1991. "The Unproductive Housewife: Her Evolution in Nineteenth-Century Economic Thought." *Signs* 16(3): 42–63.

———. 2004. "A Theory of the Misallocation of Time." In *Family Time: The Social Organization of Care,* edited by Nancy Folbre and Michael Bittman. New York: Routledge.

———. 2006a. "Chicks, Hawks, and Patriarchal Institutions." In *Handbook of Behavioral Economics,* edited by Morris Altman. Armonk, N.Y.: M. E. Sharpe.

———. 2006b. "Demanding Quality: Worker/Consumer Coalitions and 'High Road' Strategies in the Care Sector." *Politics and Society* 34(1): 1–21.

———. 2008a. *Valuing Children: Rethinking the Economics of the Family.* Cambridge, Mass.: Harvard University Press.

———. 2008b. "Time Use and Inequality in the Household." In *Oxford Handbook of Economic Inequality,* edited by Wiemer Salverda, Brian Nolan, and Timothy Smeeding. New York: Oxford University Press.

———. 2008c. "When a Commodity Is Not Exactly a Commodity." *Science* 319(5871): 1769–70.

———. 2009. *Greed, Lust, and Gender: A History of Economic Ideas.* New York: Oxford University Press.

Folbre, Nancy, and Elissa Braunstein. 2001. "To Honor or Obey: The Patriarch as Residual Claimant." *Feminist Economics* 7(1): 25–54.

Folbre, Nancy, and Janet C. Gornick, Helen Connolly, and Teresa Munzi. 2010. "Women's Employment, Unpaid Work, and Economic Well-being: A Cross-National Analysis." Paper presented to the "Luxembourg Income Study Conference on Inequality and the Middle Class." Walferdange, Luxembourg (June).

Folbre, Nancy, and Julie Nelson. 2002. "For Love or Money?" *Journal of Economic Perspectives* 14(4): 123–40.

———. 2006. "Why a Well-Paid Nurse Is a Better Nurse!" *Journal of Nursing Economics* 24(3): 127–30.

Folbre, Nancy, and Thomas Weisskopf. 1998. "Did Father Know Best? Families, Markets, and the Supply of Caring Labor." In *Economics, Values, and Organization,* edited by Avner Ben-Ner and Louis Putterman. Cambridge: Cambridge University Press.

Folbre, Nancy, and Jayoung Yoon. 2007a. "The Value of Unpaid Child Care in the U.S. in 2003." In *How Do We Spend Our Time? Recent Evidence from the American Time-Use Survey,* edited by Jean Kimmel. Kalamazoo, Mich.: W. E. Upjohn Institute for Employment Research.

———. 2007b. "What Is Child Care? Lessons from Time Use Surveys of Major English-Speaking Countries." *Review of Economics of the Household* 5(3): 223–48.

Folbre, Nancy, Jayoung Yoon, Kade Finnoff, and Allison Fuligni. 2005. "By What Measure? Family Time Devoted to Children in the U.S." *Demography* 42(2): 373–90.

Forhan, Lisa. 2010. "Summary of Comments Regarding Department of Labor Proposed Amendments to 29CFR Part 552: Application of the Fair Labor Standards Act to Domestic Service." Unpublished paper, University of Massachusetts at Amherst, Center for Public Policy and Administration.

Fortin, Nicole. 2008. "The Gender Wage Gap Among Young Adults in the United States: The Importance of Money Versus People." *Journal of Human Resources* 43(4): 886–920.

François, Patrick. 2000. " 'Public Service Motivation' as an Argument for Government Provision." *Journal of Public Economics* 78(3): 275–99.

———. 2003. "Not-for-Profit Provision of Public Services." *Economic Journal* 113(486): C53–61.

Frazis, Harley, and Jay Stewart. 2006. "How Does Household Production Affect Earnings Inequality? Evidence from the American Time Use Survey." Levy Institute Working Paper 454. Annandale-on-Hudson, N.Y.: Bard College (April).

Freedman, Vicki A., Eileen Crimmins, Robert F. Schoeni, Brenda C. Spillman, Hakan Aykan, Ellen Kramarow, Kenneth Land, James Lubitz, Kenneth Manton, Linda G. Martin, Diane Shinberg, and Timothy Waidmann. 2004. "Resolving Inconsistencies in Trends in Old-Age Disability: Report from a Technical Working Group." *Demography* 41(3): 417–41.

Freedman, Vicki A., Douglas Wolf, Beth J. Soldo, and Elizabeth Hervey Stephen. 1991. "Intergenerational Transfers: A Question of Perspective." *The Gerontologist* 31(5): 640–47.

Frey, Bruno S. 1998. "Institutions and Morale: The Crowding-Out Effect." In *Economics, Values, and Organization,* edited by Avner Ben-Ner and Louis Putterman. Cambridge: Cambridge University Press.

Frey, Bruno S., and Reto Jegen. 2001. "Motivation Crowding Theory: A Survey of Empirical Evidence." *Journal of Economic Surveys* 15(5): 589–611.

Friedman, Esther M., and Judith Seltzer. 2010. "Providing for Older Parents: Is It a Family Affair?" Paper (revised) presented to the Population Association of America. Dallas, Tex. (April).

Fuller-Thomson, Esme, Bin Yu, Amani M. Nuru-Jeter, Jack M. Guralnik, and Meredith Minkler. 2009. "Basic ADL Disability and Functional Limitation Rate Among Older Americans from 2000–2005: The End of the Decline?" *Journal of Gerontology: Medical Sciences* 64(12): 1333–36.

Furtado, Delia, and Heinrich Hock. 2010. "Low-Skilled Immigration and Work-Fertility Trade-offs Among High-Skilled U.S. Natives." *American Economic Review* 100(2): 224–28.

Gallo, Joseph J. 2006. "Activities of Daily Living and Instrumental Activities of Daily Living." In *Handbook of Geriatric Assessment,* edited by Joseph J. Gallo, Hillary R. Bogner, Terry Fulmer, and Gregory J. Paveza. Sudbury, Mass.: Jones and Bartlett.

Gardiner, Jean. 1997. *Gender, Care, and Economics.* Basingstoke, U.K.: Macmillan.

Gautié, Jérôme, and John Schmitt, eds. 2010. *Low-Wage Work in the Wealthy World.* New York: Russell Sage Foundation.

Geen, Rob, ed. 2003. *Kinship Care: Making the Most of a Valuable Resource.* Washington, DC: Urban Institute.

———. 2004. "The Evolution of Kinship Care Policy and Practice." *The Future of Children* 14(1): 131–50.

Generations United. 2010. *Family Matters: Public Policy and the Interdependence of Generations.* Available at: http://www2.gu.org/LinkClick.aspx?fileticket=3eJS8MxzD9Q%3D&tabid=157&mid=606 (accessed January 2, 2011).

George, Robert M., Lucy Mackey Bilaver, Bong Joo Lee, Barbara Needell, Alan Brookhart, William Jackman. 2002. "Employment Outcomes for Youth Aging Out of Foster Care." Washington: U.S. Department of Health and Human Services, Office of the Assistant Secretary for Planning and Evaluation (May). Available at: http://aspe.hhs.gov/hsp/fostercare-agingout02 (accessed May 21, 2011).

Georgetown University. National Long-Term Care Financing Project. 2007. "National Spending for Long-Term Care: Fact Sheet." February. Available at: http://ltc.georgetown.edu/pdfs/natspendfeb07.pdf (accessed May 25, 2010).

Gerson, Kathleen. 2010. *The Unfinished Revolution.* New York: Oxford University Press.

Gerstel, Naomi. 2011. "Rethinking Families and Community: The Color, Class, and Centrality of Extended Kin Ties." *Sociological Forum* (26)1: 1–20.

Gerstel, Naomi, and Amy Armenia. 2009. "Giving and Taking Family Leaves: Right or Privilege." *Yale Journal of Law and Feminism* 21(1): 161–84.

Gerstel, Naomi, and Natalia Sarkisian. 2008. "The Color of Family Ties: Race, Class, Gender, and Extended Family Involvement." In *It's American Families: A Multicultural Reader,* edited by Stephanie Coontz, Maya Parson, and Gabrielle Rayley, 2d ed. New York: Routledge.

Giannelli, Giana C., Lucia Mangiavacchi, and Luca Piccoli. 2010. "GDP and the Value of Family Caretaking: How Much Does Europe Care?" IZA Discussion Paper 5046. Bonn: Forschungsinstitut zur Zukunft der Arbeit (Institute for the Study of Labor).

Gibson, Mary Jo, and Ari Houser. 2007. "Valuing the Invaluable: A New Look at the Economic Value of Family Caregiving." Washington, D.C.: AARP Public Policy Institute.

Gill, Thomas M., Evelyne A. Gahbauer, Ling Han, and Heather G. Allore. 2010. "Trajectories of Disability in the Last Year of Life." *New England Journal of Medicine* 362(13): 1173–80.

Glenn, Evelyn Nakano. 2010. *Forced to Care: Coercion and Caregiving in America.* Cambridge, Mass.: Harvard University Press.

Gneezy, Uri, and Aldo Rustichini. 2000. "Pay Enough or Don't Pay at All." *Quarterly Journal of Economics* 115(3): 791–801.

Golberstein, Ezra, David C. Grabowski, Kenneth M. Langa, and Michael E. Chernew. 2009. "Effects of Medicare Home Health Care Payment on Informal Care." *Inquiry* 46(1): 58–71.

Goldscheider, Frances, and Linda Waite. 1991. *New Families, No Families: The Transformation of the American Home.* Berkeley: University of California Press.

Goleman, Daniel. 1995. *Emotional Intelligence.* New York: Bantam.

Goodwin, Paula Y., William D. Mosher, and Anjani Chandra. 2010. "Marriage and Cohabitation in the United States: A Statistical Portrait Based on Cycle 6 (2002) of the National Survey of Family Growth." *Vital Health Statistics* 23(28): 1–45. Hyattsville, Md.: National Center for Health Statistics.

Gornick, Janet C., and Marcia K. Meyers. 2003. *Families That Work: Policies for Reconciling Parenthood and Employment.* New York: Russell Sage Foundation.

Gornick, Janet C., and Marcia K. Meyers, and Erik Olin Wright. 2009. *Gender Equality: Transforming Family Divisions of Labor.* London: Verso.

Granovetter, Mark. 2005. "The Impact of Social Structure on Economic Outcomes." *Journal of Economic Perspectives* 19(1): 33–50.

Grant, Adam M. 2008. "Does Intrinsic Motivation Fuel the Prosocial Fire? Motivational Synergy in Predicting Persistence, Performance, and Productivity." *Journal of Applied Psychology* 93(1): 48–58.

Gregory, Stephen R. 2004. "Disability: Federal Survey Definitions, Measurements, and Estimates." *Data Digest* 98: 1–8. Washington, D.C.: AARP Public Policy Institute.

Grimm, Bill, and Julian Darwall. 2005. "Foster Parents: Who Are They and What Are Their Motivations?" *Journal of National Center for Youth Law* 16(3): 1–8. Available at: http://www.youthlaw.org/fileadmin/ncyl/youthlaw/publications/yln/2005/issue_3/05_yln_3_grimm_darwall.pdf (accessed May 21, 2011).

Gronau, Reuben. 1977. "Leisure, Home Production, and Work—The Theory of the Allocation of Time Revisited." *Journal of Political Economy* 85(6): 1099–1123.

Hackman, Richard J., and Greg R. Oldham. 1980. *Work Re-Design*. Reading, Mass.: Addison-Wesley.

Hall, Douglas T., and Dawn E. Chandler. 2005. "Psychological Success: When the Career Is a Calling." *Journal of Organizational Behavior* 26(2): 155–76.

Hamilton, Brady E., Joyce A. Martin, and Stephanie J. Ventura. 2009. "Births: Preliminary Data for 2007." *National Vital Statistics Reports* 57(12). Hyattsville, Md.: National Center for Health Statistics.

Harkness, Susan. 2010. "The Contribution of Women's Employment and Earnings to Household Income Inequality: A Cross-Country Analysis." Luxembourg Income Survey (LIS) Working Paper 531 (June).

Harrington, Charlene, Helen Carrillo, and Brandee Wolesagle Blank. 2009. "Nursing Facilities, Staffing, Residents, and Facility Deficiencies, 2003 Through 2008." San Francisco: University of California (November). Available at: http://www.nccnhr.org/sites/default/files/OSCAR%20complete%202009.pdf; data at http://www.statehealthfacts.org/compare.jsp (accessed January 18, 2010).

Harrington, Charlene, Terence Ng, Stephen H. Kaye, and Robert Newcomer. 2009. "Home and Community-Based Services: Public Policies to Improve Access, Costs, and Quality." San Francisco: University of California, Center for Personal Assistance Services (CPAS) (January). Available at: http://www.pascenter.org/documents/PASCenter_HCBS_policy_brief.pdf (accessed February 3, 2010).

Harrington, Charlene, Terence Ng, and Molly O'Malley Watts. 2009. "Medicaid Home and Community-Based Service Programs: Data Update." Issue brief for Kaiser Commission on Medicaid and the Uninsured, Publication 7720-03 (November). Available at: http://www.kff.org/medicaid/upload/7720-03.pdf (accessed November 9, 2009).

———. 2011a. "Medicaid Home- and Community-Based Service Programs: Data Update." Issue brief for Kaiser Commission on Medicaid and the Uninsured, publication 7720-04 (February). Available at: http://www.kff.org/medicaid/upload/7720-04.pdf (accessed April 29, 2012).

———. 2011b. "Medicaid Home- and Community-Based Service Programs: Data Update." Issue brief for Kaiser Commission on Medicaid and the Uninsured, publication 7720-05 (December). Available at: http://www.kff.org/medicaid/upload/7720-05.pdf (accessed April 29, 2012).

Harris, Margaret. 1995. "Quiet Care: Welfare Work and Religious Congregations." *Journal of Social Policy* 24(1): 53–71.

Hartmann, Heidi, and Vicky Lovell. 2009. "A U.S. Model for Universal Sickness and Family Leave: Gender-Egalitarian and Cross-Class Caregiving Support for All." In *Gender Equality:*

Transforming Family Divisions of Labor, edited by Janet C. Gornick, Marcia K. Meyers, and Erik Olin Wright. London: Verso.

Haskins, Catherine. 2010. "Household Employer Payroll Tax Evasion: An Exploration Based on IRS Data and on Interviews with Employers and Domestic Workers." Ph.D. diss., University of Massachusetts at Amherst, Department of Economics.

Hatch, Lynn. 2009. "Labor Turnover in the Child-Care Industry: Voice and Exit." Ph.D. diss., University of Massachusetts at Amherst, Department of Economics. Available at: http://scholarworks.umass.edu/open_access_dissertations/146 (accessed May 21, 2011).

Haveman, Robert, and Barbara Wolfe. 1984. "Schooling and Economic Well-being: The Role of Non-Market Effects." *Journal of Human Resources* 19(3): 377–407.

Heckman, James J., and Dimitriy V. Masterov. 2007. "The Productivity Argument for Investing in Young Children." *Review of Agricultural Economics* 29(3): 446–93.

Helburn, Suzanne, ed. 1995. *Cost, Quality, and Child Outcomes in Child Care Centers.* Technical report. Denver: University of Colorado.

Helburn, Suzanne, and Barbara Bergmann. 2002. *America's Child Care Problem: The Way Out.* New York: Palgrave/St. Martin's Press.

Hendershot, Gerry, Sheryl Larson, S. Charley Lakin, and Robert Doljanac. 2005. "Problems in Defining Mental Retardation and Developmental Disability: Using the NHIS." DD data brief 7(1). Minneapolis: University of Minnesota, Research and Training Center on Community Living (June). Available at: http://rtc.umn.edu/docs/dddb7-1.pdf (accessed September 22, 2010).

Henretta, John C., Martha Hill, Wei Li, Beth J. Soldo, and Douglas A. Wolf. 1997. "Selection of Children to Provide Care: The Effect of Earlier Parental Transfers." *Journal of Gerontology: Social Sciences* 52B: 110–19.

Herd, Pamela, and Madonna Harrington Meyer. 2002. "Care Work: Invisible Civic Engagement." *Gender and Society* 16(5): 665–88.

Herrera, Angelica P., Jerry Lee, Guadalupe Palos, and Isabel Torres-Vigil. 2008. "Cultural Influences in the Patterns of Long-Term Care Use Among Mexican American Family Caregivers." *Journal of Applied Gerontology* 27(2): 141–65.

Herzenberg, Stephen A., John A. Alic, and Howard Wial. 1998. *New Rules for a New Economy: Employment and Opportunity in Postindustrial America.* Ithaca, N.Y.: Cornell University Press.

Herzenberg, Stephen, Mark Price, and David Bradley. 2005. *Losing Ground in Early Childhood Education: Declining Workforce Qualifications in an Expanding Industry, 1979–2004.* Washington, D.C.: Economic Policy Institute.

Herzog, A. Regula, and Willard L. Rogers. 1988. "Interviewing Older Adults: Mode Comparisons Using Data from a Face-to-Face Survey and a Telephone Survey." *Public Opinion Quarterly* 52(1): 84–99.

Hewitt, Amy, and K. Charley Lakin. 2001. "Issues in the Direct Support Workforce and Their Connections to the Growth, Sustainability, and Quality of Community Supports." A Technical Assistance Paper of the National Project: Self-Determination for People with Developmental Disabilities, May. Minneapolis: University of Minnesota, Research and Training Center on Community Living. Available at: http://rtc.umn.edu/docs/hcfa.pdf (accessed February 21, 2012)

Hewitt, Amy S., and Sheryl A. Larson. 2007. "The Direct Service Workforce in Community Supports to Individuals with Developmental Disabilities: Issues, Implications, and Promising Practices." *Mental Retardation and Developmental Disabilities Research Reviews* 13(2): 178–87.

Heyes, Anthony. 2005. "The Economics of Vocation or 'Why Is a Badly Paid Nurse a Good Nurse?' " *Journal of Health Economics* 24(3): 561–69.

Heymann, Jody. 2001. *The Widening Gap: Why America's Working Families Are in Jeopardy—and What Can Be Done About It.* New York: Basic Books.

———. 2005. "Inequalities at Work and at Home: Social Class and Gender." In *Unfinished Work: Building Equality and Democracy in an Era of Working Families,* edited by Jody Heymann and Christopher Beem. New York: New Press.

Hill, Robert D., Marilyn K. Luptak, Randall W. Rupper, Byron Bair, Cherie Peterson, Nancy Dailey, and Bret L. Hicken. 2010. "Review of Veterans Health Administration Telemedicine Interventions." *American Journal of Managed Care* (December). Available at: http://www.ajmc.com/supplement/managed-care/2010/AJMC_10dec_HIT/AJMC_10HITdecHill_Xcls_e302to10 (accessed January 24, 2011).

Himmelweit, Susan. 1999. "Caring Labor." *Annals of the American Academy of Political and Social Science* 561(1): 27–38.

Hochschild, Arlie. 1983. *The Managed Heart: Commercialization of Human Feeling.* Berkeley: University of California Press.

Hodson, Randy. 2008. "The Ethnographic Contribution of Understanding Co-worker Relations." *British Journal of Industrial Relations* 46(1): 169–92.

Hofferth, Sandra L., Joseph Pleck, Jeffrey L. Stueve, Suzanne Bianchi, and Liana Sayer. 2002. "The Demography of Fathers: What Fathers Do." *In Handbook of Father Involvement,* edited by Natasha Cabrera and Catherine S. Tamis-LeMonde. Mahwah, N.J.: Lawrence Erlbaum Associates.

Holloway, Sue, Sandra Short, and Sarah Tamplin. 2002. *Household Satellite Account (Experimental) Methodology.* Technical report. London: Office of National Statistics.

Holmstrom, Bengt, and Paul Milgrom. 1991. "Multitask Principal-Agent Analysis: Incentive Contracts, Asset Ownership, and Job Design." *Journal of Law, Economics, and Organization* 7: 24–52.

———. 1994. "The Firm as an Incentive System." *American Economic Review* 84(4): 972–91.

Holt, Stephen D., and Jennifer Romich. 2007. "Marginal Tax Rates Facing Low- and Moderate-Income Workers Who Participate in Means-Tested Transfer Programs." *National Tax Journal* 60(2): 253–76.

Holtom, Brooks C., Thomas Lee, and Simon T. Tidd. 2002. "The Relationship Between Work Status Congruence and Work-Related Attitudes and Behaviors." *Journal of Applied Psychology* 87(5): 903–15.

Holzer, Harry J. 2009. "Workforce Development as an Antipoverty Strategy: What Do We Know? What Should We Do?" In *Changing Poverty, Changing Policies,* edited by Maria Cancian and Sheldon Danziger. New York: Russell Sage Foundation.

Holzer, Harry J., Julia I. Lane, David B. Rosenblum, and Fredrik Andersson. 2011. *Where Are All the Good Jobs Going?* New York: Russell Sage Foundation.

Horowitz, Brian T. 2010. "Cyber Care: Will Robots Help the Elderly Live at Home Longer?" *Scientific American,* June 21, 2010. Available at: http://www.scientificamerican.com/article.cfm?id=robot-elder-care (accessed May 21, 2011).

Howes, Candace. 2002. *The Impact of a Large Wage Increase on the Workforce Stability of IHSS Home Care Workers in San Francisco County.* Working paper. Berkeley: University of California at Berkeley Labor Center (November). Available at: http://laborcenter.berkeley.edu/homecare/Howes.pdf (accessed August 5, 2004).

———. 2004. "Upgrading California's Home Care Workforce: The Impact of Political Action and Unionization." *The State of California Labor 2004* (UCLA Institute for Research on Labor and Employment): 71–105. Available at: http://www.irle.ucla.edu/research/scl/2004.html (accessed May 21, 2011).

———. 2005. "Living Wages and Retention of Homecare Workers in San Francisco." *Industrial Relations* 44(1): 139–63.

———. 2008. "Love, Money, or Flexibility: What Motivates People to Work in Consumer-Directed Home Care?" *The Gerontologist* 48(supplement): 46–60.

———. 2010. "The Best and Worst State Practices in Medicaid Long-Term Care." Direct Care Alliance policy brief 3 (April). Available at: http://blog.directcarealliance.org/wp-content/uploads/2010/03/Howes-Medicaid-Policy-Brief_final.pdf (accessed May 21, 2011).

———. 2011. "Homecare Workers and the Immigrant Workforce in the U.S." Paper presented to the Feminist Economics Workshop on Migrant Labor. Bilbao, Spain (March 11–12). Connecticut College, Department of Economics.

Hrdy, Sarah. 1999. *Mother Nature: A History of Mothers, Infants, and Natural Selection.* New York: Pantheon.

Hutson, Rutledge Q. 2001. "Red Flags: Research Raises Concerns About the Impact of 'Welfare Reform' on Child Maltreatment." Washington, D.C.: Center for Law and Social Policy (CLASP) (October). Available at: http://s242739747.onlinehome.us/publications/red_flags.pdf (accessed March 7, 2012).

Hyde, Janet S., and Marcia C. Linn. 2006. "Gender Similarities in Mathematics and Science." *Science* 314(5799): 599–600.

Hyde, Lewis, 1983. *The Gift: Imagination and the Erotic Life of Property.* New York: Vintage.

Ibarra, Maria de la Luz. 2010. "Creating Intimate Boundaries: Culture and Social Relations." In *Intimate Labors: Cultures, Technologies, and the Politics of Care,* edited by Eileen Boris and Rhacel Salazar Parreñas. Stanford, Calif.: Stanford University Press.

Ingersoll-Dayton, Berit, Margaret Neal, Jung-Hwa Ha, and Leslie Hammer. 2003. "Redressing Inequity in Parent Care Among Siblings." *Journal of Marriage and the Family* 65(1): 201–12.

Institute for Women's Policy Research (IWPR). 2010. "44 Million U.S. Workers Lacked Paid Sick Days in 2010." Briefing paper. Available at: http://www.iwpr.org (accessed January 3, 2011).

Institute of Medicine (IOM). 2007. *The Future of Disability in America,* edited by Marilyn J. Field and Alan M. Jette. Washington, D.C.: National Academies Press.

———. 2008. *Retooling for an Aging America: Building the Health Care Workforce.* Washington, D.C.: National Academies Press.

Internal Revenue Service (IRS). 2009. "Publication 503: Child and Dependent Care Expenses." Available at: http://www.irs.gov/pub/irs-pdf/p503.pdf (accessed May 21, 2011).

Ironmonger, Duncan. 2004. "Bringing Up Bobby and Betty: The Inputs and Outputs of Childcare Time." In *Family Time: The Social Organization of Care,* edited by Nancy Folbre and Michael Bittman. New York: Routledge.

Jantz, Amy, Rob Geen, Roseana Bess, Cynthia Andrews, and Victoria Russell. 2002. "The Continuing Evolution of State Kinship Care Policies." Discussion paper 02-11. Washington, D.C.: Urban Institute.

Jochimsen, Marem. 2003. *Careful Economics: Integrating Caring Activities and Economic Science.* Boston: Kluwer Academic Publishers.

Joesch, Jutta M., and Ken R. Smith. 1997. "Children's Health and Their Mothers' Risk of Divorce or Separation." *Social Biology* 44(3–4): 159–69.

Johnson, Kay. 2010. "Managing the T in EPSDT Services." National Academy for State Health Policy (June). Available at: http://www.nashp.org/node/2042 (accessed May 21, 2011).

Johnson, Robert W., and Simone G. Schaner. 2005. "Many Older Americans Engage in Caregiving Activities." *The Retirement Project: Perspectives on Productive Aging* 3(July). Washington, D.C.: Urban Institute.

Johnson, Tallese. 2008. "Maternity Leave and Employment Patterns of First-Time Mothers, 1961–2003." *Current Population Reports,* P70-133. Washington: U.S. Census Bureau.

Jones, Alexandra. 2006. "About Time for Change." The Work Foundation report, in association with Employers for Work-Life Balance. Available at: http://www.thework foundation.com/assets/docs/publications/177_About%20time%20for%20change.pdf (accessed January 3, 2011).

Joshi, Heather. 1998. "The Opportunity Costs of Childbearing: More than Mothers' Business." *Journal of Population Economics* 11(2): 161–83.

Juster, Thomas F., and Frank Stafford. 1985. "Process Benefits and the Problem of Joint Production." In *Time, Goods, and Well-being,* edited by Thomas F. Juster and Frank Stafford. Ann Arbor, Mich.: ISR.

Kagan, Sharon Lynn, Kristie Kauerz, and Kate Tarrant. 2008. *The Early Care and Education Teaching Workforce at the Fulcrum.* New York: Columbia University/Teachers College Press.

Kahneman, Daniel, Alan B. Krueger, David Schkade, Norbert Schwarz, and Arthur Stone. 2004. "Toward National Well-being Accounts." *American Economic Review* 94(2): 429–34.

Kaiser Family Foundation (KFF). 2010. "State Health Facts." Available at: http://www. statehealthfacts.org (accessed May 21, 2011).

Kalleberg, Arne L. 2000. "Nonstandard Employment Relations: Part-time, Temporary, and Contract Work." *Annual Review of Sociology* 26: 341–65.

Kalleberg, Arne L., Barbara F. Reskin, and Ken Hudson 2000. "Bad Jobs in America: Standard and Nonstandard Employment Relations and Job Quality in the United States." *American Sociological Review* 65(2): 256–78.

Karasak, Robert. 1979. "Job Demands, Job Decision Latitude, and Mental Strain: Implications for Job Redesign." *Administrative Science Quarterly* 24(2): 285–311.

Karasak, Robert, and Tares Theorell. 1990. *Healthy Work: Stress, Productivity, and the Reconstruction of Working Life.* New York: Basic Books.

Kaye, H. Stephen, Susan Chapman, Robert J. Newcomer, and Charlene Harrington. 2006. "The Personal Assistance Workforce: Trends in Supply and Demand." *Health Affairs* 25(4): 1113–20.

Kaye, H. Stephen, Charlene Harrington, and Mitchell P. LaPlante. 2010. "Long-Term Care: Who Gets It, Who Provides It, Who Pays, and How Much?" *Health Affairs* 29(1): 11–21.

Kenney, Genevieve M., Victoria Lynch, Allison Cook, and Samantha Phong. 2010. "Who and Where Are the Children Yet to Enroll in Medicaid and the Children's Health Insurance Program?" *Health Affairs* 29(10): 1920–29.

Kenney, Genevieve M., Joel Ruhter, and Thomas Seldon. 2009. "Containing Costs and Improving Care for Children in Medicaid and CHIP." *Health Affairs* 28(6): w1025–36.

Keystone Research Center. 2007. "Historic Union Election Establishes Stateside Union of PA Home-Based Child Care Providers." Press release, November 1, 2007. Available at: http://keystoneresearch.org/media-center/press-releases/historic-union-election-establishes-statewide-union-pa-home-based-child- (accessed February 20, 2012).

Kiecolt-Glaser, Janice K., Ronald Glaser, Stefan Gravenstein, William B. Malarkey, and John Sheridan. 1996. "Chronic Stress Alters the Immune Response to Influenza Virus Vaccine in Older Adults." *Proceedings of the National Academy of Sciences of the United States of America* 93(7): 3043–47.

Kim, Il-Ho, Jeanne Geiger-Brown, Alison Trinkoff, and Carles Muntaner. 2010. "Physically Demanding Workloads and the Risks of Musculoskeletal Disorders in Homecare Workers in the USA." *Health and Social Care in the Community* 18(5): 445–55.

Kim, Jeounghee, and Myungkook Joo. 2009. "Work-Related Activities of Single Mothers Before and After Welfare Reform." *Monthly Labor Review* 132(12): 3–17.

Kim, Youngmee, and Barbara A. Given. 2008. "Quality of Life of Family Caregivers of Cancer Survivors." *Cancer* 112 (supplement): 2556–68.

King, Rosalind Berkowitz. 1999. "Time Spent in Parenthood Status Among Adults in the United States." *Demography* 36(3): 377–85.

King, Willford I., Wesley G. Mitchell, Frederick Macaulay, and Oswald W. Knauth. 1921. *Income in the United States, Its Amount and Distribution.* New York: Harcourt Brace.

Kinney, Jennifer M., and Mary Ann Parris Stephens. 1989. "Hassles and Uplifts of Giving Care to a Parent with Dementia." *Psychology and Aging* 4(4): 402–8.

Kittay, Eva. 1999. *Love's Labor: Essays on Women, Equality, and Dependency.* New York: Routledge.

Knight, Jack. 1992. *Institutions and Social Conflict.* Cambridge: Cambridge University Press.

Kochan, Thomas A., Eileen Appelbaum, Jody Hoffer Gittell, Carrie Leana, and Richard A. Gephardt. 2009. *Workplace Innovation and Labor Policy Leadership. A Challenge to Business, Labor, and Government.* Washington, D.C.: Center for Economic and Policy Research (April). Available at: http://www.cepr.net/index.php/publications/reports/workplace-innovation-and-labor-policy-leadership-a-challenge-to-business-labor-and-government/.

Kogan, Michael D., Stephen J. Blumberg, Kathleen M. Heyman, Bonnie B. Strickland, Gopal K. Singh, and Mary Beth Zeni. 2010. "State Variation in Underinsurance Among Children with Special Health Care Needs in the United States." *Pediatrics* 125(4): 673–80.

Kohn, Alfie. 1990. *The Brighter Side of Human Nature.* New York: Basic Books.

Kohn, Melvin L. 1989. *Class and Conformity: A Study in Values,* 2d ed. Chicago: University of Chicago Press.

Kohn, Melvin L., and Carmi Schooler. 1983. *Work and Personality: An Inquiry into the Impact of Social Stratification.* Norwood, N.J.: Ablex.

Kosfield, Michale, Markus Heinrichs, Paul J. Zak, Urs Fischbacher, and Ernst Fehr. 2005. "Oxytocin Increases Trust in Humans." *Nature* 435: 673–76.

Kreider, Rose M., and Diana B. Elliott. 2009. "America's Families and Living Arrangements 2007." *Current Population Reports,* P20-561. Washington: U.S. Census Bureau.

Kreps, David M. 1997. "Intrinsic Motivation and Extrinsic Incentives." *American Economic Review* 87(2): 359–69.

Kyrk, Hazel. 1929. *Economic Problems of the Family.* New York: Harper and Brothers.

Lake Snell Perry and Associates. 2001. Summary of "Family Caregivers Self-Awareness and Empowerment Project: A Report on Formative Focus Groups." Report prepared for the National Family Caregivers Association and the National Alliance for Caregiving (September).

Lakin, K. Charley, Sheryl A. Larson, Patricia Salmi, and Naomi Scott. 2009. *Residential Services for Persons with Developmental Disabilities: Status and Trends Through 2008.* Minneapolis: Research and Training Center on Community Living, Institute on Community Integration, University of Minnesota. Available at: http://rtc.umn.edu/docs/risp2008.pdf (accessed at April 4, 2010).

Land, Hilary, and Hilary Rose. 1985. "Compulsory Altruism for Some or an Altruistic Society for All." In *In Defense of Welfare,* edited by Phillip Bean, Jerry Ferris, and David K. Whynes. London: Tavistock.

Landefeld, Steve, and Stephanie McCulla. 2000. "Accounting for Nonmarket Household Production Within a National Accounts Framework." *Review of Income and Wealth* 46(3): 289–307.

LaPlante, Mitchell P., Charlene Harrington, and Taewoon Kang. 2002. "Estimating Paid and Unpaid Hours of Personal Assistance Services in Activities of Daily Living Provided to Adults Living at Home." *Health Services Research* 37(2): 397–413.

Larson, Sheryl A., Robert Doljanac, and K. Charlie Lakin. 2005. "United States Living Arrangements of People with Intellectual and/or Developmental Disabilities in 1995." *Journal of Intellectual and Developmental Disability* 30(4): 248–51.

Larson, Sheryl, K. Charlie Lakin, Lynda Anderson, Nohoon Kwak Lee, Jeoung Hak Lee, and Deborah Anderson. 2000. "Prevalence of Mental Retardation and/or Developmental Disabilities: Analysis of the 1994/1995 NHIS-D." DD data brief 2(1). Minneapolis: University of Minnesota, Research and Training Center on Community Living (April).

Lawton, M. Powell, Miriam Moss, Morton H. Kleban, Allen Glicksman, and Michael Rovine. 1991. "A Two-Factor Model of Caregiving Appraisal and Psychological Well-being." *Journal of Gerontology: Psychological Sciences* 46(4): P181–89.

Layard, Richard. 2005. *Happiness: Lessons from a New Science.* New York: Penguin.

Leana, Carrie, Eileen Appelbaum, and Iryna Shevchuk. 2009. "Work Process and Quality of Care: Encouraging Positive Job Crafting in Childcare Classrooms." *Academy of Management Journal* 52(6): 1169–92.

Leana, Carrie, and Gary Florkowski. 1992. "Employee Involvement Programs: Integrating Psychological Theory and Management Practice." *Research in Personnel and Human Resources Management* 25(5): 233–70.

Leana, Carrie, and Harry J. van Buren. 1999. "Organizational Social Capital and Employment Practices." *Academy of Management Review* 24(3): 538–55.

Lee, Ronald D., and Ryan D. Edwards. 2001. "The Fiscal Impact of Population Change." In *Seismic Shifts: The Economic Impact of Population Change,* edited by Jane Sneddon Little and Robert K. Triest. Boston: Federal Reserve Bank of Boston.

Lee, Sunmin, Graham A. Colditz, Lisa F. Berkman, and Ichiro Kawachi. 2003. "Caregiving and Risk of Coronary Heart Disease in U.S. Women: A Prospective Study." *American Journal of Preventive Medicine* 24(2): 113–19.

Lee, Thomas W., and Darryll R. Johnson. 1991. "The Effects of Work Schedule and Employment Status on the Organizational Commitment and Job Satisfaction of Full- Versus Part-Time Employees." *Journal of Vocational Behavior* 38(2): 208–24.

References

Leira, Arnaug. 1994. "Concepts of Caring: Loving, Thinking, and Doing." *Social Service Review* 68(2): 185–201.

Lenz-Rashid, Sonja. 2004. "Employment Experiences of Homeless Young Adults: Are They Different for Youth with a History of Foster Care?" *Children and Youth Services Review* 28(2): 235–59.

Leon, Joel, Jonas Marainen, and John Marcotte. 2001. "Pennsylvania's Frontline Workers in Long-Term Care: The Provider Organization Perspective." A Report to the Intergovernmental Council on Long-Term Care. Philadelphia: Polisher Research Institute at the Philadelphia Geriatric Center.

Levine, Carol, Deborah Helper, Ariella Peist, and David A. Gould. 2010. "Bridging Troubled Waters: Family Caregivers, Transitions, and Long-Term Care." *Health Affairs* 19(1): 116–24.

Levine, Linda. 2009. "Leave Benefits in the U.S." Congressional Research Service Report to Congress (June 5). Available at: http://www.policyarchive.org/handle/10207/bitstreams/19939.pdf (accessed May 9, 2011).

Levy, Frank, and Richard J. Murnane. 2004. *The New Division of Labor: How Computers Are Creating the Next Job Market.* New York: Russell Sage Foundation.

Lewchuk, Wayne A. 1993. "Men and Monotony: Fraternalism as a Managerial Strategy at the Ford Motor Company." *The Journal of Economic History* 53: 824–56. doi: 10.1017/S0022050700051330. Published online March 3, 2009. Available at http://journals.cambridge.org/action/displayAbstract?fromPage=online&aid=4167212 (accessed July 2, 2011).

Lilly, Meredith B., Audrey Laporte, and Peter C. Coyte. 2007. "Labor Market Work and Home Care's Unpaid Caregivers: A Systematic Review of Labor Force Participation Rates, Predictors of Labor Market Withdrawal, and Hours of Work." *Milbank Quarterly* 85(4): 641–90.

Lindsey, Duncan, and Sacha Klein Martin. 2002. "Deepening Child Poverty: The Not So Good News About Welfare Reform." *Child and Family Services Review* 25(1–2): 165–73.

Lohrmann, Christa, Ate Dijkstra, and Theo Dassen. 2003. "Care Dependency: Testing the German Version of the Care Dependency Scale in Nursing Homes and on Geriatric Wards." *Scandinavian Journal of Caring Science* 17(1): 51–56.

Lo Sasso, Anthony T., and Richard W. Johnson. 2002. "Does Informal Care from Adult Children Reduce Nursing Home Admissions for the Elderly?" *Inquiry* 39(3): 279–97.

Low, Bobbi. 2000. *Why Sex Matters: A Darwinian Look at Human Behavior.* Princeton, N.J.: Princeton University Press.

Lowes, Robert. 2010. "Nurses Rally Renews Debate over Mandatory Staffing Ratios." *Medscape Medical News,* May 12. Available at: http://www.medscape.com/viewarticle/721714 (accessed August 18, 2010).

Lundberg, Shelly, and Robert Pollak. 1993. "Separate Spheres Bargaining and the Marriage Market." *Journal of Political Economy* 101(6): 988–1010.

———. 2003. "Efficiency in Marriage." *Review of Economics of the Household* 1(3): 153–67.

Lunney, June R., Joanne Lynn, Daniel J. Foley, Steven Lipson, and Jack M. Guralnik. 2003. "Patterns of Functional Decline at the End of Life." *Journal of the American Medical Association* 289(18): 2387–92.

Maag, Elaine. 2005. "State Tax Credits for Child Care." Urban Institute Tax Note (July 11). Washington, D.C.: Urban Institute. Available at: http://www.urban.org/url.cfm?ID=1000796 (accessed May 21, 2011).

———. 2007. "The Disappearing Child Care Credit." Washington, D.C.: Urban Institute and Brookings Institution, Tax Policy Center (October 8). Available at: http://www.urban.org/UploadedPDF/1001105_child_care_credit.pdf (accessed April 29, 2012).

Maas, Meridean, and Kathleen Buckwalter. 2006. "Providing Quality Care in Assisted Living Facilities: Recommendations for Enhanced Staffing and Staff Training." *Journal of Gerontological Nursing* 32(11): 14–22.

MacDonald, Cameron. 1996. "Shadow Others: Nannies, Au Pairs, and Invisible Work." In *Working in the Service Society,* edited by Cameron MacDonald and Carmen Sirianni. Philadelphia: Temple University Press.

Macomber, Jennifer Ehrle, Rob Geen, and Regan Main. 2003. "Kinship Foster Care: Custody, Hardships, and Services." *Snapshots of America's Families* 3(14). Washington, D.C.: Urban Institute. Available at: http://www.urban.org/UploadedPDF/310893_snapshots3_no14.pdf (accessed May 21, 2011).

Manton, Kenneth G., Xi Liang Gu, and Vicki L. Lamb. 2006. "Change in Chronic Disability from 1982 to 2004–2005 as Measured by Long-Term Changes in Function and Health in the U.S. Elderly Population." *Proceedings of the National Academy of Sciences of the United States of America* 103(48): 18374–79.

Marini, Margaret Mooney, and Pi-Ling Fan. 1997. "The Gender Gap in Earnings at Career Entry." *American Sociological Review* 62(4): 588–604.

Marks, Nadine F. 1996. "Caregiving Across the Lifespan: National Prevalence and Predictors." *Family Relations* 45(1): 27–36.

Masi, C. G. 2009. "Personal Robots to Monitor Elderly Vital Signs." EyeOnTechnology (June 16). Available at: http://www.cgmasi.com/eyeontechnology/2009/06/personal-robots-to-monitor-elderly-vital-signs.html (accessed April 29, 2012).

Mason, Karen Oppenheim, John L. Czajka, and Sara Arber. 1976. "Change in U.S. Women's Sex-Role Attitudes, 1964–1974." *American Sociological Review* 41(4): 573–96.

Mason, Karen Oppenheim, and Yu-Hsia Lu. 1988. "Attitudes Toward Women's Familial Roles: Changes in the United States, 1977–1985." *Gender and Society* 2(1): 39–57.

Matthews, Hannah. 2009. "Child Care Assistance: A Program That Works." Washington, D.C.: Center for Law and Social Policy (January 23). Available at: http://www.clasp.org/admin/site/publications/files/0452.pdf (accessed March 7, 2012).

Matthews, Sarah H. 2002. *Sisters and Brothers/Daughters and Sons: Meeting the Needs of Old Parents.* Bloomington, Ind.: Unlimited Publishing.

Mayer, Susan. 1998. *What Money Can't Buy: Family Income and Children's Life Chances.* Cambridge, Mass.: Harvard University Press.

McCaughey, Dierdre, Jungyoon Kim, Gwen McGhan, Rita Jablonski, and Diane Brannon. 2010. "Who Needs Caring? We Do! Workplace Injury and Its Effect on Home Health Aides." In *Best Paper Proceedings of the 2010 Academy of Management Meeting.* Montreal, Canada (August 6–10).

McGarry, Kathleen. 1998. "Caring for the Elderly: The Role of Adult Children." In *Inquiries in the Economics of Aging,* edited by David A. Wise. Chicago: University of Chicago Press.

McKenna, Christine. 2010. "Child Care Subsidies in the United States: Government Funding to Families (2010)." Sloan Work and Family Research Network, Boston College (July). Available at: http://wfnetwork.bc.edu/encyclopedia_entry.php?id=17275&area=All (accessed May 21, 2011).

McLanahan, Sara. 2004. "Diverging Destinies: How Children Are Faring Under the Second Demographic Transition." *Demography* 41(4): 607–27.

McLanahan, Sara S., and Renee A. Monson. 1990. "Caring for the Elderly: Prevalence and Consequences." National Survey of Families and Households Working Paper 18. Madison: University of Wisconsin, Department of Sociology.

McNeil, John M. 1999. "Preliminary Estimates on Caregiving from Wave 7 of the 1996 Survey of Income and Program Participation." Survey of Income and Program Participation Working Paper No. 231, December 10, 1999. Washington: U.S. Bureau of the Census. Available at: http://www.census.gov/prod/www/abs/sipp_wp.html (accessed March 7, 2012).

Mendell, Marjorie, and Nancy Neamtan. 2008. "The Social Economy in Quebec: Towards a New Political Economy." In *Why the Social Economy Matters,* edited by Laurie Mook, Jack Quarter, and Sherida Ryan. Toronto: University of Toronto Press.

Menjivar, Cecilia. 2000. *Fragmented Ties: Salvadoran Immigrant Networks in America.* Berkeley: University of California Press.

Metlife Mature Market Institute (MMMI). 2009. "2009 Metlife Mature Market Survey of Nursing Home, Assisted Living, Adult Day Services Costs, and Home Care Costs." Accessed May 21, 2011, at: http://www.metlife.com/mmi/research/09-market-survey.html#findings (no longer available).

Meyer, John D., and Carles Muntaner. 1999. "Injuries in Home Healthcare Workers: An Analysis of Occupational Morbidity from a State Compensation Database." *American Journal of Industrial Medicine* 35(3): 295–301.

Meyer, Madonna Harrington, Pam Herd, and Sonya Michel. 2000. "Introduction." In *Care Work: Gender, Labor, and the Welfare State,* edited by Madonna Harrington Meyer. New York: Routledge.

Meyers, Marcia, Sarah Bruch, Laura Peck, and Janet Gornick. 2011. State Safety Net Policy (data set). Seattle: University of Washington, West Coast Poverty Center.

Meyers, Marcia K., Dan Rosenbaum, Christopher Ruhm, and Jane Waldfogel. 2004. "Inequality in Early Childhood Education and Care: What Do We Know?" In *Social Inequality,* edited by Kathryn M. Neckerman. New York: Russell Sage Foundation.

Milkman, Ruth, and Eileen Appelbaum. 2004. "Paid Family Leave in California: New Research Findings." *The State of California Labor* 4: 45–67.

Mittal, Vikas, Jules Rosen, and Carrie Leana. 2009. "A Dual-Driver Model of Turnover and Retention in the Direct Care Workforce." *The Gerontologist* 49(5): 623–34.

Mollica, Robert L., Kristin Simms-Kastelein, Michael Cheek, Candace Baldwin, Jennifer Farnham, Susan Reinhard, and Jean Assius. 2009. *Building Adult Foster Care: What States Can Do.* Washington, D.C.: AARP Public Policy Institute.

Moody, Anissa L., Susan Morgello, Pieter Gerits, and Desiree Byrd. 2009. "Vulnerabilities and Caregiving in an Ethnically Diverse HIV-Infected Population." *AIDS and Behavior* 13(2): 337–47.

Moon, Jennifer, and John Burbank. 2004. *The Early Childhood Education Career and Wage Ladder: A Model for Improving Quality in Early Learning and Care Programs.* Seattle: Economic Opportunity Institute.

Morgan, Jennifer Craft, Janette Dill, Emmeline Chuang, Brandy Farrar, Kendra Jason, and Thomas R. Konrad. 2010. *UNC Evaluation of the Jobs to Careers Program.* Synthesis report, round 1. Chapel Hill: University of North Carolina Institute on Aging.

Morris, Lisa. 2009. "Quits and Job Changes Among Home Care Workers in Maine." *The Gerontologist* 49(5): 635–50.

Morrissey, Taryn, and Patti Banghart. 2007. "Family Child Care in the United States." New York: Columbia University, National Center for Children in Poverty.

Mulvey, Janemarie, and Christine Scott. 2010. "Dependent Care: Current Tax Benefits and Legislative Issues." Congressional Research Service (January 29). Available at: http://assets.opencrs.com/rpts/RS21466_20100129.pdf (accessed January 3, 2011).

Muraco, Anna, and Karen Fredrikson-Goldsen. 2011. " 'That's What Friends Do': Informal Caregiving for Chronically Ill Midlife and Older Lesbian, Gay, and Bisexual Adults." *Journal of Social and Personal Relationships,* published online March 23, 2011, doi:10.1177/0265407511402419.

Murray, Kasia O'Neill. 2004. "The Federal Legal Framework for Child Welfare." Washington, D.C.: Pew Commission on Children in Foster Care. Available at: http://www.pewfostercare.org (accessed May 21, 2011).

Musil, Carol M., and Muayyad Ahmad. 2002. "Health of Grandmothers: A Comparison by Caregiver Status." *Journal of Aging and Health* 14(1): 96–121.

Muszynska, Magdalena, Yeonjoo Yi, and Roland Rau. 2010. "Old-Age Health Dependency Ratio in Europe." Paper presented to the annual meeting of the Population Association of America. Dallas (April).

National Alliance for Caregiving (NAC). American Association of Retired Persons (AARP). 2009a. *Caregiving in the U.S. 2009.* Bethesda, Md., and Washington, D.C.: NAC and AARP (November). Available at: http://www.caregiving.org/data/Caregiving_in_the_US_2009_full_report.pdf (accessed October 18, 2010).

———. 2009b. "Caregivers of Children: A Focused Look at Those Caring for a Child with Special Needs Under the Age of Eighteen." November. Available at: http://www.caregiving.org/data/Report_Caregivers_of_Children_11-12-09.pdf (accessed May 21, 2011).

National Alliance for Caregiving (NAC). Metlife Mature Market Institute (MMMI). 2006. *The Metlife Caregiving Cost Study: Productivity Losses to U.S. Business.* Available at: http://www.caregiving.org/data/Caregiver%20Cost%20Study.pdf (accessed March 7, 2012).

National Association of Child Care Resource and Referral Agencies (NACCRRA). 2009. "Dependent Care Tax Credit." Available at: http://www.naccrra.org/policy/background_issues/dctc (accessed May 21, 2011).

National Association of Public Child Welfare Administrators (NAPCWA). 2007. "Basic Family Foster Care Maintenance Rates Survey: Summary of Findings." Available at: http://www.childrensrights.org/wp-content/uploads/2008/06/foster_care_rate_survey_may_2007.pdf (accessed May 21, 2011).

National Direct Service Workforce Resource Center (NDSWRC). 2008. "A Synthesis of Direct Service Workforce Demographics and Challenges Across Intellectual/Developmental Disabilities, Aging, Physical Disabilities, and Behavioral Health." Report prepared by Amy Hewitt, Sheryl Larson, Steve Edelstein, Dorie Seavey, Michael A. Hoge, and John Morris (November). Available at: http://rtc.umn.edu/docs/Cross-Disability SynthesisWhitePaperFinal.pdf (accessed January 11, 2010).

National Family Caregivers Association (NFCA). Family Caregiver Alliance (FCA). 2006. "Estimated Prevalence and Economic Value of Family Caregiving, by State (2004)." Available at: www.caregiver.com/2004_State_Caregiving.pdf (accessed May 25, 2011).

National Partnership for Women & Families. 2012. *Expecting Better: A State By State Analysis of Laws That Help New Parents.* Washington, D.C.: National Partnership for Women & Families.

National Resource Center for Health and Safety in Child Care and Early Education. n.d. "Individual States Child Care Licensure Regulations." Available at: http://nrckids.org/STATES/states.htm (accessed February 20, 2012).

National Women's Law Center. 2006. "Making Care Less Taxing: Improving State Child and Dependent Care Tax Provisions." April. Available at: http://www.nwlc.org/sites/default/files/pdfs/MakingCareLessTaxing2006.pdf (accessed January 10, 2010).

Neal, Margaret B., and Leslie B. Hammer. 2009. "Dual-Earner Couples in the Sandwiched Generation: Effects of Coping Strategies Over Time." *The Psychologist-Manager Journal* 12(4): 205–234.

Nelson, Julie. 2011. "For Love or Money: Current Issues in the Economics of Care." *Journal of Gender Studies* (Ochanomizu University, Japan) 1(March): 1–19.

Nelson, Margaret K. 2006. "Single Mothers 'Do' Family." *Journal of Marriage and Family* 68(4): 781–95.

Newman, Katherine. 2000. "On the High Wire: How the Working Poor Juggle Job and Family Responsibilities." In *Balancing Acts: Easing the Burdens and Improving the Options for Working Families,* edited by Eileen Appelbaum. Washington, D.C.: Economic Policy Institute.

Ng, Terence, Alice Wong, and Charlene Harrington. 2009. "Home- and Community-Based Services: Introduction to Olmstead Lawsuits and Olmstead Plans." San Francisco: University of California, National Center for Personal Assistance Services (August). Available at: http://www.pascenter.org/olmstead/downloads/Olmstead8_4_09.pdf (accessed February 3, 2010).

Noah, Timothy. 2010. "The Great Divergence." *Slate* (September 3–14). Available at: http://www.slate.com/articles/news_and_politics/the_great_divergence.html (accessed February 17, 2012).

O'Brien, Ellen, and Mark Merlis. 2007. "Medicaid's Spousal Impoverishment Protections." Fact Sheet, Washington, D.C.: Georgetown University Long-Term Care Financing Project, February. Available at: http://ltc.georgetown.edu/pdfs/spousal0207.pdf (accessed February 16, 2012).

Ochsner, Michele, Carrie Leana, and Eileen Appelbaum. 2009. "Improving Direct Care Work: Integrating Theory, Research, and Practice." Alfred P. Sloan Foundation White Paper (July 29).

Okamoto, Dina, and Paula England. 1999. "Is There a Supply Side to Occupational Sex Segregation?" *Sociological Perspectives* 42(4): 557–82.

Oliker, Stacey J. 2000. "Examining Care at Welfare's End." In *Care Work: Gender, Class, and the Welfare State,* edited by Madonna Harrington Meyer. New York: Routledge.

Osborne, Melissa. 2000. "The Power of Personality: Labor Market Rewards and the Transmission of Earnings." Ph.D. diss., Department of Economics, University of Massachusetts at Amherst.

O'Shaughnessy, Carol V. 2009. "The Older Americans Act of 1965: The Basics." Washington, D.C.: National Health Policy Forum (October 8). Available at: http://www.nhpf.org/library/the-basics/Basics_OlderAmericansAct_07-09-10.pdf (accessed May 21, 2011).

Ostrom, Elinor. 1990. *Governing the Commons: The Evolution of Institutions for Collective Action.* New York: Cambridge University Press.

Parrish, Thomas. 2010. "Policy Alternatives for Special Education Funding in Illinois." Report submitted to Illinois State Board of Education. Palo Alto, Calif.: Center for Special Education Finance, American Institutes for Research (June 30).

Parrish, Thomas, Jenifer Harr, Jennifer Anthony, Amy Merickel, and Phil Esra. 2003. "State Special Education Finance Systems, 1999–2000, Part 1." Palo Alto, Calif.: Center for Special Education Finance, American Institutes of Research (May). Available at: http://csef.air.org/publications/csef/state/statpart1.pdf (accessed May 21, 2011).

Parrish, Thomas, Jenifer Harr, Jean Wollman, Jennifer Anthony, Amy Merickel, and Phil Esra. 2004. "State Special Education Finance Systems, 1999–2000, Part II: Special Education Revenues and Expenditures." Palo Alto, Calif.: Center for Special Education Finance, American Institutes of Research (March). Available at: http://csef.air.org/publications/csef/state/statepart2.pdf (accessed May 21, 2011).

Paxson, Christina, and Jane Waldfogel. 1999. "Parental Resources and Child Abuse and Neglect." *American Economic Review* 89(2): 239–44.

PHI (formerly Paraprofessional Healthcare Institute). 2003. "The Personal Assistance Services and Direct-Support Workforce: A Literature Review." Direct Care Clearinghouse (June 12). Available at: http://www.directcareclearinghouse.org/download/CMS_Lit_Rev_FINAL_6.12.03.pdf (accessed June 2, 2010).

———. 2010. "Who are Direct Care Workers?" *Facts 3*, February update. Available at: http://www.directcareclearinghouse.org/download/NCDCW%20Fact%20Sheet-1.pdf. (accessed May 15, 2010).

PHI (formerly Paraprofessional Healthcare Institute). Direct Care Workers Association of North Carolina (DCWA-NC). 2009. *The 2007 National Survey of State Initiatives on the Direct Care Workforce: Key Findings.* December. Available at: http://directcareclearinghouse.org/l_art_det.jsp?res_id=297910 (accessed April 3, 2010).

Phipps, Shelly, Peter Burton, and Lynn Lethbridge. 2001. "In and Out of the Labour Market: Long-Term Income Consequences of Child-Related Interruptions to Women's Paid Work." *Canadian Journal of Economics* 34(2): 411–29.

Pierret, Charles R. 2006. "The 'Sandwich Generation': Women Caring for Parents and Children." *Monthly Labor Review* (September): 3–9.

Pineau, Joelle, Michael Montemerlo, Martha Pollack, Nicholas Roy, and Sebastian Thrun. 2003. "Towards Robotic Assistants in Nursing Homes: Challenges and Results." *Robotics and Autonomous Systems* 42(3–4): 271–81.

Pinker, Susan. 2008. *The Sexual Paradox.* New York: Scribner.

Pinquart, Martin, and Silvia Sörensen. 2005. "Caregiving Distress and Psychological Health of Caregivers." In *Psychology of Stress,* edited by Kimberly V. Oxington. New York: Nova Biomedical Books.

———. 2007. "Correlates of Physical Health of Informal Caregivers: A Meta-Analysis." *Journal of Gerontology: Psychological Sciences* 62B: P126–37.

Polachek, Solomon. 1981. "Occupational Self-Selection: A Human Capital Approach to Sex Differences in Occupational Structure." *Review of Economics and Statistics* 63(1): 60–69.

Pozzilli, Carlo, Laura Palmisano, Catarina Mainero, Valentina Tomassini, Fiorenzo Marinelli, Giovanni Ristori, Claudio Gasperini, Monica Fabiani, and Mario Alberto Battaglia. 2004. "Relationship Between Emotional Distress in Caregivers and Health Status in Persons with Multiple Sclerosis." *Multiple Sclerosis* 10(4): 442–46.

References

Presser, Harriet. 2003. *Working in a 24/7 Economy: Challenges for American Families.* New York: Russell Sage Foundation.

Prouty, Robert W., Kathryn Alba, and K. Charlie Lakin, eds. 2008. *Residential Services for Persons with Developmental Disabilities: Status and Trends Through 2007.* Minneapolis: University of Minnesota, Research and Training Center on Community Living, Institute on Community Integration (August). Available at: http://rtc.umn.edu/docs/risp2007.pdf (accessed April 4, 2010).

Putnam, Robert D. 2000. *Bowling Alone: The Collapse and Revival of American Community.* New York: Simon & Schuster.

Quinn, Catherine, Linda Clare, and Robert T. Woods. 2010. "The Impact of Motivation and Meanings on the Well-being of Caregivers of People with Dementia: A Systematic Review." *International Psychogeriatrics* 22(1): 43–55.

Rabiner, Donna J., Galina Khatutsky, Joshua M. Wiener, Deborah S. Osber, David W. Brown, and Beth Koetse. 2006. "Evaluation of the Select Consumer, Program, and System Characteristics Under the Supportive Service Program (Title III-B) of the Older Americans Act, AoA, Interim Quantitative Report." Research Triangle Park, N.C.: RTI International (June). Available at: http://www.aoa.gov/AoARoot/Program_Results/docs/Program_Eval/TitleIIIB_quantitative-report_6-1-06_psgFINAL.pdf (accessed May 21, 2011).

Radin, Martha. 1996. *Contested Commodities.* Cambridge, Mass.: Harvard University Press.

Raley, Sara, Suzanne M. Bianchi, and Wendy Wang. Forthcoming. "When Do Fathers Care? Mothers' Economic Contribution and Fathers' Involvement in Childcare." *American Journal of Sociology* 117(5): 1422–59.

Rankin, Nancy. 2002. "Fixing Social Insecurity: A Proposal to Finance Parenthood." In *Taking Parenting Public: The Case for a New Social Movement,* edited by Sylvia Ann Hewlett, Nancy Rankin, and Cornel West. New York: Rowman and Littlefield.

Raschick, Michael, and Berit Ingersoll-Dayton. 2004. "The Costs and Rewards of Caregiving Among Aging Spouses and Adult Children." *Family Relations* 53(3): 317–25.

Razavi, Shahra. 2007. "The Political and Social Economy of Care in a Development Context: Contextual Issues, Research Questions, and Policy Options." Gender and Development Program Paper 3. United Nations Research Institute for Social Development (June). Available at: http://www.unrisd.org/80256B3C005BCCF9/(httpAuxPages)/2DBE6A93350A7783C12573240036D5A0/$file/Razavi-paper.pdf (accessed May 23, 2011).

Reid, Margaret. 1934. *Economics of Household Production.* New York: John Wiley and Sons.

Reidel, Sara E., Lisa Fredman, and Pat Langenberg. 1998. "Associations Among Caregiving Difficulties, Burden, and Rewards in Caregivers to Older Post-Rehabilitation Parents." *Journal of Gerontology: Psychological Sciences* 53B: P165–74.

Reskin, Barbara, and Patricia Roos. 1990. *Job Queues, Gender Queues.* Philadelphia: Temple University Press.

Rizzolo, Mary C. 2009. "Family Support Services in the United States: 2008." *Policy Research Brief* 20(2): 1–11. Minneapolis: Research and Training Center on Community Living, Institute on Community Integration, University of Minnesota, May. Available at http://ici.umn.edu/products/prb/202/202.pdf (accessed June 2, 2011).

Rose, Stephen J., and Heidi I. Hartmann. 2004. *Still a Man's Labor Market.* Washington, D.C.: Institute for Women's Policy Research.

Rosenbaum, Sara. 2008. "CMS' Medicaid Regulations: Implications for Children with Special Health Care Needs." Policy brief (March). Washington, D.C.: George Washington University School of Public Health and Health Care Services. Available at: http://www.gwumc.edu/sphhs/departments/healthpolicy/dhp_publications/pub_uploads/dhpPublication_63E70BAC-5056-9D20-3DEBBD5D6D824B25.pdf (accessed May 21, 2011).

Rosenbaum, Sara, Sara Wilensky, and Kamala Allen. 2008. "EPSDT at Forty: Modernizing a Pediatric Health Policy to Reflect a Changing Health Care System." Resource paper. Washington, D.C.: Center for Health Care Strategies (July). Available at: http://www.chcs.org/usr_doc/EPSDT_at_40.pdf (accessed May 21, 2011).

Ross Phillips, Katherin. 2004. "Getting Time Off: Access to Leave Among Working Parents." Washington, D.C.: Urban Institute (April). Available at: http://www.urban.org/UploadedPDF/310977_B-57.pdf (accessed May 21, 2011).

Rossin, Maya. 2011. "The Effects of Maternity Leave on Children's Birth and Infant Health Outcomes in the United States." *Journal of Health Economics* 30(2): 221–39.

Roth, David L., William E. Haley, Virginia G. Wadley, Olivio J. Clay, and George Howard. 2007. "Race and Gender Differences in Perceived Caregiver Availability for Community-Dwelling Middle-Aged and Older Adults." *The Gerontologist* 47(6): 721–29.

Rothstein, Bo. 2005. *Social Traps and the Problem of Trust.* Cambridge: Cambridge University Press.

Rubin, Rose, and Shelley White-Means. 2009. "Informal Caregiving: Dilemmas of Sandwiched Caregivers." *Journal of Family Economic Issues* 20(3): 252–67.

Ryan, Jennifer. 2009. "Children's Health Insurance Program: The Fundamentals." Background paper 68. Washington, D.C.: National Health Policy Forum (April 23). Available at: http://www.nhpf.org/library/background-papers/BP68_CHIPFundamentals_04-23-09.pdf (accessed May 24, 2011).

Santos-Eggimann, Brigitte, Frank Zobel, and Annick Clerc Bérod. 1999. "Functional Status of Elderly Home Health Users: Do Subjects, Informal and Professional Caregivers Agree?" *Journal of Clinical Epidemiology* 52(3): 181–86.

Sarkisian, Natalia, Mariana Gerena, and Naomi Gerstel. 2006. "Extended Family Ties Among Mexicans, Puerto Ricans, and Whites: Superintegration or Disintegration?" *Family Relations* 55(3): 331–44.

Sarkisian, Natalia, and Naomi Gerstel. 2004a. "Explaining the Gender Gap in Help to Parents: The Importance of Employment." *Journal of Marriage and the Family* 66(2): 431–51.

———. 2004b. "Kin Support Among Blacks and Whites: Race and Family Organization." *American Sociological Review* 69(6): 812–37.

Satterly, Faye. 2004. *Where Have All of the Nurses Gone? The Impact of the Nursing Shortage on American Health Care.* Amherst, N.Y.: Prometheus Books.

Sayer, Liana C., Philip Cohen, and Lynn M. Casper. 2004. "Women, Men, and Work." In *The American People Census 2000 Series.* New York: Russell Sage Foundation and Population Reference Bureau.

Schmitt, John, 2008. "The Union Wage Advantage for Low-Wage Workers." Washington, D.C.: Center for Economic and Policy Research (May). Available at: http://www.cepr.net/index.php/publications/reports/the-union-wage-advantage-for-low-wage-workers/ (accessed April 29, 2012).

———. 2009. "Unions and Upward Mobility for Service-Sector Workers." Washington, D.C.: Center for Economic and Policy Research (April). Available at: http://www.cepr. net/index.php/publications/reports/unions-and-upward-mobility-for-service-sector-workers (accessed April 29, 2012).

Schmitt, John, Margy Waller, Shawn Fremstad, and Ben Zipperer. 2007. "Unions and Upward Mobility for Low-Wage Workers." Washington, D.C.: Center for Economic and Policy Research (August). Available at: http://www.cepr.net/documents/publications/UnionsandUpwardMobility.pdf (accessed April 29, 2012).

Schulz, Richard, and Scott R. Beach. 1999. "Caregiving as a Risk Factor for Mortality: The Caregiver Health Effects Study." *Journal of the American Medical Association* 282(23): 2215–19.

Schulz, Richard, Paul Visintainer, and Gail M. Williamson. 1990. "Psychiatric and Physical Morbidity Effects of Caregiving." *Journal of Gerontology: Psychological Sciences* 45(5): P181–91.

Schweinhart, Lawrence J. 2002. "How the HighScope Perry Preschool Study Grew: A Researcher's Tale." Published online by Phi Delta Kappa Center for Evaluation, Development, and Research, no. 32 (June); reprinted at HighScope, http://www.highscope.org/Content.asp?ContentId=232 (accessed October 12, 2010).

Seavey, Dorie. 2004. "The Cost of Frontline Turnover in Long-Term Care." A Better Jobs, Better Care Practice and Policy Report, October. Washington, D.C.: Institute for Aging Services, American Association of Homes and Services for the Aging. Available at: http://www.directcareclearinghouse.org/download/TOCostReport.pdf (accessed February 17, 2012).

Seavey, Dorie, and Abby Marquand. 2011. "Caring in America: A Comprehensive Analysis of the Nation's Fastest Growing Jobs—Home Health and Personal Care Aides." December. New York: PHI National. Available at: http://www.directcareclearinghouse.org/download/caringinamerica-20111212.pdf (accessed February 20, 2012).

Seavey, Dorie, and Vera Salter. 2006. "Paying for Quality Care: State and Local Strategies for Improving Wages and Benefits for Personal Care Assistants." AARP/PHI 2006-18. Washington, D.C.: AARP Public Policy Institute (October). Available at: http://assets.aarp.org/rgcenter/il/2006_18_care.pdf (accessed May 21, 2011).

Seeman, Teresa E., Sharon S. Merkin, and Arun S. Karlamangla. 2010. "Disability Trends Among Older Americans: National Health and Nutrition Examination Surveys, 1988–1994 and 1999–2004." *American Journal of Public Health* 100(1): 100–107.

Shapiro, Adam. 2003. "Later Life Divorce and Parent–Adult Child Contact and Proximity." *Journal of Family Issues* 24(2): 264–85.

Shih, Anthony, and Stephen C. Schoenbaum. 2007. "Measuring Hospital Performance: The Importance of Process Measures." Commonwealth Fund data brief (July). Available at: http://www.commonwealthfund.org/Publications/Data-Briefs/2007/Jul/Measuring-Hospital-Performance--The-Importance-of-Process-Measures.aspx (accessed November 8, 2011).

Sigle-Rushton, Wendy, and Jane Waldfogel. 2004. "Family Gaps in Income: A Cross-National Comparison." Paper presented to the conference "Supporting Children: English-Speaking Countries in International Context." Princeton University (January 8–9).

Simon, Herbert A. 1990. "A Mechanism for Social Selection and Successful Altruism." *Science* 250(4988): 1665–68.

———. 1992. "Altruism and Economics." *Eastern Economic Journal* 18(1): 73–83.

Simon-Rusinowitz, Lori, Kevin J. Mahoney, Dawn M. Loughly, and Michele DeBarthe Sadler. 2005. "Paying Family Caregivers: An Effective Policy Option in the Arkansas Cash and Counseling Demonstration and Evaluation." *Marriage and Family Review* 37(1–2): 83–105.

Simpson, Brent. 2003. "Sex, Fear, and Greed: A Social Dilemma Analysis of Gender and Cooperation." *Social Forces* 82(1): 35–52.

Sloan Foundation. 2009. "Work-Family Information for State Legislators." Policy briefing series 17. Available at: http://www.worklifelaw.org/pubs/policybrieffrd.pdf (accessed April 29, 2012).

Small, Mario Luis. 2009. *Unanticipated Gains: Origins of Network Inequality in Everyday Life.* New York: Oxford University Press.

Smith, Kristin. 2012. "Home Care Workers Lack Protections: Overtime Pay and Minimum Wage." Issue brief 43. Durham, N.H.: Carsey Institute, University of New Hampshire.

Smith, Kristin, and Reagan Baughman. 2007a. "Caring for America's Aging Population: A Profile of the Direct-Care Workforce." *Monthly Labor Review* (September): 20–26.

———. 2007b. "Low Wages Prevalent in Direct Care and Child Care Workforce." Policy brief 7. Durham, N.H.: University of New Hampshire, Carsey Institute.

Smith, Kristin, and Allison Churilla. 2010. "Low-Income Status Among Female Direct Care and Child Care Workers: The Intersection of Race and Other Family Income." Unpublished paper, University of New Hampshire, Department of Sociology.

Smith, Kristin, Barbara Downs, and Martin O'Connell. 2001. "Maternity Leave and Employment Patterns: 1961–1995." *Current Population Reports* (November). Washington: U.S. Census Bureau.

Smith, Peggie. 2008. "The Publicization of Home-Based Care Work in State Labor Law." 92 Minn. L. Rev. 1390–1423. Available at: http://www.minnesotalawreview.org/wp-content/uploads/2012/01/Smith_FinalPDF.pdf (accessed February 21, 2012).

———. 2009a. "Protecting Home Care Workers Under the Fair Labor Standards Act." Direct Care Alliance policy brief 2 (June). Available at: http://blog.directcarealliance.org/wp-content/uploads/2009/06/6709-dca_policybrief_2final.pdf (accessed May 21, 2011).

———. 2009b. "Union Representation of Child-Care Workers in the United States." In *Comparative Patriarchy and American Institutions: The Language, Culture, and Politics of Liberalism,* edited by M. Francis McCollum Feeley. Chambery, Fr.: Université de Savoie Press.

Sober, Elliott, and David Sloan Wilson. 1998. *Unto Others: The Evolution and Psychology of Unselfish Behavior.* Cambridge, Mass.: Harvard University Press.

Social Security Administration (SSA). 2011. "Benefits for Children with Disabilities." Publication 05-10026. ICN 455360 (June). Available at: http://www.ssa.gov/pubs/10026.html (accessed April 29, 2012).

Sonn, Paul K., and Stephanie Luce. 2008. "New Directions for the Living Wage Movement." In *The Gloves-Off Economy: Workplace Standards at the Bottom of America's Labor Market,* edited by Annette Bernhardt, Heather Boushey, Laura Dresser, and Chris Tilly. Urbana-Champaign, Ill.: Labor and Employment Relations Association.

Spence, Janet T., and Camille E. Buckner. 2000. "Instrumental and Expressive Traits, Trait Stereotypes, and Sexist Attitudes: What Do They Signify?" *Psychology of Women Quarterly* 24(1): 44–62.

Spillman, Brenda C. 2004. "Changes in Elderly Disability Rates and the Implications for Health Care Utilization and Cost." *Milbank Quarterly* 82(1): 157–94.

Spillman, Brenda, and Kirsten Black. 2008. "The Size of the Long-Term Care Population in Residential Care: A Review of Estimates and Methodology." Washington, D.C.: Urban Institute (August 4). Available at: http://www.urban.org/health_policy/url.cfm?ID=1001202 (accessed May 25, 2011).

Spillman, Brenda C., and Liliana Pezzin. 2000. "Potential and Active Family Caregivers: Changing Networks and the 'Sandwich Generation.' " *Milbank Quarterly* 78(3): 347–74.

Spitze, Glenna, and Katherine Trent. 2006. "Gender Differences in Adult Sibling Relations in Two-Child Families." *Journal of Marriage and Family* 68(4): 977–92.

Spreitzer, Gretchen M., and Scott Sonenshein. 2003. "Positive Deviance and Extraordinary Organizing." In *Positive Organizational Scholarship,* edited by Jane E. Dutton, Robert E. Quinn, and Kim S. Cameron. San Francisco: Berrett-Koehler.

Stacey, Clare L. 2011. *The Caring Self: The Work Experiences of Home Care Aides.* Ithaca, N.Y.: Cornell University Press.

Stack, Carol B. 1974. *All Our Kin: Strategies for Survival in a Black Community.* New York: Harper & Row.

State of California. Employment Development Department (EDD). 2010a. "Paid Family Leave." Available at: http://www.edd.ca.gov/disability/Paid_Family_Leave.htm (accessed May 21, 2011).

———. 2010b. Paid family leave and disability insurance program statistics, SFY 2009–2010 and CY2010 (unpublished data).

State of New Jersey. Department of Labor and Workforce Development (DOLWD). 2010a. "Family Leave Insurance—Program Statistics." Available at: http://lwd.state.nj.us/labor/fli/content/monthly_report_fli.html (accessed May 21, 2011).

———. 2010b. "Family Leave Insurance: Frequently Asked Questions." Available at: http://lwd.dol.state.nj.us/labor/fli/content/fli_faq.html#3 (accessed May 21, 2011).

———. 2010c. Data provided by Christopher Longo, director, Temporary Disability and Family Leave Insurance, December 2010.

State of New Jersey. Employers' Pensions and Benefits Administration Manual (EPBAM). 2010. "New Jersey Family Leave Act and Family and Medical Leave Act of 1993: Frequently Asked Questions and Answers." Available at: http://www.state.nj.us/treasury/pensions/epbam/additional/fmla-qa.htm (accessed May 21, 2011).

Still, Mary C. 2006. "Litigating the Maternal Wall: U.S. Lawsuits Charging Discrimination Against Workers with Family Responsibilities." San Francisco: Center for Work Life Law. Available at: http://www.worklifelaw.org/pubs/FRDreport.pdf (accessed January 2, 2010).

Stone, Deborah. 2000a. "Caring by the Book." In *Care Work: Gender, Labor, and the Welfare State,* edited by Madonna Harrington Meyer. New York: Routledge.

———. 2000b. "Why We Need a Care Movement." *The Nation,* March 13.

Stone, Philip J. 1972. "Child Care in Twelve Countries." In *The Use of Time: Daily Activities of Urban and Suburban Populations in Twelve Countries,* edited by Alexander Szalai. Paris: Mouton.

Stone, Robyn, and Steve Dawson. 2008. "The Origins of Better Jobs, Better Care." *The Gerontologist* 48(Suppl 1): 5–13.

Stukes Chipungu, Sandra, and Tricia Bent-Goodley. 2004. "Meeting the Challenges of Contemporary Foster Care." *The Future of Children* 14(1): 75–94.

Summer, Laura. 2005. "Strategies to Keep Consumers Needing Long-Term Care in the Community and Out of Nursing Facilities." Report prepared for the Kaiser Commission on Medicaid and the Uninsured (October). Available at: http://www.kff.org/medicaid/upload/Strategies-to-Keep-Consumers-Needing-Long-Term-Care-in-the-Community-and-Out-of-Nursing-Facilities-Report.pdf (accessed April 29, 2012).

Sweeney, Megan M., and Maria Cancian. 2004. "The Changing Importance of White Women's Economic Prospects for Assortative Mating." *Journal of Marriage and Family* 66(4): 1015–28.

Swidler, Ann. 1986. "Culture in Action: Symbols and Strategies." *American Sociological Review* 51(2): 273–86.

Taylor, Lowell J. 2007. "Optimal Wages in the Market for Nurses: An Analysis Based on Heyes' Model." *Journal of Health Economics* 26(5): 1027–30.

Taylor, Shelley E. 2002. *The Tending Instinct: Women, Men, and the Biology of Our Relationships.* New York: Henry Holt.

Thompson, James D. 2003. *Organizations in Action: Social Science Bases of Administrative Theory.* New Brunswick, N.J.: Transaction Publishers.

Thompson, W. Grant. 2005. *The Placebo Effect and Health: Combining Science and Compassionate Care.* New York: Prometheus.

Thornton, Arland, Duane F. Alwin, and Donald Camburn. 1983. "Causes and Consequences of Sex-Role Attitudes and Attitude Change." *American Sociological Review* 48(2): 211–27.

Thornton, Arland, and Deborah Freedman. 1979. "Changes in the Sex-Role Attitudes of Women, 1962–1977: Evidence from a Panel Study." *American Sociological Review* 44(5): 831–42.

Todorov, Alexander, and Corrine Kirchner. 2000. "Bias in Proxies' Reports of Disability: Data from the National Health Interview Survey on Disability." *American Journal of Public Health* 90(8): 1248–1453.

Tomassini, Cecilia, and Douglas A. Wolf. 2000. "Shrinking Kin Networks in Italy Due To Sustained Low Fertility." *European Journal of Population* 16(4): 353–72.

Trivers, Robert. 1972. "Parental Investment and Sexual Selection." In *Sexual Selection and the Descent of Man,* edited by Bernard G. Campbell. Chicago: Aldine.

Turkle, Sherry. 2011. *Alone Together: Why We Expect More from Technology and Less from Each Other.* New York: Basic Books.

Turnham, Hollis, and Steven L. Dawson. 2003. "Michigan's Care Gap: Our Emerging Direct-Care Workforce Crisis." Bronx, N.Y.: Paraprofessional Health Care Institute (PHI), National Clearing House on the Direct Care Workforce. Available at: http://directcareclearinghouse.org/download/MI%20Care%20Gap%20Publicn.pdf (accessed May 21, 2011).

Tweddle, Ann. 2007. "Youth Leaving Care: How Do They Fare?" *New Directions for Youth Development* 2007(113): 15–31.

Twenge, Jean. 1997. "Attitudes Toward Women, 1970–1995." *Psychology of Women Quarterly* 21(1): 35–51.

Uhlenberg, Peter. 2005. "Historical Forces Shaping Grandparent-Grandchild Relationships: Demography and Beyond." *Annual Review of Gerontology and Geriatrics* ("Intergenerational Relations Across Time and Place," edited by Merril Silverstein) 24: 77–119. New York: Springer Verlag.

Ungerson, Clare. 1997. "Social Politics and the Commodification of Care." *Social Politics* 4(3): 362–81.

———. 2004. "Whose Empowerment and Independence? A Cross-National Perspective on 'Cash for Care' Schemes." *Ageing and Society* 24(2): 189–212. doi:10.1017/S0144686X03001508.

University of Michigan, Institute for Social Research. Various years, a. *Health and Retirement Study.* Available at: http://hrsonline.isr.umich.edu/ (accessed February 27, 2012).

University of Michigan, Institute for Social Research. Various years, b. *Panel Study of Income Dynamics.* Available at: http://psidonline.isr.umich.edu/ (accessed February 27, 2012).

University of Pittsburgh. 2006. *The State of the Homecare Industry in Pennsylvania.* Prepared for the Pennsylvania Homecare Association.

Urban Institute. 2003. "Children in Kinship Care." Assessing the New Federalism. Available at: http://www.urban.org/UploadedPDF/900661.pdf (accessed May 21, 2011).

U.S. Bureau of Labor Statistics (BLS). Various years. *American Time Use Survey.* Available at: http://www.bls.gov/tus/ (accessed February 27, 2012).

———. 2010a. "Nonfatal Occupational Injuries and Illnesses Requiring Days Away from Work, 2006." News release (November 8). http://www.bls.gov/news.release/History/osh2.txt (accessed February 23, 2008).

———. 2010b. "U.S. Occupational Outlook Handbook, 2010–2011 Edition: Home Health Aides and Personal and Home Care Aides." Available at: http://www.bls.gov/oco/ocos326.htm (accessed March 23, 2011).

———. 2012. "Employment Projections 2010–2020." News release (February 1). Available at: http://www.bls.gov/news.release/pdf/ecopro.pdf (accessed February 20, 2012).

U.S. Bureau of Labor Statistics (BLS), Current Population Survey (CPS). 2010a. *Household Data Annual Averages: 2010,* "Table 11: Employed Persons by Detailed Occupation, Sex, Race and Hispanic or Latino Ethnicity." Available at: stats.bls.gov/cps/cpsaat11.pdf (accessed February 20, 2012).

———. 2010b. *Household Data Annual Averages: 2010,* "Table 16: Employed Persons in Non-agricultural Industries by Sex and Class of Worker." Available at: stats.bls.gov/cps/cpsaat16.pdf (accessed February 20, 2012).

———. 2010c. *Household Data Annual Averages: 2010,* "Table 18: Employed Persons by Detailed Industries by Sex, Race and Hispanic or Latino Ethnicity." Available at: stats.bls.gov/cps/cpsaat18.pdf (accessed February 20, 2012).

———. 2010d. *2010 Annual Social and Economic (ASEC) Supplement* [machine-readable data file]. Conducted by the Bureau of the Census for the Bureau of Labor Statistics. Washington: U.S. Census Bureau [producer and distributor].

U.S. Census Bureau. 1975. "Historical Statistics of the United States, Colonial Times to 1970, Part 1." Washington: Government Printing Office.

———. 1997. "Statistical Abstract of the United States, 1997." Washington: Government Printing Office.

———. 2000. "2000 Decennial Census SF-1." Available at: http://www.census.gov/prod/cen2000/doc/sf1.pdf (accessed May 21, 2011).

———. 2006. *2005 American Community Survey.* Available at: http://www.census.gov/acs/www (accessed May 21, 2011).

———. 2007. *2006 American Community Survey.* Available at: http://www.census.gov/acs/www (accessed May 21, 2011).

———. 2008a. *2005–2007 American Community Survey.* Available at: http://www.census.gov/acs/www (accessed May 21, 2011).

————. 2008b. "Table C1: Household Relationship and Family Status of Children Under 18 Years, by Age and Sex: 2011." Available at: http://www.census.gov/population/www/socdemo/hh-fam/cps2011.html (accessed February 22, 2011).

————. 2008c. "Tables 1B and 2B: Who's Minding the Kids? Child Care Arrangements: Spring 2005." Housing and Household Economic Statistics Division, Fertility and Family Statistics Branch (February). Available at: http://www.census.gov/hhes/childcare/data/sipp/2005/tables.html (accessed May 21, 2011).

————. 2009a. *2008 American Community Survey.* Available at: http://www.census.gov/acs/www (accessed May 21, 2011).

————. 2009b. "Annual Estimates of the Resident Population for the United States, Regions, States, and Puerto Rico: April 1, 2000 to July 1, 2009." NST-EST2009-01. December. Available at: http://www.census.gov/popest/states/NST-ann-est.html (accessed May 21, 2011).

————. 2010a. "S2601B. Characteristics of the Group Quarters Population by Group Quarters Type, 2009 American Community Survey 1-Year Estimates." Available at: http://factfinder2.census.gov/faces/tableservices/jsf/pages/productview.xhtml?pid=ACS_09_1YR_S2601B&prodType=table (accessed February 17, 2012).

————. 2010b. "Statistical Abstract of the United States, 2010." Washington: Government Printing Office.

————. 2011a. "Who's Minding the Kids? Child Care Arrangements: Spring 2010—Detailed Tables." Available at: http://www.census.gov/hhes/childcare/data/sipp/2010/tables.html (accessed March 1, 2012).

————. 2011b. *2010 American Community Survey.* Available at: http://www.census.gov/acs/www (accessed May 21, 2011).

U.S. Department of Education (DOE). National Center for Education Statistics (NCES). 2011. *Digest of Education Statistics, 2010.* "Table 188: Total Expenditures for Public Elementary and Secondary Education, by Function and Subfunction, Selected Years, 1990–91 Through 2007–08." NCES 2011-015. Available at: http://nces.ed.gov/programs/digest/d10/tables/dt10_188.asp?referrer=list.

U.S. Department of Education (DOE). National Center for Education Statistics (NCES). Institute of Education Services (IES). 2009. "Digest of Education Statistics: 2009." October. Available at: http://nces.ed.gov/programs/digest/d09/tables/dt09_378.asp?referrer=list. (accessed May 21, 2011).

U.S. Department of Education (DOE). Office of Special Education and Rehabilitative Services (OSERS). Office of Special Education Programs (OSEP). 2009. "Twenty-Eighth Annual Report to Congress on the Implementation of the Individuals with Disabilities Education Act, 2006, Vol. 2." Available at: http://www2.ed.gov/about/reports/annual/osep/2006/parts-b-c/index.html (accessed February 18, 2012).

U.S. Department of Education (DOE). Office of Special Education and Rehabilitative Services (OSERS). Rehabilitation Services Administration (RSA). 2009. *Annual Report, Fiscal Year 2005, Report on Federal Activities Under the Rehabilitation Act.* Available at: http://www2.ed.gov/about/reports/annual/rsa/2005/rsa-2005-annual-report.pdf (accessed May 24, 2011).

U.S. Department of Health and Human Services (DHSS). Administration for Children and Families (ACF). 2010. "National Survey of Child and Adolescent Well-Being (NSCAW), No. 2: Foster Children's Caregivers and Caregiving Environments." Research brief.

U.S. Department of Health and Human Services (DHHS). Administration for Children and Families (ACF). Administration on Children, Youth, and Families (ACYF), Children's Bureau (CB). 2008. *The AFCARS Report: Preliminary FY 2008 Estimates as of October 2009.* Available at: http://www.acf.hhs.gov/programs/cb/stats_research/afcars/tar/report16.htm (accessed May 21, 2011).

———. 2009a. "Foster Care FY 2002–FY 2008 Entries, Exits, and Numbers of Children in Care on the Last Day of Each Federal Fiscal Year." Available at: http://www.acf.hhs.gov/programs/cb/stats_research/afcars/statistics/entryexit2008.htm (accessed May 21, 2011).

———. 2009b. "The AFCARS Report: Preliminary FY 2008 Estimates as of October 2009." Available at: http://www.acf.hhs.gov/programs/cb/stats_research/afcars/tar/report16.htm (accessed May 21, 2011).

———. 2010. "Children in Public Foster Care on September 30 of Each Year Who Are Waiting to Be Adopted: FY 2002–FY 2009." August. Available at: http://www.acf.hhs.gov/programs/cb/stats_research/afcars/waiting2009.pdf (accessed May 21, 2011).

U.S. Department of Health and Human Services (DHHS). Administration for Children and Families (ACF). Child Care Bureau (CCB). 2008. "FFY 2007 CCDF Data Tables." October. Available at: http://www.acf.hhs.gov/programs/ccb/data/ccdf_data/07acf800_preliminary/table1.htm (accessed May 21, 2011).

U.S. Department of Health and Human Services (DHHS). Administration for Children and Families (ACF). Office of Community Services (OCS). 2007. "SSBG Focus Reports 2007: Child Care." Available at: http://www.acf.hhs.gov/programs/ocs/ssbg/reports/ssbg_focus_2007/child_care.html (accessed May 21, 2011).

———. 2008. "SSBG Focus Reports 2008: Child Care." Available at: http://www.acf.hhs.gov/programs/ocs/ssbg/reports/ssbg_focus_2008/child_care.html (accessed May 21, 2011).

U.S. Department of Health and Human Services (DHSS). Administration for Children and Families (ACF). Office of Head Start (OHS). 2010. "Head Start Program Fact Sheet: 2010." Available at: http://eclkc.ohs.acf.hhs.gov/hslc/mr/factsheets/fHeadStartProgr.htm (accessed May 21, 2011).

U.S. Department of Health and Human Services (DHHS). Office of the Assistant Secretary for Policy Evaluation (ASPE). Office of Disability, Aging, and Long-Term Care Policy (DALTCP). 2000. "Understanding Medicaid Home and Community Services: A Primer." October. Available at: http://aspe.hhs.gov/daltcp/reports/primer.pdf (accessed January 12, 2010).

———. 2006. "The Supply of Direct Support Professionals Serving Individuals with Intellectual Disabilities and Other Developmental Disabilities: Report to Congress." January. Available at: http://aspe.hhs.gov/daltcp/reports/2006/DSPsupply.pdf (accessed May 21, 2011).

———. 2011. "Understanding Direct Care Workers: A Snapshot of Two of America's Most Important Jobs—Certified Nursing Assistants and Home Health Aides." Report prepared by Galina Khatutsky, Joshua Wiener, Wayne Anderson, Valentina Akhmerova, and E. Andrew Jessup of RIT International and Marie R. Squillace of DHHS (March). Available at: http://aspe.hhs.gov/daltcp/reports/2011/CNAchart.htm (accessed December 14, 2011).

U.S. Department of Health and Human Services (DHHS). Health Resources and Services Administration (HRSA). Maternal and Child Health Bureau. 2007. "The National Survey of Children with Special Health Care Needs: Chartbook 2005–2006." Rockville, Md.: DHHS.

U.S. Department of Health and Human Services (DHHS). Office of the Inspector General (OIG). 2007. "Enrollment Levels in Head Start." April. Available at: http://oig.hhs.gov/oei/reports/oei-05-06-00250.pdf (accessed May 21, 2011).

U.S. Department of Labor (DOL). 2000. "Balancing the Needs of Families and Employers: The Family and Medical Leave Surveys, 2000 Update." Executive summary available at: http://www.dol.gov/whd/fmla/cover-statement.pdf (accessed May 21, 2011).

———. 2007. "Family and Medical Leave Act Regulations: A Report on the Department of Labor's Request for Information." *Federal Register* 72(124): 35550–638.

———. 2010. "Administrator's Interpretation 2010-3" (June 22). Available at: http://www.dol.gov/whd/opinion/adminIntrprtn/FMLA/2010/FMLAAI2010_3.htm (accessed May 21, 2011).

U.S. General Accountability Office (GAO). 1999. "Foster Care: Challenges in Helping Youths Live Independently." Washington, D.C.: Committee on Ways and Means.

———. 2003. *Nursing Home Quality: Prevalence of Serious Problems, While Declining, Reinforces Importance of Enhanced Oversight.* GAO 03-061. Washington: GAO (July). Available at: http://www.gao.gov/new.items/d03561.pdf (accessed May 21, 2011).

———. 2004. "Child Care: State Efforts to Enforce Safety and Health Requirements." GAO-04-786 (September). Available at: http://www.gao.gov/new.items/d04786.pdf (accessed May 21, 2011).

———. 2010a. "Older Americans Act: Preliminary Observations on Services Requested by Seniors and Challenges Providing Assistance." Testimony by Kate E. Brown, Director, Education, Workforce, and Income Security Issues, before the Special Committee on Aging, U.S. Senate (September 7).

———. 2010b. "Undercover Testing Finds Fraud and Abuse at Selected Head Start Centers." Statement of Gregory D. Kutz, Managing Director, Forensic Audits and Special Investigations, before the House Committee on Education and Labor. GAO-10-733T (May 18). Available at: http://www.gao.gov/new.items/d10733t.pdf (accessed April 29, 2012).

———. 2011. "Older Americans Act: More Should Be Done to Measure the Extent of Unmet Need for Services." Report to the Chairman, Special Committee on Aging, U.S. Senate. Washington: GAO (February). Available at: http://www.gao.gov/new.items/d11237.pdf (accessed December 3, 2011).

U.S. Small Business Administration (SBA). Office of Advocacy. 2010. "Employer Firms, Establishments, Employment, and Annual Payroll Small Firm Size Classes, 2007." Data drawn from the U.S. Census Bureau, "Statistics of U.S. Businesses." Available at: http://www.sba.gov/advo/research/us_07ss.pdf (accessed May 21, 2011).

Uttal, Lynet, and Mary Tuominen. 1999. "Tenuous Relationships: Exploitation, Emotion, and Racial Ethnic Significance in Paid Child Care Work." *Gender and Society* 13(6): 758–80.

Van Houtven, Harold Courtney, and Edward C. Norton. 2004. "Informal Care and Health Care Use of Older Adults." *Journal of Health Economics* 23(6): 1159–80.

van Staveren, Irene. 2001. *The Values of Economics: An Aristotelian Perspective.* London: Routledge.

Vandell, Deborah Lowe, Jay Belsky, Margaret Burchinal, Laurence Steinberg, and Nathan Vandergrift. 2010. "Do Effects of Early Child Care Extend to Age Fifteen Years? Results from the NICHD Study of Early Child Care and Youth Development." *Child Development* 81(3): 737–56.

References

Vedhara, Kav, Nigel K. M. Cox, Gordon K. Wilcock, Paula Perks, Moira Hunt, Stephen Anderson, Stafford L. Lightman, and Nola M. Shanks. 1999. "Chronic Stress in Elderly Carers of Dementia Patients and Antibody Response to Influenza Vaccination." *The Lancet* 353(9153): 627–31.

Verbrugge, Lois M., and Alan M. Jette. 1994. "The Disablement Process." *Social Science and Medicine* 38(1): 1–14.

Verbrugge, Lois M., and Li-Shou Yang. 2002. "Aging with Disability and Disability with Aging." *Journal of Disability Policy Studies* 12(4): 253–267.

Vickery, Claire. 1977. "The Time-Poor: A New Look at Poverty." *Journal of Human Resources* 12(1): 27–48.

Vitaliano, Peter P., Jinaping Zhang, and James M. Scanlan. 2003. "Is Caregiving Hazardous to One's Physical Health? A Meta-Analysis." Psychological Bulletin 129(6): 946–72.

Wachter, Kenneth. 1997. "Kinship Resources for the Elderly." *Philosophical Transactions of the Royal Society* 352(1363): 1811–17.

Waerness, Kari. 1987. "On the Rationality of Caring." In *Women and the State: The Shifting Boundaries of Public and Private,* edited by Ann Showstack Sassoon. London: Hutchinson.

Wagman, Barnet, and Nancy Folbre. 1996. "Household Services and Economic Growth in the United States, 1870–1930."q *Feminist Economics* 2(1): 43–66.

Wagner, John A., III, Carrie R. Leana, Edwin A. Locke, and David M. Schweiger. 1997. "Cognitive and Motivational Frameworks in U.S. Research on Participation: A Meta-Analysis of Primary Effects." *Journal of Organizational Behavior* 18(1): 49–65.

Waldfogel, Jane. 1997. "The Effect of Children on Women's Wages." *American Sociological Review* 62(2): 209–17.

———. 1998. "Understanding the 'Family Gap' in Pay for Women with Children." *Journal of Economic Perspectives* 12(1): 137–56.

———. 2000. "Child Welfare Research: How Adequate Are the Data?" *Children and Youth Services Review* 22(9–10): 705–41.

———. 2010. *Britain's War on Poverty.* New York: Russell Sage Foundation.

Walker, Alexis J., Clara C. Pratt, and Linda Eddy. 1995. "Informal Caregiving to Aging Family Members: A Critical Review." *Family Relations* 44(4): 402–11.

Walls, Jenna, Kathleen Gifford, Catherine Rudd, Rex O'Rourke, Martha Roherty, Lindsey Copeland, and Wendy Fox-Grage. 2011. *Weathering the Storm: The Impact of the Great Recession on Long-Term Services and Supports.* AARP Public Policy Institute research report 2011-11. Washington, D.C.: AARP Public Policy Institute. Available at: http://assets.aarp.org/rg center/ppi/ltc/CURRENT__Budget_Paper_v9Jan6.pdf (accessed January 23, 2011).

Weiss, Carlos O., Hector M. González, Mohammed U. Kabeto, and Kenneth M. Langer. 2005. "Differences in Amount of Informal Care Received by Non-Hispanic Whites and Latinos in a Nationally Representative Sample of Older Americans." *Journal of the American Geriatrics Society* 53(1): 146–51.

Weiss, Yoram, and Robert J. Willis. 1985. "Children as Collective Goods and Divorce Settlements." *Journal of Labor Economics* 3(3): 268–92.

West, Candace, and Don H. Zimmerman. 1987. "Doing Gender." *Gender and Society* 1(2): 125–51.

White, Carole L., Sylvie Lauzon, Mark J. Yaffe, and Sharon Wood-Dauphinee. 2004. "Toward a Model of Quality of Life for Family Caregivers of Stroke Survivors." *Quality of Life Research* 13(3): 625–38.

Whitebook, Marcy, and Laura Sakai. 2004. *By a Thread: How Child Care Centers Hold on to Teachers, How Teachers Build Lasting Careers.* Kalamazoo, Mich.: W. E. Upjohn Institute for Employment Research.

Whitebook, Marcy, Fran Kipnis, and Dan Bellm. 2007. "Disparities in California's Child Care Subsidy System: A Look at Teacher Education, Stability, and Diversity. Berkeley, Calif.: Center for the Study of Child Care Employment, University of California at Berkeley. Available at: http://www.irle.berkeley.edu/cscce/wp-content/uploads/2007/01/subsidy_system07.pdf (accessed February 20, 2012).

Wiener, Joshua M., Raymond J. Hanley, Robert Clark, and Joan F. van Nostrand. 1990. "Measuring the Activities of Daily Living: Comparisons Across National Surveys." *Journal of Gerontology: Social Sciences* 45(6): S229–37.

Wilde, Elizabeth Ty, Lily Batchelder, and David T. Ellwood. 2010. "The Mommy Track Divides: The Impact of Childbearing on Wages of Women of Differing Skill Levels." Working paper 16582. Cambridge, Mass.: National Bureau of Economic Research (December). Available at: http://www.nber.org/papers/w16582 (accessed January 30, 2010).

Williams, Joan C., and Stephanie Bornstein. 2008. "The Evolution of 'FReD': Family Responsibilities Discrimination and Developments in the Law of Stereotyping and Implicit Bias." *Hastings Law Journal* 59(6): 1311–58.

Williams, Joan C., and Heather Boushey. 2010. "The Three Faces of Work-Family Conflict." Center for American Progress (January 25). Available at: http://www.americanprogress.org/issues/2010/01/three_faces_report.html (accessed May 21, 2011).

Wilson, Julie, Jeff Katz and Robert Geen. 2005. "Listening to Parents: Overcoming Barriers to the Adoption of Children from Foster Care." KSG Working Paper RWP05-005 (February). Available at http://ssrn.com/abstract=663944 (accessed April 29, 2012).

Winston, Gordon C. 1999. "Subsidies, Hierarchy, and Peers: The Awkward Economics of Higher Education." *Journal of Economic Perspectives* 13(1): 13–36.

Wistow, Gerald, Martin Knapp, Brian Hardy, Julien Forder, Jeremy Kendall, and Rob Manning. 1996. *Social Care Markets: Progress and Prospects.* Philadelphia: Open University Press.

Wolf, Douglas A. 1999. "The Family as Provider of Long-Term Care: Efficiency, Equity, and Externalities." *Journal of Aging and Health* 11(3): 30–82.

———. 2001. "Population Change: Friend or Foe of the Chronic-Care System?" *Health Affairs* 20(6): 28–42.

———. 2004. "Valuing Informal Care." In *Family Time: The Social Organization of Care,* edited by Nancy Folbre and Michael Bittman. New York: Routledge.

Wolf, Douglas, Vicki Freedman, and Beth Soldo. 1997. "The Division of Family Labor: Care for Elderly Parents." *Journal of Gerontology: Social Sciences* 52B: 102–9.

Wolf, Douglas A., Ronald D. Lee, Timothy Miller, Gretchen Donehower, and Alexandre Genest. 2010. "Fiscal Externalities of Becoming a Parent." Paper presented to the annual meeting of the Population Association of America. Dallas (April 15–17).

Wolf, Douglas A., Carlos F. Mendes de Leon, and Thomas A. Glass. 2007. "Trends in Rates of Onset of and Recovery from Disability at Older Ages: 1982–1994." *Journal of Gerontology: Social Sciences* 62B: S3–10.

References

Wolf, Douglas A., and Beth J. Soldo. 1994. "Married Women's Allocation of Time to Employ-ment and Care of Elderly Parents." *Journal of Human Resources* 29(4): 1259–76.

Wolf, Douglas A., Beth Soldo, and Vicki Freedman. 1996. "The Demography of Family Care for the Elderly." In *Aging and Generational Relations over the Life Course,* edited by Tamara Hareven. Hawthorne, N.Y.: Walter de Gruyter.

Wolff, Jennifer L., and Judith D. Kasper 2006. "Caregivers of Frail Elders: Updating a National Profile." *The Gerontologist* 46(3): 344–56.

Yoshikawa, Hirokazu, Thomas S. Weisner, and Edward D. Lowe, eds. 2006. *Making It Work: Low-Wage Employment, Family Life, and Child Development.* New York: Russell Sage Foundation.

Young, Jeffrey R. 2011. "Programmed for Love." *Chronicle of Higher Education* (January 14). Available at: http://chronicle.com/article/Programmed-for-Love-The/125922 (accessed January 24, 2011).

Zarit, Steven H. 1989. "Do We Need Another 'Stress and Caregiving' Study?" *The Gerontologist* 29(2): 147–48.

Zelizer, Viviana. 2005. *The Purchase of Intimacy.* Princeton, N.J.: Princeton University Press.

Index

Boldface numbers refer to figures and tables.

Index

HRS (Health and Retirement Survey), 46–47, 64n7, 212–13, 219
HRSA (Health Resources and Services Administration), 19n6
human capital, 100, 104, 187

IADLs (instrumental activities of daily living). *See* instrumental activities of daily living (IADLs)
ICF (International Classification of Functioning, Disability, and Health), 207–8
ID/DD (intellectual and developmental disabilities), 128, 130–32, 134, 135, 174–78. *See also* adults with disabilities; children with disabilities
IDEA (Individuals with Disabilities Education Act), 127, 128, **129**, 130, 147
IEPs (individualized education programs), 131, 147
Illinois: special education, 131; unionization of family day care providers, 198
immigrants: adult care work, 83, **84;** child care work, **77;** interactive care work, **68,** 74–75; low-paid care work, 4
immigration reform, 199
immune system, 59
income: adult care workers, **84;** child care workers, **77;** disparate impacts of care policy by, 141–49, 178–79; and family resilience, 200; interactive care workers, **68.** *See also* wages and earnings
income inequality, 106
independent contractors. *See* self-employment
independent living centers, 134
indirect care, 19n1
individualized education programs (IEPs), 131, 147
Individuals with Disabilities Education Act (IDEA), 127, 128, **129**, 130, 147
industry data, 221–25
inequality, 4, 106. *See also* disparate impacts of care policy
infants, 7–8, 11, 145

informal caregiving. *See* unpaid care work
informal child care sector, 75
information technology, 188–89
injuries, work-related, 85–86
Institute of Medicine, 86
institutions providing care: cost-cutting strategies, 33; gender discrimination, 29; motivations of care providers, 14–18, 33–36; types of, 14–16. *See also specific institutions*
instrumental activities of daily living (IADLs): assistance with, 48, 132; disability definition, 45; needs assessments, 11–12; prevalence of those unable to perform, 13; survey disability scales, 212–13; survey question importance, 221
insurance, 28. *See also* health insurance
insurance companies, 14, **15**
intellectual and developmental disabilities (ID/DD), 128, 130–32, 134, 135, 174–78. *See also* adults with disabilities; children with disabilities
intensity of work, 103–4
interactive care: activities, 50, **51;** for children, 55; data sources, 221; definition of, 1, 4–7; features of, 2–4; occupational employment statistics, 66–67; time spent providing, 51–53; worker characteristics, 67–75
Internal Revenue Service (IRS), 74–75
International Classification of Functioning, Disability, and Health (ICF), 207–8
Interstate Compact on the Placement of Children, 127
interviews, 214
intrinsic motivation: importance of, 1, 5, 188; matching consumer needs with, 17–18; paid care providers, 33–34; sources of, 25–31; typology of, 22–25
Iowa: maternity leave, 154; unionization of family day care providers, 198
IRS (Internal Revenue Service), 74–75

job crafting, 10
job growth, 70
job quality, 76–80, 83–88, 188, 195–200
job tenure, 35
job training, 36, 86, 134, 196
job turnover, 9, 78–79, 85–87
Jochimsen, Maren, 19n2
joint production, 226

Kaiser Family Foundation, **165**
Kaye, Stephen, 136
Keeping Children and Families Safe Act (KCFSA), 125, **126**
Kenney, Genevieve, 131, 181n6
kindergarten, 75–76, 116, **117**
kin foster care placements, xiv, 146, 162–63, 194–95
Kittay, Eva, 32
Kohn, Melvin, 27
Kyrk, Hazel, 102

labor costs, 100
Labor Department, 197
labor force, definition of, 95. *See also* employment issues
labor force participation, of women, 41–42, 187
labor force surveys, 221–25
labor law, 199
labor process of care, 5, 33–36
Lake Research Partners, 189
Lakin, K. Charley, **177**
Land, Hilary, 29
LaPlante, Mitchell, 136
Latinos. *See* Hispanics
laws and legislation: Adoption and Safe Families Act (ASFA), 125, **126;** Affordable Healthcare for Americans Act (2009), 203; American Recovery and Reinvestment Act (ARRA), 189–90; Americans with Disabilities Act (ADA), 208; Child Abuse Prevention and Treatment Act (CAPTA), 125, **126;** Community Living Assistance Services and Supports Act (CLASS Act), 203; Fair Labor Standards Act (FLSA), 85, 199, 224; Family and Medical Leave Act (FMLA), 121–23, 143–45, 154, 191; Fostering Connections to Success and Increasing Adoptions Act (2008), 138n4; Health Care and Education